The Sjögren's Book

The Sjögren's Book

Fifth Edition

Edited by

Daniel J. Wallace, MD

Associate Editors

Alan N. Baer, MD
Steven E. Carsons, MD
Nancy L. Carteron, MD
Katherine M. Hammitt, MA
Matthew A. Makara, MPH

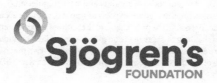

and

OXFORD
UNIVERSITY PRESS

OXFORD
UNIVERSITY PRESS

Oxford University Press is a department of the University of Oxford. It furthers the University's objective of excellence in research, scholarship, and education by publishing worldwide. Oxford is a registered trade mark of Oxford University Press in the UK and certain other countries.

Published in the United States of America by Oxford University Press
198 Madison Avenue, New York, NY 10016, United States of America.

Library of Congress Cataloging-in-Publication Data
Names: Wallace, Daniel J. (Daniel Jeffrey), 1949– editor.
Title: The Sjögren's book / Daniel J. Wallace.
Description: 5th edition. | New York, NY : Oxford University Press, [2022] |
Includes bibliographical references and index.
Identifiers: LCCN 2022000249 (print) | LCCN 2022000250 (ebook) |
ISBN 9780197502112 (hardback) | ISBN 9780197502136 (epub) | ISBN 9780197650417
Subjects: LCSH: Sjögren's syndrome—Popular works.
Classification: LCC RC647.5.S5 N49 2022 (print) |
LCC RC647.5.S5 (ebook) | DDC 616.7/75—dc23/eng/20220203
LC record available at https://lccn.loc.gov/2022000249
LC ebook record available at https://lccn.loc.gov/2022000250

DOI: 10.1093/oso/9780197502112.001.0001

Printed by Sheridan Books, Inc., United States of America

The manufacturer's authorised representative in the EU for product safety is Oxford University Press España S.A. of El Parque Empresarial San Fernando de Henares, Avenida de Castilla, 2 – 28830 Madrid (www.oup.es/en or product.safety@oup.com). OUP España S.A. also acts as importer into Spain of products made by the manufacturer.

Contents

PART VI   TAKING CHARGE OF YOUR SJÖGREN'S

PART VII   THE FUTURE

Contributors

Soo Kim Abboud, MD
Associate Professor
Chief, Otorhinolaryngology, Penn
Presbyterian Hospital
Clinical Director of Otolaryngology, Penn
Medicine University City
Philadelphia, PA, USA

Alan N. Baer, MD
Professor of Medicine
Director, Jerome L. Greene Sjögren's
Syndrome Center
Johns Hopkins University School of
Medicine
Baltimore, MD, USA

Margaret Baim, MS, ANP-BC
Clinical Director, Center for Training
Director, Stress Management and
Resiliency Training Program, Benson-
Henry Institute for Mind Body
Medicine, Massachusetts General Hospital
Boston, MA, USA

Chiara Baldini, MD, PhD
Associate Professor
Rheumatology Unit
University of Pisa
Pisa, Italy

Santanu Banerjee, PhD
Assistant Professor, Department of Surgery
University of Miami Miller School of
Medicine
Miami, FL, USA

Simon J. Bowman, MBBS, PhD
Professor, University Hospitals
Birmingham, UK
Biomedical Resource Centre, University of
Birmingham, UK
Milton Keynes University Hospital, UK
Birmingham, UK

Richard D. Brasington Jr., MD
Emeritus Professor of Medicine
Washington University in St. Louis School
of Medicine
St. Louis, MO, USA

E. Sherwood Brown, MD, PhD
Professor of Psychiatry
Vice Chair for Clinical Research
Chief of the Division of Clinical
Neuroscience
Director of the Psychoneuroendocrine
Research Program
The University of Texas Southwestern
Medical Center
Dallas, TX, USA

Anne E. Burke, MD, MPH
Associate Professor of Gynecology and
Obstetrics
Director, Family Planning Division
Johns Hopkins University School of
Medicine, Bayview Medical Center
Baltimore, MD, USA

Steven E. Carsons, MD, FACR
Professor, Department of Medicine at
NYU Long Island School of Medicine
Program Director, Rheum Fellowship
Program
Senior Associate Dean, Translational
Science Integration, NYU Long Island
School of Medicine
Chief of Rheumatology, Allergy and
Immunology, NYU Langone Hospital-
Long Island
Mineola, NY, USA

Nancy L. Carteron, MD
Associate Clinical Professor
Department of Medicine, Rheumatology
University of California, San Francisco &
Berkeley
San Francisco, CA, USA

Kara M. Cavuoto, MD
Associate Professor of Clinical
Ophthalmology
Bascom Palmer Eye Institute
University of Miami Miller School of
Medicine
Miami, FL, USA

Lan Chen, MD, PhD
Former Clinical Associate of Medicine and
Attending Rheumatologist
Division of Rheumatology, Penn
Presbyterian Medical Center
Penn Sjögren's Center, University of
Pennsylvania School of Medicine
Philadelphia, PA, USA

Janet E. Church
President & Chief Executive Officer
Sjögren's Foundation
Reston, VA, USA

Reza Dana, MD, MPH, MSc
Professor of Ophthalmology
Director of Cornea Service, Massachusetts
Eye and Ear Infirmary, Harvard
Medical School
Boston, MA, USA

Troy E. Daniels, DDS, MS
Professor of Oral Medicine and Pathology
School of Dentistry and Medicine,
University of California, San Francisco
San Fransciso, CA, USA

Cintia S. de Paiva, MD, PHD
Associate Professor of Ophthalmology
Baylor College of Medicine—Ocular
Surface Center
Houston, TX, USA

Peter Donshik, MD
Ophthalmologist (Retired)
Bloomfield, CT, USA

Kieron Dunleavy, MD
Chair, Division of Hematology
Director, Lymphoma Program
Lombardi Cancer Center
Georgetown University
Washington, DC, USA

Lynn C. Epstein, MD, DLFAPA, FAACAP
Clinical Professor of Psychiatry
Tufts University School of Medicine
Boston, MA, USA

Benjamin Fisher, MD(Res)
Senior Lecturer in Clinical Rheumatology
University Hospitals Birmingham, UK
Biomedical Resource Centre, University of
Birmingham, UK
Institute of Inflammation and Ageing,
University of Birmingham
Birmingham, UK

H. Kenneth Fisher, MD, FCCP
Professor of Clinical Medicine (Retired)
University of California
Los Angeles, CA, USA

Gary N. Foulks, MD, FACS
Emeritus Professor of Ophthalmology
University of Louisville School of Medicine
Louisville, KY, USA

Robert I. Fox, MD, PhD
Chief of Rheumatology, Scripps Memorial
Hospital and Research Foundation
La Jolla, CA, USA

Anat Galor, MD, MSPH
Staff Physician, Miami Veterans Affairs
Medical Center
Associate Professor of Clinical
Ophthalmology
Bascom Palmer Eye Institute University of
Miami Miller School of Medicine
Miami, FL, USA

Leila M. Haddad
Clinical Assistant
Penn Medicine, University of Pennsylvania
Health System
Philadelphia, PA, USA

Katherine M. Hammitt, MA
Vice President of Medical & Scientific
Affairs
Sjögren's Foundation
Reston, VA, USA

Chadwick R. Johr, MD
Director, Penn Sjögren's Center
Associate Program Director, Combined
Internal Medicine and Pediatrics
Residency Program
Associate Professor of Clinical Medicine,
Division of Rheumatology
Perelman School of Medicine at the
University of Pennsylvania
Philadelphia, PA, USA

Malin V. Jonsson, DMD, PhD
Professor
Department of Clinical Dentistry
Section for Oral and Maxillofacial
Radiology
University of Bergen
Bergen, Norway

Efstathia K. Kapsogeorgou, PhD
Assistant Professor of Immunology
Department of Pathophysiology
School of Medicine, National and
Kapodistrian University of Athens
Athens, Greece

Stuart S. Kassan, MD, FACP, MACR
Distinguished Clinical Prof of Medicine
University of Colorado School of Medicine
Denver, CO, USA

Theresa Lawrence Ford, MD
CEO & Medical Director
North Georgia Rheumatology Group, PC
Lawrenceville, GA, USA

Augustine S. Lee, MD
Pulmonologist, Critical Care Specialist
Mayo Clinic
Jacksonville, FL, USA

Christine H. Lee, MD, MPH
Attending Physician
Cedars-Sinai Medical Center
Beverly Hills, CA, USA

Janet Lewis, MD
Associate Professor
Chief of the Division of Rheumatology
University of Virginia
Charlottesville, VA, USA

Scott M. Lieberman, MD, PhD, FACR
Associate Professor of Pediatrics
Division of Rheumatology, Allergy, and
Immunology
University of Iowa Carver College of
Medicine
Iowa City, IA, USA

Valerie G. Loehr, PhD
Assistant Professor
Department of Psychiatry
The University of Texas Southwestern
Medical Center at Dallas
Dallas, TX, USA

Shalini Mahajan, MD
Assistant Professor
Department of Neurology
Cedars Sinai Medical Center
Los Angeles, CA, USA

Edward Maitz, PhD
Clinical Neuropsychologist
Clinical Neuropsychologist Associates
Philadelphia, PA, USA

Stephen Maitz, PsyD
Neuropsychology Postdoctoral Fellow
Penn Medicine, University of Pennsylvania
Health System
Philadelphia, PA, USA

Matthew Makara, MPH
Director of Research & Scientific Affairs
Sjögren's Foundation
Reston, VA, USA

Steven Mandel, MD
Clinical Professor of Neurology
Donald and Barbara Zucker School of
Medicine at Hofstra/Northwell
Adjunct Professor of Medicine
New York Medical College
New York City, NY, USA

Thomas Mandl, MD, PhD
Associate Professor of Rheumatology
Lund University
Malmö, Sweden

Nancy McNamara, OD, PhD
Professor, UC Berkeley School of
Optometry
Associate Dean for Academic Affairs
Chief, UC Berkeley Sjögren's Clinic
Co-Chief, UC Berkeley Dry Eye Clinic
Berkeley, CA, USA

Jay Mehta, MD, MS
Attending Physician, Division of
Rheumatology
Associate Program Director of the
Pediatrics Residency Program
Children's Hospital of Philadelphia
Philadelphia, PA, USA

Rita Melkonian, MD, FACOG
Physician, Marin Health
Marin County, CA, USA

Richa Mishra
Rheumatology Fellow
University of Pennsylvania
Philadelphia, PA

Haralampos M. Moutsopoulos
Professor and Director
Department of Pathophysiology, School of
Medicine
National University of Athens
Athens, Greece

Ghaith Noaiseh, MD
Associate Professor of Medicine
Division of Allergy, Clinical Immunology
& Rheumatology
University of Kansas
Kansas City, KS, USA

Peter Olsson, MD, PhD
Department of Clinical Sciences
Lund University
Malmö, Sweden

Pantelis P. Pavlakis, MD, PhD
Assistant Attending
Department of Neurology
Hospital for Special Surgery
New York, NY, USA

Astrid Rasmussen, MD, PhD
Research Associate Member
Genes and Human Disease Research
Program
Oklahoma Medical Research Foundation
Oklahoma City, OK, USA

Teri P. Rumpf, PhD
Psychologist
Newton Highlands, MA, USA

Vidya Sankar, DMD, MHS
Associate Professor and Division Director
for Oral Medicine
Department of Diagnostic Sciences
Tufts University School of Dental
Medicine
Boston, MA, USA

R. Hal Scofield, MD, FACR
Member, Arthritis & Clinical Immunology
Program
Oklahoma Medical Research Foundation
Oklahoma City, OK, USA
Professor, Department of Medicine,
College of Medicine
University of Oklahoma Health
Sciences Center
Oklahoma City, OK, USA

Staff Physician, Associate Chief of Staff for Research, Medical Service
United States Department of Veterans Affairs Medical Center
Oklahoma City, OK, USA

Katerina Shetler, MD
Physician
Division of Gastroenterology
Palo Alto Medical Foundation
Mountain View, CA, USA

Mabi Singh, DMD, MS
Associate Professor
Assistant Director, Oral Medicine Service
Department of Diagnostic Sciences
Tufts University School of Dental Medicine
Boston, MA, USA

Kathy L. Sivils, PhD
Former Member, Arthritis & Clinical Immunology Research Program
Former Adjunct Associate Professor, Department of Pathology, University of Oklahoma Health Sciences Center
Director, Oklahoma Sjögren's Center of Research Translation
Former Director, OMRF Sjögren's Research Clinic
Oklahoma, OK, USA

Kathrine Skarstein, DMD, PhD
Professor, Department of Clinical Medicine—Gade Laboratory for Pathology, University of Bergen
Department of Pathology, Haukeland University Hospital
Bergen, Norway

Fotini C. Soliotis, MD, MRCP
Rheumatologist, Euroclinic
Athens, Greece

Sara M. Stern, MD
Associate Professor of Pediatrics
University of Utah School of Medicine
Salt Lake City, UT, USA

Thomas D. Sutton, Esq.
Partner, Leventhal Sutton & Gornstein
Bucks County, PA, USA

Donald E. Thomas Jr., MD, FACP, FACR, RhMSUS
Arthritis and Pain Associates of PG County
Associate Professor of Clinical Medicine
Uniformed Services University of the Health Sciences
Bethesda, MD, USA

Athanasios G. Tzioufas, MD
Professor
Department of Pathophysiology, School of Medicine
National and Kapodistrian University of Athens
Athens, Greece

Jolien F. van Nimwegen, MD, PhD
Department of Rheumatology and Clinical Immunology
University of Groningen and University Medical Center Groningen
Groningen, The Netherlands

Arun Varadhachary, MD, PhD
Associate Professor of Neurology
Washington University School of Medicine in St. Louis
Saint Louis, MO, USA

Frederick B. Vivino, MD, MS, FACR
Former Chief, Division of Rheumatology, Penn Presbyterian Medical Center
Former Director, Penn Sjögren's Center
Philadelphia, PA, USA

Michael Voulgarelis, MD
Professor
Department of Pathophysiology, School of Medicine
National and Kapodistrian University of Athens
Athens, Greece

Daniel J. Wallace, MD, FACP, MACR
Associate Director, Rheumatology
Fellowship Program
Board of Governors, Cedars-Sinai
Medical Center
Professor of Medicine, Cedars-Sinai
Medical Center
David Geffen School of Medicine Center
at UCLA
Beverly Hills, CA, USA

Jeffrey W. Wilson, MD
Rheumatologist (Retired)
Lynchburg, VA, USA

Ava J. Wu, DDS
Clinical Professor, Orofacial Sciences
Sjögren's Clinic
University of California, San Francisco &
Berkeley
San Francisco, CA, USA

Introduction: Why Write a Book on Sjögren's?

One American in 83 has a mysterious condition known as Sjögren's. Named after a Swedish ophthalmologist who described its salient features nearly 80 years ago, Sjögren's, until recently, resided in a nosologic purgatory, with its manifestations misunderstood, underappreciated, and ignored. An international consensus has finally been derived regarding what the term *Sjögren's* means. Now that organized science has finally come to terms (literally) with the disease, a number of insights elucidated by Sjogrenologists have been rapidly forthcoming. The collective wisdom of these investigators has continued to result in the publication of prescient findings that serve to emphasize the importance of research into this area and will have implications far beyond Sjögren's itself. It is our hope that researchers, clinicians, physicians, and allied health professionals as well as patients and their families will be able to use this resource.

Why should we write a book on Sjögren's? It is an autoimmune condition that affects the whole body, especially musculoskeletal and glandular tissues. It can exist as a primary condition or concomitantly with rheumatoid arthritis, systemic lupus erythematosus, scleroderma, or other rheumatic disorders. According to the most recent report from the National Institutes of Health, 14.7 to 23.5 million people in the United States have an autoimmune condition, and 150 such conditions have been identified to date. Up to 4 million of these individuals have conditions related to Sjögren's according to the National Arthritis Data Workshop estimates, which would make the perception that it is uncommon incorrect. Its prevalence varies internationally from 0.1% to 4.8% of a general population. Sjögren's does not have a strong focus in medical education. Its symptoms are subtle and can be intermittent or nonspecific. It has been estimated that symptoms are present for a mean of nearly 3 years before it is properly diagnosed. While this is an improvement from where we were a decade ago, this is unfortunate because a delayed diagnosis drastically alters quality of life. For example:

- Patients report greater fatigue, pain, and depression and diminished cognitive function compared with their peers.

- A survey showed that Sjögren's impacts patients in the following ways: 97% experience physical symptoms; 59% experience an impact on their sex life; work life is impacted for 54%; 71% experience an impact on daily life, and; 63% experience a negative impact on relationships with family and friends.
- The majority have serious dental complications (e.g., caries) as well as fatigue and significant musculoskeletal impairments.

More importantly, 5% to 10% of those with Sjögren's develop a lymphoproliferative malignancy. Sjögren's is almost unique among autoimmune disorders in its ability to result in lymphoma in certain cases. This link could be exploited by researchers to help us understand many of the common immunologic features shared by cancer and autoimmune disorders.

Although Sjögren's is the second most common autoimmune condition affecting the musculoskeletal system, it ranks eighth in terms of research funding. Studies aimed at finding the cause of and cure for Sjögren's will ultimately save taxpayers billions of dollars in lost wages and productivity, as well as improve the lives of many. We hope that our efforts will result in increased awareness and greater understanding of this underappreciated disease.

Finally, another reason to write a book on Sjögren's relates to presenting the figurative tsunami of new advances and insights that have been published in the last decade. Investigators now have a validated criteria set for Sjögren's, improved metrics for measuring disease activity, greater understanding of its genetics and pathogenesis, and new biomarkers that are of clinical and prognostic value. These discoveries will lead to improved treatments, which, in addition to being lifesaving, greatly enhance the quality of life of millions of afflicted individuals throughout the world. This writer is grateful to the Sjögren's Foundation for their hard work in helping to complete this task.

The editor gratefully acknowledges the help of Katherine M. Hammitt, Vice President of Medical and Scientific Affairs, and Matt Makara, Director of Research and Scientific Affairs, at the Sjögren's Foundation, along with our section editors for their assistance in putting together this manuscript.

Daniel J. Wallace, MD, FACP, MACR
Professor of Medicine
Cedars-Sinai Medical Center
David Geffen School of Medicine at the
University of California, Los Angeles

PART I

WHAT IS SJÖGREN'S AND WHO IS THE SJÖGREN'S PATIENT?

1
The Sjögren's Foundation

The Patients' and Professionals' Key Resource and Advocate

Janet E. Church

The Sjögren's Foundation was founded in 1983 by a patient, for the patient, and continues to serve as the only nonprofit organization in the United States that is solely focused on Sjögren's.

The Foundation's mission, as seen in Box 1.1, shows our commitment to ensuring that patients and healthcare professionals have the education, resources, and services they need to help conquer the complexities of Sjögren's.

Being diagnosed with Sjögren's can be overwhelming and frightening. However, many patients also feel relief after having spent years seeking an answer for what was causing all their symptoms. To help patients cope with the daunting challenge of learning about the complexities of Sjögren's, the Foundation provides multiple avenues of education and support, including a comprehensive review of the disease in this fifth edition of *The Sjögren's Book*, which holds the latest information about the disease and recognizes Sjögren's as serious, systemic, and prevalent.

For healthcare professionals, Sjögren's can be especially challenging to diagnose, treat, and monitor. Patients often present differently and are at risk for a multitude of complications, and until recently, no guidance on management and treatment was available. However, the Sjögren's Foundation is helping to change that with continued investment for educating medical professionals.

Patient Resources

The Sjögren's Foundation is continually developing and updating materials to help patients understand their disease and its potential complications and to help educate their family and friends. The Foundation's website, www.sjogrens. org, has a wide selection of downloadable materials, including education

Janet E. Church, *The Sjögren's Foundation* In: *The Sjögren's Book*. Edited by: Daniel J. Wallace, Oxford University Press.
© Sjögren's Foundation 2022. DOI: 10.1093/oso/9780197502112.003.0001

Box 1.1 Sjögren's Foundation Mission Statement

- Support Sjögren's patients and their loved ones through education, resources, and services.
- Provide credible resources and education for healthcare professionals.
- Serve as the voice for all Sjögren's patients through advocacy and awareness initiatives.
- Lead, encourage, and fund innovative research projects to better understand, diagnose, and treat Sjögren's.

---

sheets on the many symptoms patients might encounter, brochures, tips for living with Sjögren's, and information on how to sign up for the Foundation's monthly patient-focused newsletter, *Conquering Sjögren's*.

On the site, you will also learn about the Foundation's nearly 70 support groups in the United States, each led by a local patient. In addition, you will find information about a number of other Foundation activities and educational conferences for patients in cities around the United States. These additional programs provide attendees first-hand opportunities to learn from leading Sjögren's experts.

Annually, the Sjögren's Foundation hosts a two-day national patient conference with more than 10 speakers, covering the various manifestations of Sjögren's. Beyond expanding one's knowledge at these conferences, patients and family members find it to be a great way to meet and collaborate with other patients and families who share similar circumstances.

Professional Resources

Similar to our patient resources and materials just mentioned, the Foundation focuses on expanding resources and education for healthcare professionals.

In 2006, in an effort to raise awareness and provide education and updates on the latest Sjögren's research and clinical findings, the Foundation introduced our newsletter for healthcare professionals, *Sjögren's Quarterly*. This newsletter, published four times per year, is distributed free to any healthcare professional, worldwide, who is interested in learning about Sjögren's. Each issue reviews the latest in Sjögren's research and clinical news, features a healthcare professional's experience in treating various aspects of Sjögren's, and provides updates on new products and industry news. Here, the foundation also recaps scientific conferences and updates professionals on clinical trials in Sjögren's.

The Foundation's website, www.sjogrens.org, also hosts a section for professionals with a variety of resources, ranging from downloadable patient materials to research information.

Most impressively, the Foundation has invested more than $2.5 million in Sjögren's research since 2005. The Foundation has helped to fund programs in genetics, gene expression, biomarkers, the immune system, and potential regeneration of glands and cognitive symptoms, just to name a few topics. We have supported projects at institutions around the United States to encourage new researchers to enter the field of Sjögren's, as well as offering continued support to current researchers devoted to Sjögren's. This focus on maintaining current relationships and developing new researchers is key to sparking novel ideas that all researchers can build upon.

Perhaps most helpful to Sjögren's clinicians is the Foundation's major initiative to develop clinical practice guidelines for treating Sjögren's. These guidelines are the first of their kind for the disease and provide a comprehensive overview on a range of important topics and manifestations of Sjögren's.

To date, the Foundation has completed clinical practice guidelines on the following key topics: dental caries prevention, dry eye, inflammatory musculoskeletal pain, fatigue, use of biologics, and pulmonary manifestations. Additional topics that are being addressed include peripheral nervous and autonomic nervous system involvement, lymphoma, and vasculitis. For this work, the Foundation has been reaching out to specialists beyond those in rheumatology and oral and ocular medicine to ensure that neurologists, pulmonologists, oncologists, and others participate in management guidelines and subsequently share information on Sjögren's with colleagues through their respective professional societies. Watch the Foundation website and/or *Sjögren's Quarterly* for regular updates as this important initiative progresses.

Advocate for Patients

The Sjögren's Foundation regularly advocates for Sjögren's patients by representing their voice and telling their story in Washington, DC, on Capitol Hill and to federal and state regulatory agencies. The Foundation furthers this work by participating and leading numerous coalitions to increase awareness of Sjögren's and its seriousness and the need for increased government-funded research that will help expand knowledge and lead to new therapies.

Sjögren's patients face a high burden of illness every day, and the Foundation works to find opportunities to ease this burden. This includes, but is not limited to, working to increase access to knowledgeable healthcare professionals, reducing the high cost of over-the-counter and prescription products, and ensuring that Sjögren's patients are able to secure affordable and quality health insurance.

In addition to our coalition work, the Foundation has been invited to serve on prestigious committees and boards, including those managed by the National Institutes of Health, National Health Council, professional societies, and other government and private agencies. Through our work and representation of the Sjögren's community, the Foundation has increased awareness for Sjögren's as well as ensured that our disease is represented in legislative bills, government guidelines, and research appropriations.

The Foundation also organizes community events to increase awareness for Sjögren's. These events include participating in local health fairs throughout the United States as well as hosting more than 15 additional special events to help raise funds for our research and education programs.

Patient advocacy is a critical mission, and the Foundation participates in annual professional conferences, including those for rheumatology, ocular, and dental professionals to ensure patients' voices are represented. At such events, the Foundation coordinates presentations, panels, and other opportunities to help educate professionals on Sjögren's.

Finally, in early 2018, the Foundation announced that its work to increase awareness and education among healthcare professionals led to a major reduction in the time it takes to receive a proper diagnosis of Sjögren's. The time has now been reduced from 6 years in 2012 to only 2.8 years! This decrease will help those suffering from the symptoms of Sjögren's to receive an accurate diagnosis and begin the proper treatment they need to improve their quality of life.

Hope for the Future

In 1983, when Elaine Harris founded the Sjögren's Foundation, she believed in the basic premise that the organization would always help Sjögren's patients by providing education, increasing awareness, and supporting research. Now, almost 40 years later, the Foundation operates under the same guiding principle.

The Foundation staff and volunteers, both past and present, have always approached every project and initiative with one question in mind: "How will this help patients?" The Foundation continues to focus on finding answers on what is causing Sjögren's while working hard to ensure that patients receive a prompt diagnosis, have options for treatment, and are being treated by healthcare professionals who are knowledgeable about Sjögren's. Together, we will achieve the Foundation's vision of creating a community where patients, healthcare professionals, and researchers come together to conquer the complexities of Sjögren's.

2
What Is Sjögren's?

Frederick B. Vivino

This chapter provides a general overview of Sjögren's, including disease definition and history, information about the presenting signs and symptoms, approach to diagnosis, classification criteria, and an explanation regarding why a proper diagnosis is important. Many of these topics will be covered in greater detail in the chapters that follow. See the list of suggested reading at the end of this chapter for further information.

Definition and Terminology

Sjögren's can be defined as a chronic autoimmune, rheumatic disease characterized by lymphocytic infiltration (inflammation) of the exocrine (moisture-producing) glands in association with the production of autoantibodies in the blood that causes dry eyes, dry mouth, and less commonly inflammation of the internal organs.

Sjögren's is considered *autoimmune* because the antibodies that appear in the blood are directed against components of the body's own cells or tissues. The *lymphocytes* (white blood cells that participate in immune reactions) that invade and attack the glands are also considered another prominent sign of autoimmunity. *Exocrine glands* are glands that empty through ducts and produce body fluids. For that reason, they are sometimes nicknamed the *moisture-producing* glands. Examples include the lacrimal glands that make tears and the salivary glands that produce saliva. We have exocrine glands all over the body, and therefore Sjögren's can sometimes cause whole-body dryness. The word "sicca" (derived from the Latin word *siccus*, meaning dry or thirsty) is frequently used to describe dryness symptoms in connection with Sjögren's. The term "sicca syndrome," however, is no longer used because it is now widely recognized that Sjögren's is a systemic disease not confined to sicca symptoms.

Sjögren's is considered a *rheumatic disease* because it frequently causes musculoskeletal pain and sometimes arthritis (joint pain associated with swelling and

Frederick B. Vivino, *What Is Sjögren's?* In: *The Sjögren's Book*. Edited by: Daniel J. Wallace, Oxford University Press. © Sjögren's Foundation 2022. DOI: 10.1093/oso/9780197502112.003.0002 other signs of inflammation). Sjögren's can occur alone or with another connective tissue or autoimmune disease. In the past, medical professionals used the terms "primary" to indicate the former and "secondary" to indicate the latter. We no longer use these terms, because just as with rheumatoid arthritis, systemic lupus, and scleroderma, someone either has these diseases or does not have them.

Sjögren's Syndrome or Disease?

The Sjögren's Foundation has dropped "syndrome" from its name because its Medical and Scientific Advisory Committee and Board of Directors agreed that calling Sjögren's a syndrome was inaccurate. Nowadays, both descriptors are used interchangeably even though these terms have different connotations. A *syndrome* is defined as a group of signs and symptoms that usually occur together and characterize a particular medical condition. The term *disease* implies three main features: well-defined symptoms, alterations in the structure and/or function of the target organ, and a specific etiology or cause. The dryness symptoms in Sjögren's arise when the moisture-producing glands are slowly damaged by inflammation (i.e., lymphocytic infiltration) and become dysfunctional. This occurs in part because over time normal glands become replaced by scar tissue and fat. Although the exact cause of Sjögren's remains unknown, scientific evidence points to genetics, hormones, and environmental agents (e.g., viral infections) as the most likely causes. The Foundation now is simply using "Sjögren's" or "Sjögren's disease" and is encouraging the international community to adopt this language as well.

History

Although one can find case reports of people who had Sjögren's dating back to the European medical literature of the late 19th century, Henrik Sjögren, a Swedish ophthalmologist, is credited with "discovering" the disease because he published the first comprehensive description of Sjögren's as a disease in a large group of patients. This occurred in 1933 when, while working on his PhD thesis, he described 19 women, all of whom had severe dryness of the eyes and mouth and two-thirds of whom had chronic arthritis. He was the first person to recognize the classic triad of symptoms in Sjögren's: dry eyes, dry mouth, and arthritis. Dr. Sjögren was also the first physician to emphasize the systemic nature of the disease, and he coined the term *keratoconjunctivitis sicca* (KCS) to describe dry eyes with ocular surface damage. Nowadays, the term KCS has become synonymous with dry eyes. Dr. Sjögren was also one of the first ophthalmologists to use a vital dye, rose bengal, to study the surface of the eye for damage due to dryness. Thus, for these and other contributions, the disease still bears his name.

In the years that followed Dr. Sjögren's initial description, Sjögren's was considered quite rare and was listed in the National Organization of Rare Disorders (NORD) registry. However, in the late 1990s the pendulum regarding prevalence began to swing in the opposite direction when new research suggested a higher prevalence of Sjögren's than previously recognized. This disease is now considered to be quite common and, among the autoimmune rheumatic diseases, Sjögren's ranks second, only behind rheumatoid arthritis, in prevalence.

Clinical Presentations

Like most autoimmune diseases, Sjögren's preferentially affects women and less commonly occurs in children and men. About 80% of the overall patient group present with the insidious onset of dryness of the eyes, mouth, and other body parts that evolves slowly over months to years. Among the various scenarios, dry eyes is typically the most common presenting manifestation. Less commonly, dry mouth can be the presenting manifestation, or all the sicca symptoms develop simultaneously. In the remaining 20% of patients Sjögren's begins in an unusual or atypical fashion. In these cases, one of the internal organ manifestations will predominate and, when the patient is first seen by a healthcare provider, the dryness symptoms may be minimal or nonexistent. This scenario is particularly common among individuals who present with a neurologic complication of the disease. Other common symptoms include fatigue and swelling of the salivary glands, which can occasionally be the initial manifestations as well. Table 2.1 summarizes "atypical" clinical

Table 2.1 Atypical Presentations of Sjögren's

Rheumatoid-like arthritis	Multiple cavities
Polymyalgia rheumatica	Interstitial lung disease
Leukocytoclastic vasculitis	Fever of unknown origin
Multiple sclerosis–like disease	Chronic fatigue syndrome
Peripheral neuropathy	Renal tubular acidosis
Autonomic neuropathy	Elevated ESR or positive ANA or RF in an asymptomatic patient
Inflammatory myositis	Corneal melt or perforation
Salivary gland swelling	

presentations seen in adults diagnosed with Sjögren's over a 30-year period at a large university medical center. In children the most common presentation is parotitis, recurrent swelling and pain of the parotid gland (major salivary gland in the cheeks).

Approach to Diagnosis

Sjögren's is often considered one of the most challenging autoimmune disorders to diagnose. There is typically a lag time of 3 to 5 years between the onset of symptoms and the time of diagnosis. The explanations for this delay are numerous and include the disease's gradual onset, variety of presentations and organ manifestations, disagreement among healthcare professionals over diagnostic criteria and diagnostic tests, and, in general, a decreased famil-iarity of Sjögren's among the public and healthcare community compared to other diseases. A variety of conditions, including medication use, can cause dryness and mimic other Sjögren's symptoms (Table 2.2). For that reason, a comprehensive evaluation is required for accurate diagnosis.

Since the 1960s, physicians and scientists have proposed at least 13 dif-ferent sets of diagnostic and/or classification criteria to help identify and define patients with Sjögren's. In one way or another these criteria have usu-ally tried to satisfy three basic objectives: (1) documentation of objective evi-dence of dry eyes, (2) documentation of objective evidence of dry mouth, and (3) proof of autoimmunity. Since no one test provides an abnormal result in

Table 2.2 Differential Diagnosis of Sjögren's

Amyloidosis	Lacrimal-auriculo-dental-digital syndrome (LADD)
Anxiety/depression	Medication-related dryness
Chronic sialadenitis	Mouth breathing
Diabetes mellitus	Multiple sclerosis
Eosinophilia-myalgia syndrome	Radiation injury
Fibromyalgia	Sarcoidosis
Graft-versus-host disease	Sialadenosis
Hepatitis C	Silicone breast implant disease
HIV-related diffuse infiltrative lymphocytosis syndrome (DILS)	Systemic lupus
IgG4 syndrome	Rheumatoid arthritis
Vitamin A deficiency	Type V hyperlipidemia

every patient, a variety of diagnostic studies are required. These studies include blood tests, tests for dry eyes and dry mouth, and, frequently, a biopsy of the lower lip. At the present time, no universally accepted diagnostic criteria exist, and the physician's judgment remains the gold standard for diagnosis.

Ideally, any new diagnostic criteria developed in the future should be highly sensitive in order to help clinicians identify as many early cases of Sjögren's as possible, since this is when currently available treatments are likely to be most effective. However, the trade-off for high diagnostic sensitivity is sometimes the loss of diagnostic accuracy, since many diseases look alike in the early stages. This sometimes leads to false-positive diagnoses and the need to revise the final diagnosis at a later time.

Evolution of Classification Criteria

In more recent years, researchers have focused their attention exclusively on the development of classification criteria. Classification criteria are different from diagnostic criteria and are designed for research purposes rather than clinical practice. The goal of classification criteria is to define homogeneous populations of patients for clinical trials and other research studies. Classification criteria sometimes sacrifice sensitivity in favor of specificity or higher diagnostic accuracy. Therefore, some individuals who fail to meet classification criteria may be ineligible for a research study but could still have Sjögren's. To make matters even more confusing, different classification criteria are used in different parts of the world to define Sjögren's.

The first breakthrough occurred in 2002 following publication of the American–European Consensus Group (AECG) classification criteria (Vitali et al., 2002). These criteria were widely embraced because they offered a definition or classification of Sjögren's using a combination of symptoms and diagnostic tests. They allowed Sjögren's patients to be classified without a lip biopsy and also provided a pathway for the identification of Sjögren's even in patients who had no dryness symptoms. In 2012, an alternative set of classification criteria derived from data gathered through the international Sjögren's tissue registry was developed in the United States and later came to be known as the American College of Rheumatology (ACR)- Sjögren's International Collaborative Clinical Alliance (SICCA) criteria (Shiboski et al., 2012).

The new criteria facilitated the classification of Sjögren's based entirely on results of objective tests and were simpler to follow. Both criteria had advantages and disadvantages. However, in order to move research forward and promote uniformity of classification criteria around the world, in 2016 an international group of experts sponsored by the ACR and the European League Against Rheumatism (EULAR), the two major rheumatology professional societies, eventually developed a hybrid model (Table 2.3) derived from the best parts of the 2002 and 2012 criteria. The new 2016 ACR–EULAR Classification Criteria for Sjögren's have been endorsed by both professional societies and are likely to remain with us for a long time.

The 2016 criteria assign different weights to different tests according to perceived level of importance. Among the various autoantibodies produced in Sjögren's, only the anti-SSA (a.k.a. anti-Ro) antibody is included because this blood test is considered the most specific for the disease. A positive lip biopsy is also given equal weight. The two tests for dry eyes include the unanesthetized Schirmer's test (measures tear production) and vital dye (e.g., fluorescein, rose bengal, lissamine green, or some combination thereof) staining of the eye surface to look for dry spots. The recommended test to screen for dry mouth is simply measurement of the salivary flow rate. If all tests are positive, then a maximum total score of 9 is obtained. However, only a score of 4 or more is required to define a patient as having Sjögren's.

Table 2.3 2016 ACR-EULAR Classification Criteria for Sjögren's Syndrome

Inclusions
- Anyone with dry eyes or dry mouth as defined by the 2002 criteria
- Anyone with at least one extraglandular manifestation as defined by the ESSDAI questionnaire

Test Items	Weight
Positive lip biopsy (FS > 1 / 4 mm^2)[1]	3
Anti-SSA (Ro)+	3
OSS[2] > 5 (van Bijsterfeld[3] > 4) 1 eye	1
Schirmer's (without topical anesthesia) < 5 mm/5 min. 1 eye	1
Unstimulated salivary flow < 0.1 ml/min	1

Positive score for Sjögren's ≥ 4

[1] A positive biopsy is defined as focal lymphocytic sialadenitis with a focus score ≥1/ 4 mm^2 tissue surface area.

[2] Ocular surface staining score for dry eyes using fluorescein/ lissamine green

[3] van Bijsterfeld score for dry eyes utilizing rose bengal dye

Source: Shiboski CH, Shiboski SC, Seror R, et al. 2016 American College of Rheumatology/European League Against Rheumatism Classification Criteria for Primary Sjögren's Syndrome: A Consensus and Data-Driven Methodology Involving Three International Patient Cohorts. Arthritis Rheumatol. 2017 Jan;69(1):35-45. doi: 10.1002/art.39859.

Value of a Correct Diagnosis

Despite the challenges of diagnosis, most people eventually do receive an answer. All of the aforementioned criteria have a sensitivity and specificity of approximately 90% to 95%. Therefore, anyone who meets the 2002, 2012, or 2016 criteria, in this author's opinion, should carry a diagnosis of Sjögren's. Additionally, in a clinical setting, even those who only partially fulfill criteria can be diagnosed with Sjögren's as long as they have objective evidence of dry eyes and dry mouth and either test positive for anti-SSA or have a positive lip biopsy.

Any individual who fails to undergo a complete medical evaluation and receive a correct diagnosis of Sjögren's will be left at a distinct disadvantage. It is now generally accepted that dry eyes and dry mouth in the Sjögren's population are not trivial symptoms and, when unrecognized or untreated, can lead to some devastating and costly medical and dental complications (Table 2.4). Since Sjögren's is a systemic disease, the physician's evaluation and management of any new medical problem will frequently be impacted by awareness of this diagnosis. About 5% to 10% of the Sjögren's population will go on to develop non-Hodgkin's B-cell lymphoma, usually about 10 years after diagnosis. Not surprisingly, lumps and bumps that arise from the salivary glands or lymph nodes are taken much more seriously in Sjögren's patients than others due to an increased vigilance for this complication. Several novel treatments for Sjögren's are currently under study and may prove to be "game changers" in the future; perhaps, someday, there will even be a cure. Given the anticipated expense and potential toxicities of new and stronger therapies, in today's healthcare environment, only individuals with established diagnoses are likely to have access to these drugs.

Table 2.4 Complications of Untreated Dry Eyes and Dry Mouth

Oral	Ocular
Accelerated caries	Corneal melting
Loss of dentition	Corneal ulcers
Weight loss	Corneal perforation
Oral candidiasis	Bacterial conjunctivitis
Sialolithiasis	Bacterial interstitial keratitis
Sleep disruption	Vision loss
Fibromyalgia	

Summing Up

Sjögren's is an autoimmune rheumatic disease that causes dry eyes, dry mouth, arthritis, and fatigue and, less commonly, affects the internal organs. Proper evaluation usually requires a whole battery of tests to look for objective evidence of dry eyes, objective evidence of dry mouth, and proof of autoimmunity. A correct diagnosis will facilitate more comprehensive treatment in order to help individuals avoid costly and devastating medical and dental complications.

For Further Reading

Seror R, Bowman SJ, Brito-Zeron P, et al. EULAR Sjögren's Syndrome Disease Activity Index (ESSDAI): A user guide. *RMD Open.* 2015;1:e000022.

Shiboski CH, Shiboski SC, Seror R, et al. 2016 American College of Rheumatology/European League Against Rheumatism classification criteria for primary Sjögren's syndrome: A consensus and data-driven methodology involving three international patient cohorts. *Arthritis Rheumatol.* 2017;69:35–45.

Shiboski SC, Shiboski CH, Criswell LA, et al. American College of Rheumatology classification criteria for Sjögren's syndrome: A data-driven, expert consensus approach in the Sjögren's International Collaborative Clinical Alliance Cohort. *Arthritis Care Res.* 2012;64(4):475–487.

Vitali C, Bombardieri S, Jonsson R, et al. Classification criteria for Sjögren's syndrome: A revised version of the European criteria proposed by the American-European consensus group. *Ann Rheum Dis.* 2002;61:554–558.

Vivino F. Sjögren's syndrome: Clinical aspects. *Clin Immunol.* 2017;182:48–54.

3

Who Develops Sjögren's?

Christine H. Lee and Daniel J. Wallace

Since Sjögren's was long considered a syndrome and a disease, ascertaining how many people have it and elucidating its epidemiologic features have proven to be difficult undertakings. Although there are a variety of reasons for this, the most important is that an international consensus on how to define Sjögren's has only recently been agreed upon. This chapter will review how many people have Sjögren's and the principal identifying features of those individuals as well as issues relating to genetic predisposition.

How Many People Have Sjögren's?

Most professionals trained in estimating the numbers of people with a disorder do so in terms of prevalence or incidence. *Prevalence* is defined as the number of individuals in a population with a condition, both new and preexisting, in a given timeframe. *Incidence* is the number of individuals in a population who are newly diagnosed in a given timeframe. Typically, incidence and prevalence rates use populations of 100,000 or 1 million to show how common or rare something is.

Some papers have published figures based upon self-reported dry eye or dry mouth with arthritis. Others have relied upon older definitions of Sjögren's, which could include dry eye, dry mouth, and arthritis; some of these cases could have occurred as a consequence of viral infections such as HIV or hepatitis. If we restrict ourselves to autoimmune Sjögren's, as opposed to nonimmunologic sicca syndrome, the Sjögren's Foundation estimates that more than 4 million people in the United States (out of 330 million) have it. This breaks down to one person in 83.

Where did these numbers come from? In the United States, approximately 0.5% of the population, or one person in 200, has immune features seen in Sjögren's. To these 1.4 million Americans, we next add the numbers of those who fulfill the criteria for other autoimmune conditions and who

Christine H. Lee and Daniel J. Wallace, *Who Develops Sjögren's?* In: *The Sjögren's Book*. Edited by: Daniel J. Wallace, Oxford University Press. © Sjögren's Foundation 2022. DOI: 10.1093/oso/9780197502112.003.0003

also have Sjögren's. Overall, approximately 30% of individuals with rheumatoid arthritis (3 million), systemic lupus erythematosus (<1 million), and
scleroderma-related disorders fulfill definitions for Sjögren's, as do other
musculoskeletal conditions that are autoimmune diseases (1 million). Thus,
1.5 million of these 5 million cases brings the total to 2.9 million. How does
one account for the remaining 1.1 million? The answer is simply because
Sjögren's is underreported. Many people (especially those with mild Sjögren's)
never bother to speak to their doctor about their symptoms, or their healthcare professional may attribute their symptoms to other causes. It is estimated
that there are between 53,000 (if we consider only cases fulfilling classification
criteria) and 248,000 (considering all physician-diagnosed cases) Sjögren's
patients living in the United States who don't have an associated autoimmune
rheumatic disease.

Age, Race, Geography, Sex, and the Environment

The majority of those with Sjögren's are diagnosed in the fourth or fifth decade
of life. Less than 5% of Sjögren's patients are under the age of 20, and nearly all
of these have anti-Ro/SSA antibodies. Onset of disease in the sixth or seventh
decade is not uncommon; prevalence has been found to be five to eight times
higher, though several confounding factors must be taken into account. There
is a higher rate of comorbid conditions and use of drying medications, which
can exacerbate sicca symptoms, as well as an increased prevalence of autoantibodies in the elderly.

Sjögren's is likely found in all races and ethnicities to a similar extent, although this has not been well studied. In the past decade, published studies
estimating the prevalence of the disease in China, Spain, Slovenia, Finland,
Greece, and the United States have demonstrated strikingly similar results.
In all of these surveys, 90% to 95% of people with Sjögren's without another major rheumatic, autoimmune disease were female. The percentage
is slightly lower in those without another related disease, but for all practical purposes, signs and symptoms of Sjögren's in males and females are the
same. More recently, data from a Manhattan registry has shown that incidence of Sjögren's (presented as per 100,000 person-years) was statistically
higher among Asian (10.5) and White women (6.2) compared with Black
(3.3) and Latina women (3.2). While prevalence rates were not statistically
significant among all groups, prevalence was found to be two times higher
for non-Europeans.

Studies indicate that there is a relationship between hormones and auto-immunity. Hormonal influences no doubt play a role in the female predominance of the disease, but this issue has not been adequately explored. The strong sex bias may potentially be explained by an X chromosome dose effect.

While chemical or environmental exposures play a role in other rheumatic disorders associated with Sjögren's, with the exception of sun sensitivity (which is directly related to antibodies to anti-Ro/SSA), no specific chemical or occupational exposure correlates definitively with the presence of Sjögren's. One exception would be increased symptoms of Sjögren's among individuals residing in regions with a dry climate.

Primary and Secondary Sjögren's

The terms "primary" and "secondary" were traditionally used when referring to Sjögren's, but their use is diminishing as Sjögren's is increasingly viewed as a distinct disease entity by itself and, while it can occur alone or in conjunction with other autoimmune, rheumatic diseases, may simply be termed "Sjögren's." Because these terms are still sometimes used by physicians and researchers, the distinction can be explained as follows.

Patients with primary Sjögren's by definition lack the obvious distinguishing features of rheumatoid arthritis, systemic lupus erythematosus, or scleroderma. These include deforming arthritis, malar and discoid rashes, and tight skin. However, compared to individuals with secondary Sjögren's, there are certain features noted more commonly in primary Sjögren's. These consist of Raynaud's phenomenon (color changes in the hands with cold exposure), salivary gland enlargement, swollen lymph nodes, anti-Ro/SSA and anti-La/SSB positivity, central nervous system dysfunction, and the potential for developing lymphoma (44 times greater than in healthy individuals). The most common subjective complaints include not only dry eyes and dry mouth but also fatigue.

Sjögren's, Genetics, and Other Autoimmune Diseases

Like all autoimmune diseases, Sjögren's can run in families. The prevalence of Sjögren's patients whose relatives have the disease is 12 times higher than in the general population. One Sjögren's patient in eight will have a relative (usually female) with the condition. Only a handful of reports of identical twins with Sjögren's have been published, generally with similar phenotypic findings. Genetic distance also plays a role, with higher relative risks in siblings compared to parents or offspring.

Clearly the genetic factors regulating inheritance of the disease are complex and multifactorial. A first-degree relative (parent, sibling, or child) of someone with Sjögren's has a 1% to 3% risk of developing the disease. Actually, these relatives have a much higher risk for being diagnosed with autoimmune thyroid disease or lupus than Sjögren's. In some studies, up to 30% of Sjögren's patients have Hashimoto's thyroiditis or are hypothyroid. Other autoimmune conditions found in 1% to 30% of Sjögren's patients include lupus, rheumatoid arthritis, scleroderma, inflammatory myositis, type 1 diabetes, and multiple sclerosis. Occasionally, family members of Sjögren's patients have antinuclear antibodies, rheumatoid factor, and anti-Ro/SSA on blood testing without any symptoms or evidence of autoimmune disease. Certain members of a series of genetic markers present on the surface of cells known as human leukocyte antigen (HLA) haplotypes, which also predispose individuals to Sjögren's. However, these subtypes are more so associated with anti-Ro/SSA and anti-La/SSB antibodies than the disease itself. This suggests that a genetic predisposition along with an environmental trigger leads to a benign, subclinical autoimmunity prior to the development of clinically apparent disease.

Summing Up

- One American in 83 has Sjögren's features. This population is overwhelmingly female and middle-aged.
- Sjögren's patients are at increased risk of having another autoimmune disorder (mostly autoimmune thyroid disease), developing lymphoma, or having a family member with an autoimmune disease.
- No geographic, racial, environmental, or ethnic risk factors have been associated with Sjögren's.

For Further Reading

Bolstad AI, Skarstein K. Epidemiology of Sjögren's syndrome—from an oral perspective. *Current Oral Health Reports.* 2016;3(4):328–336. doi:10.1007/s40496-016-0112-0

Izmirly PM, Buyon JP, Wan I, et al. The incidence and prevalence of adult primary Sjögren's syndrome in New York County. *Arthritis Care Res.* 2019;71(7):949–960. doi:10.1002/acr.23707

Kuo C, Grainge MJ, Valdes AM, et al. Familial risk of Sjögren's syndrome and co-aggregation of autoimmune diseases in affected families: A nationwide population study. *Arthritis Rheumatol.* 2015;67(7):1904–1912. doi:10.1002/art.39127

Maciel G, Crowson CS, Matteson EL, Cornec D. Incidence and mortality of physician-diagnosed primary Sjögren's syndrome: Time trends over a 40-year period in a population-based cohort in the United States. *Mayo Clinic Proc.* 2017;92(5):734–743. doi:10.1016/j.mayocp.2017.01.020

Maciel G, Crowson CS, Matteson EL, Cornec D. Prevalence of primary Sjögren's syndrome in a US population-based cohort. *Arthritis Care Res.* 2017;69:1612–1616. doi:10.1002/acr.23173

Patel R, Shahane A. The epidemiology of Sjögren's syndrome. *Clin Epidemiol.* 2014;6:247–255.

Theander E, Jonsson R, Sjöström B, et al. Prediction of Sjögren's syndrome years before diagnosis and identification of patients with early onset and severe disease course by autoantibody profiling. *Arthritis Rheumatol.* 2015;67(9):2427–2436. doi:10.1002/art.39214

4

The Impact of Living with Sjögren's

Matthew Makara

Sjögren's is a complex, multifaceted disease that can affect the body in many ways. However, the total effect of this disease goes far beyond the physical manifestations. Many patients experience notable impacts to their daily living, often experiencing mental, emotional, and financial burdens due to living with Sjögren's, in addition to the physical symptoms. Both individually and combined, these variables can cause and increase stress, which can then exacerbate disease symptoms. With that in mind, it's important to note that these burdens can play into and build upon one another and are not mutually exclusive, potentially creating a cycle that is difficult to break. An example of what this may look like is in Figure 4.1.

This chapter will recognize the different ways in which Sjögren's patients are impacted by this disease, with subsequent chapters in this book exploring these topics in greater detail.

Sjögren's Foundation Patient Survey

In 2016, the Harris Poll, on behalf of the Sjögren's Foundation, conducted a survey titled "Living with Sjögren's." Its purpose was to gain an understanding of all the ways in which Sjögren's impacts the lives of patients. In all, 2,962 Sjögren's patients aged 18 and older provided responses about their experiences with Sjögren's and its impact on their quality of life. We will discuss select results from the survey here. As already mentioned, each variable can easily impact a patient in multiple ways.

Impact of Symptoms

Although the most common Sjögren's symptoms are dry eyes, dry mouth, and fatigue, the disease can affect the entire body, and neuropathy, major

Matthew Makara, *The Impact of Living with Sjögren's* In: *The Sjögren's Book*. Edited by: Daniel J. Wallace, Oxford University Press. © Sjögren's Foundation 2022. DOI: 10.1093/oso/9780197502112.003.0004

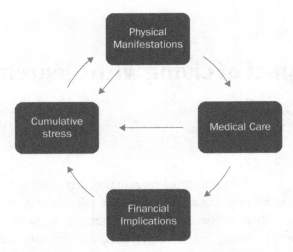

Figure 4.1 Hypothetical interactions of physical, financial, mental, and emotional burdens.

organ involvement, chronic pain, and more are also frequently experienced by patients. The survey found that there were 40 different symptoms experienced by at least 15% of respondents, 30 of which were experienced by more than 50% of this group. The top 10 most frequently experienced symptoms are listed in Table 4.1.

Table 4.1 Symptoms Most Frequently Experienced by Sjögren's Patients

Symptom	% of Patients*
Dry eyes	92
Dry mouth	92
Fatigue	80
Dry or itchy skin	76
Morning stiffness	69
Trouble sleeping	67
Joint pain	64
Dry nose	63
Forgetfulness	60
Brain fog	57

* Experienced almost weekly or more frequently during the previous 12 months at time of "Living with Sjögren's" survey completion (2016)

Impact on Daily Activities

A large majority of patients indicated that Sjögren's has a significant impact on their daily lives. Notably, 86% of patients agreed with the statement, "Living with Sjögren's makes every day a challenge." Furthermore, 71% of patients reported that Sjögren's gets in the way of their day-to-day lives. Some examples of affected activities were participating in hobbies and social and extracurricular activities (81%), performing activities of daily living (70%), traveling or taking vacations (69%), and the ability to be independent (51%). Seventy-four percent of respondents indicated they had to either stop or cut back on performing housework, and 22% had to modify their living space to accommodate limitations in mobility.

Financial Impact

The financial impact of Sjögren's on patients can be immense, with a variety of factors, including direct and indirect costs, playing a role. Two-thirds of patients who responded to the Foundation's survey stated that living with Sjögren's adds a significant financial burden to their life. Fifty-nine percent indicated that they see between two and 10 healthcare practitioners at least once per year. Specific costs, listed in order of highest, on average, for patients during a 12-month period were dental care, prescription medications, healthcare appointments and/or co-payments, over-the-counter medications/products, and alternative therapies. In total, the average amount spent on treatment was reported at $2,593.30.

Importantly, many respondents indicated that they had to adjust their work schedule, if not stop working altogether. Thirty percent of patients indicated that they had to take days off due to Sjögren's, and 28% had to either stop working or reduce their hours.

For a more detailed review and specific examples of financial implications, see Chapter 5.

Mental Impact

Cognitive impairment is commonly seen in Sjögren's. As seen in Table 4.1, "forgetfulness" and "brain fog" were two of the symptoms most frequently experienced by Sjögren's patients. Notably, 57% of respondents indicated that they experience "brain fog" weekly, if not more frequently. Speech difficulty is also common. Eighty-two percent of patients indicated that they had difficulty finding the correct word during conversations. Seventy-four percent of patients indicated that they had difficulty trying to concentrate on a task; this number increased to 77% when trying to concentrate on more than one task at a time.

Emotional Impact

As with the areas mentioned previously in this chapter, Sjögren's can greatly impact a person's emotional health. Nearly three-quarters of patients living with Sjögren's indicated that the disease adds a significant emotional burden to their lives, with 67% claiming that they struggle to cope with their disease. A large majority of Sjögren's patients indicated that living with the disease has a negative impact on their mood as well. This feeling is more apparent in younger populations (aged 60 years or less), where 89% indicated they felt a negative impact on mood. However, a large percentage (78%) of their older counterparts felt a negative impact on mood as well.

Lastly, Sjögren's patients indicated that living with Sjögren's had a negative impact on various types of relationships: 60% experienced a negative impact on their sex life, 63% experienced a negative impact with friends and family, and 55% experienced a negative impact with their spouse or partner.

Summing Up

Sjögren's is a complex disease that can impact patients in numerous ways, including physically, mentally, emotionally, and financially. These burdens are often interconnected, with an impact in one area potentially having an impact in another. A better understanding of how Sjögren's can impact a patient's life can help inform optimal healthcare decisions, assist loved ones in better understanding what is happening, and help patients cope and live their best lives possible.

For Further Reading

Hammitt KM, Naegeli AN, van den Broek RWM, Birt JA. Patient burden of Sjögren's: A comprehensive literature review revealing the range and heterogeneity of measures used in assessments of severity. *RMD Open*. 2017;3(2):e000443. doi:10.1136/rmdopen-2017-000443

McCoy SS, Bartels CM, Saldanha IJ, et al. National Sjögren's Foundation survey: burden of oral and systemic involvement on quality of life. *J Rheumatol.* 2021 Jul;48(7):1029–1036. doi:10.3899/jrheum.200733.

Saldanha IJ, Bunya VY, McCoy SS, Makara M, Baer AN, Akpek EK. Ocular manifestations and burden related to Sjögren Syndrome: results of a patient survey. *Am J Ophthalmol.* 2020 Nov;219:40–48. doi:10.1016/j.ajo.2020.05.043.

Sjögren's Foundation. Living with Sjögren's. https://www.sjogrens.org/files/articles/SSFLivingwithSjogrens.pdf

5

The Cost of Living with Sjögren's

Simon J. Bowman and Benjamin Fisher

Sjögren's is characterized on tissue biopsy by localized collections ("focal infiltrates") of white cells (lymphocytes) clustering around the ducts that move secretions, such as saliva, from secretory glands onto surfaces such as the lining of the mouth. This in turn, due to mechanisms that we don't fully understand, seems to inhibit the production of glandular secretions, leading to dryness—particularly of dry eyes and dry mouth. Sjögren's is also associated with high levels of fatigue and, in some patients, with other features affecting a variety of body systems. This can include mucosa-associated lymphoid tissue (MALT) lymphoma, but Sjögren's is not associated with a general increase in all-cause mortality. Health-related quality of life (HRQoL), however, is significantly reduced in patients with Sjögren's. Sjögren's is an area of large unmet need, with no drugs proven to modify the course of the disease (as opposed to drugs capable of improving symptoms such as eye drops, artificial saliva, and secretory stimulants such as pilocarpine or cevimeline).

Understanding the financial burden of Sjögren's is important to motivate drug development, to provide a basis for regulators and funders to license and approve any resulting therapies, and to justify the set-up of specialist multidisciplinary clinics to optimize care for patients with Sjögren's. Most of the available data on costs has been derived by studying patients who have Sjögren's in the absence of another connective tissue disease such as rheumatoid arthritis (RA), systemic lupus erythematosus, or systemic sclerosis.

In "costing" any disease there are two main aspects: direct and indirect costs. Direct costs are related to the value of resources used in the diagnosis, treatment, and rehabilitation of patients. This might include the costs of outpatient visits; blood, urine, and other tests; imaging studies; nursing care; physiotherapy; visits to the emergency room; dental and optometry care; surgery; hospital admissions; and so forth. One way that this data can be collected is by self-reporting through questionnaires. Following this approach, using the Stanford Health Questionnaire Economic Component, a study

Simon J. Bowman and Benjamin Fisher, *The Cost of Living with Sjögren's* In: *The Sjögren's Book*. Edited by: Daniel J. Wallace, Oxford University Press. © Sjögren's Foundation 2022. DOI: 10.1093/oso/9780197502112.003.0005 carried out in Birmingham, UK, calculated that the mean annual total direct costs per Sjögren's patient in the United Kingdom were 81% of those of RA at 2004–2005 prices, before the widespread introduction of biologics for RA (Table 5.1).

In the United States, a 2009 study showed that health care utilization was higher in patients over a 5-year period when compared with controls, and this included greater out-of-pocket dental expenses (on average $1,473.30 for Sjögren's patients vs. $503.60 for controls), a greater number of dental visits (4.0 vs. 2.3) and current treatments (6.6 vs. 2.5), and more hospitalizations (53% of Sjögren's patients admitted to hospitals over the 5-year period vs. 40% of controls). Fox et al. also showed higher oral healthcare costs in Sjögren's patients, with an annual out-of-pocket dental care spending two to three times higher than controls. Patients had more frequent dental visits, more decayed teeth, and more dental restorations. In East China, the medical cost of treating dry eye in Sjögren's has been reported to have a heavy economic burden on both patients and the healthcare system, with an average annual per patient total expenditure of 7,637.2 Chinese yuan (approximately $1,173.80), with about a third of this being paid by patients themselves. Higher medical expenses for dry eye were associated with poorer mental health in Sjögren's patients.

A second approach to measure direct costs, which can be used in health-care systems that automatically collect electronic data, is to extract the direct healthcare costs from the provider/insurer/national database. In a more recent U.S. study, all-cause healthcare costs were 40% higher for patients in the 12 months after diagnosis versus the 12 months before diagnosis, with costs averaging $20,416 per patient. Outpatient visits were required by nearly 100%

Table 5.1 Annual Indirect and Direct Costs of Sjögren's, RA, and Controls

	Indirect Costs		Direct Costs	Total Costs
	Low Range	High Range	(not including cost of biologic agents)	
Control group	£892 (~US$1,418)	£3,382 (~US$5,353)	£949 (~US$1,509)	£1,841–£4,331 (~US$2,927–$6,886)
Sjögren's patients	£7,677 (~US$12,150)	£13,502 (~US$16,530)	£2,188 (~US$3,479)	£9,865–£15,690 (~US$15,685–$24,947)
RA patients	£10,444 (~US$16,530)	£17,070 (~US$27,016)	£2,693 (~US$4,282)	£13,137–£19,763 (~US$20,887–$31,423)

Table reprinted from the *Sjögren's Quarterly*, Summer 2010, U.S. comparables added.

of Sjögren's patients to various providers, with almost four visits on average per patient over a 1-year period.

Healthcare costs, however, are not the only costs of a disease. Perhaps even more important are the broader societal and individual costs—the indirect costs. These include the consequences of loss of work as a result of developing a disease and more subtle versions of this, such as only being able to work part-time; having to take time off to attend medical or other appointments; leaving work early; family/friends having to take time off work to accompany the patient or care for them; needing additional help with housework or child-care; and so forth. In addition, patients and their families face potential loss of health insurance or excessively high premiums; may have more difficulty than their healthy counterparts in securing life, health, or disability insurance; and, because of their unpredictable health and employment status, may face difficulty securing loans such as mortgages. Often these costs are estimates—future salaries or other lost opportunity costs are inevitably speculative, so often a range of costs can be calculated depending on how various estimates are modeled.

In a UK study based on the same patient group mentioned earlier, the estimated total annual indirect costs, at 2004–2005 prices, including lost economic productivity, housework, and childcare, were £7,677 for Sjögren's patients, £10,444 for RA patients, and £892 (95% confidence interval: £307–£1,478) for controls. Using a model that maximizes the estimates, the equivalent figures were £13,502, £17,070, and £3,382, respectively (see Table 5.1).

Similar to the findings in the UK study, the 2009 study by Segal et al. also showed that Sjögren's patients were more likely to be unemployed due to disability. In Germany, there is a greater frequency of physician visits for patients with Sjögren's and lower levels of gainful employment; these findings were associated with depression, fatigue, and a lack of stamina.

An interesting study from Sweden linked data from a Sjögren's register with that from the Swedish Social Insurance Agency. The authors showed that work disability increased in the first 2 years after diagnosis of Sjögren's. They found an initial increase in sick leave that was followed by a rising number of patients receiving a disability pension. At diagnosis, 26% of patients were work-disabled, compared with 37% at 12 months after diagnosis and 41% at 24 months. Similarly, a higher percentage of Sjögren's patients received disease compensation (47%) versus the general Dutch population (2%). Patients were less often employed, worked fewer hours, and were less frequently employed full time. Having disease compensation in this study was associated with a number of factors that may indicate more severe disease, such as having a greater number of extraglandular manifestations and needing artificial saliva and the prescription of hydroxychloroquine.

Treatment for Sjögren's is currently limited, essentially, to symptomatic approaches, with modest exceptions. As a consequence, there is currently considerable interest in developing biologic or other novel therapies to address the unmet need in Sjögren's. The best-studied therapy to date is rituximab (a humanized anti-CD20 monoclonal antibody that targets B lymphocytes). In the UK TRACTISS study, however, this was found to be neither clinically effective nor cost-effective for the management of Sjögren's.

Summing Up

Although Sjögren's does not, in general, impair life expectancy and is often inappropriately considered a benign condition, the financial burden and the work disability associated with it, as assessed across multiple countries and continents, are striking. This strongly supports the economic argument for the development of new therapies to treat this disease.

Acknowledgments and Conflicts of Interest

Both authors are part-funded through the National Institute of Health Research Birmingham Biomedical Research Centre. Simon Bowman has consulted for the following companies in the field of Sjögren's: Astra Zeneca, Biogen, BMS, Celgene, Eli Lilly, Genentech, Glenmark, GSK, Medimmune, MT Pharma, Novartis, Ono, Pfizer, Roche, Servier, UCB, xtlbio. Benjamin Fisher has consulted for Novartis, Roche, BMS and Astra Zeneca/Medimmune.

For Further Reading

Birt JA, Tan Y MN. Sjögren's syndrome: Managed care data from a large United States population highlight real-world health care burden and lack of treatment options. *Clin Exp Rheumatol.* 2017;35:98–107.

Bowman S, Colin C, O'Dwyer J, et al. Randomized controlled trial of rituximab and cost-effectiveness analysis in treating fatigue and oral dryness in primary Sjögren's syndrome. *Arthritis Rheumatol.* 2017;69:1440–1450.

Bowman SJ, St Pierre Y, Sutcliffe N, et al. Estimating indirect costs in primary Sjögren's syndrome. *J Rheumatol.* 2010;37:1010–1015.

Callaghan R, Prabu A, Allan RB, et al. UK Sjögren's Interest Group. Direct healthcare costs and predictors of costs in patients with primary Sjögren's syndrome. *Rheumatology.* 2007;46(1):105–111.

Fox PC, Bowman SJ, Segal B, et al. Oral involvement in primary Sjögren syndrome. *J Am Dent Assoc.* 2008;139:1592–1601.

Lendrem D, Mitchell S, McMeekin P, et al. Health-related utility values of patients with primary Sjögren's syndrome and its predictors. *Ann Rheum Dis.* 2014;73:1362–1368.

Mandl T, Jørgensen TS, Skougaard M, et al. Work disability in newly diagnosed patients with primary Sjögren syndrome. *J Rheumatol.* 2017;44:209–215.

Meijer JM, Meiners PM, Huddleston Slater JJR, et al. Health-related quality of life, employment and disability in patients with Sjögren's syndrome. *Rheumatology.* 2009;48:1077–1082.

Segal B, Bowman SJ, Fox PC, et al. Primary Sjögren's syndrome: Health experiences and predictors of health quality among patients in the United States. *Health & Quality of Life Outcomes.* 2009;7:46.

Theander E, Manthorpe R, Jacobsson LT. Mortality and causes of death in primary Sjögren's syndrome: A prospective cohort study. *Arthritis Rheumatol.* 2004;50:1262–1269.

Westhoff G, Dörner T, Zink A. Fatigue and depression predict physician visits and work disability in women with primary Sjögren's syndrome: Results from a cohort study. *Rheumatology.* 2012;51(2):262–269.

Yao W, Le Q. Social-economic analysis of patients with Sjogren's syndrome dry eye in East China: A cross-sectional study. *BMC Ophthalmol.* 2018;18:23.

PART II
THE SCIENCE OF SJÖGREN'S

6

Sjögren's and the Immune System

Robert I. Fox and Steven E. Carsons

Sjögren's is an autoimmune disorder that develops when one's *genetic predisposition* combines with *environmental or infectious factors*. Further, *neural* and *hormonal factors* influence the onset and severity of the disease.

The immune process involves the salivary, lacrimal, and other moisture-producing glands (leading to dryness) and may involve additional organs, including nerves, muscles, joints, lung, kidney, gastrointestinal organs, and/or skin. There is a high frequency of associated fibromyalgia, a poorly understood condition that has symptoms of fatigue and vague cognitive changes. Although the pathogenesis of Sjögren's remains unclear, it involves the immune system in a manner that leads to an imbalance of inflammatory transmitters in the glands, tissues, and nerve fibers. Chapter 8 outlines recent advances on specific genes associated with Sjögren's.

This chapter reviews the two basic parts of the immune system:

1. The *acquired* (HLA-DR dependent) immune system associated with autoantibody production
2. The *innate* (HLA-DR independent) system responsible for many of the symptoms occurring in Sjögren's.

We will also review how genetic factors interact with environmental factors to alter the hormonal and neural system and thus produce the symptoms of Sjögren's.

There are several important take-home points regarding the immune system and of Sjögren's that will help us understand symptoms, current therapies, and approaches to develop new therapies:

1. On biopsy of the salivary or lacrimal gland, only about 50% of the ducts and acini are destroyed, so one of the key questions is: *Why are the residual glands not functioning at optimal level?*
2. Salivary and lacrimal functions, namely the production of tears and saliva, are part of a "functional" circuit that includes the central nervous

Robert I. Fox and Steven E. Carsons, *Sjögren's and the Immune System* In: *The Sjögren's Book*. Edited by: Daniel J. Wallace, Oxford University Press. © Sjögren's Foundation 2022. DOI: 10.1093/oso/9780197502112.003.0006 system (midbrain and cortex of the brain), which in turn controls the blood vessels and glandular function.

3. Saliva and tears are more than just water; they contain a complex mixture of proteins, carbohydrates, and mucins to provide the lubrication required for movement of the mucosal membranes (including the eyelids and tongue).

4. Complex interactions of immune cells release a series of inflammatory factors that interfere with normal glandular function of the moisture-producing glands and of extraglandular tissues. Type I interferon is an important part of this process.

5. Sjögren's patients have more aggressive lymphocytes compared to patients with other autoimmune disorders. This factor is reflected in an elevated frequency of lymphomas or infiltration into other organs such as nerves, lung, or kidney.

Interaction of Genetic and Environmental Factors

Inherited genes are important—but not enough to explain why patients develop Sjögren's. In this chapter, we will often "lump together" certain results of studies in Sjögren's and systemic lupus erythematosus (SLE), since the genetic and non-genetic factors appear to have a great deal in common, and the "data banks" for SLE are more extensive than those available for Sjögren's at present. Indeed, the symptoms and pattern of autoantibodies often overlap, and the medications used for management are frequently similar. However, the differences between Sjögren's and SLE will also be discussed.

Physicians and patients have long recognized that simply having susceptibility genes is not enough to guarantee the emergence of clinical disease. The simplest example is the lack of "concurrence" of Sjögren's or SLE in identical twins:

- Each identical twin shares the same genome but has different exposure to environmental agents and slightly different ways in which their genes are activated (or rearranged) as they respond to infections and hormonal changes.
- If only genetic factors were required, we would expect that if one twin develops Sjögren's, then the other twin would always develop Sjögren's as well.
- Although the second identical twin does have an increased risk for development of Sjögren's (which is called the "concordance rate"), the

observed frequency of Sjögren's (or SLE) in the other twin is only about 15% to 20%.

- Roughly speaking, only about 20% of the disease can be considered strictly genetic (i.e., encoded by a person's genome), with the other 80% due to other factors such as environmental influence, including exposure to infections or hormonal changes.
- Recently, there has been much excitement regarding the field of epigenetics, which involves inheritable changes in gene expression by factors outside of the individual's DNA sequence. It has been postulated that prenatal exposures, a person's diet, and environmental factors such as pollution can induce epigenetic changes. Thus, epigenetics may explain differences between the occurrence of Sjögren's in genetically identical individuals

Even though there is a great deal of enthusiasm surrounding "genomic sequencing," we must remember that the best we will do in terms of prediction is what nature has provided us in the form of identical twins.

We do not want to minimize the important role of advances in genetics, and Chapter 8 will outline advances in identifying important genes and the interaction of genes (a field called proteomics).

To summarize, the study of genetics of Sjögren's has allowed the identification of different genes that vary from "very important" to those that seem to play a much weaker role, as assessed by a genetic measure termed *relative risk association*. Each individual will have some combination of these genes, and, in the presence of an environmental trigger, an "immune mistake" will occur in which the body attacks some portion of glands or other tissues in a pattern characteristic for each Sjögren's patient.

Long before we ever started genetic studies, it was clear that *one of the most important genes was gender, as 90% of Sjögren's patients are female*. However, specific genes on the X chromosome have been difficult to identify. One of the important genes identified in animal models was called the "Toll receptor," a molecule that helps link immune response to different environmental antigens (discussed in more details later in the chapter). An important role also exists for sex hormones in modulating the effect of many other genes involved in inflammation. In males who have Sjögren's, there is an increased frequency of an extra X chromosome (a condition called Klinefelter's syndrome). However, only a small percentage of males with Sjögren's have the extra chromosome, so that cannot be the whole story. Researchers are trying to identify the specific mechanisms of hormonally responsive genes (particularly because of their role in progression of certain cancers), but this task has remained difficult to translate into useful therapies for Sjögren's or other auto-immune diseases.

The second strongest gene (or cluster of genes) is located on chromosome 6 in a region that was first identified during the early days of organ transplantation. These genes are termed "human lymphocyte antigen" (HLA) genes and control the body's immune response to foreign cells or proteins. When a person is "typed" for donation of an organ (such as liver or kidney), both the donor and recipient are tested for their HLA genes, since a match will greatly decrease the chance of organ rejection by the immune system. Subsequent studies have identified a series of additional genes on chromosome 6 that also contribute by encoding additional proteins, including one that was named "complement" (since it complemented the activity of antibodies), and other inflammatory mediators or receptors for those mediators.

The take-home lesson here is that each Sjögren's patient has a series of genes, and when a genetically predisposed individual encounters certain environmental and hormonal stimulation, a "mistake" may be made that leads to activation of the immune system and the initiation and perpetuation of clinical symptoms of Sjögren's or SLE. Figure 6.1 is a schematic showing the timeline. The patient starts with the genetic tendency (i.e., female and perhaps HLA-DR3, discussed later in the chapter). This predisposes the patient to make a particular set of autoantibodies that we measure in blood tests, such as the *anti-nuclear antibody* (ANA) and the antibody to *Sjögren's-associated antigen A* (SS-A), which we now recognize as actually two different proteins with molecular weight 60,000 and 52,000 respectively. Some patients make antibodies against only the 60,000 molecule, others only against the 52,000 molecule, but most patients make antibodies against both. In some patients, a second Sjögren's-associated antigen termed SS-B, with molecular weight 45,000, is also found. These are detected in clinical blood tests run for the diagnosis of Sjögren's. The ability of each patient to make particular antibodies is closely correlated with the particular HLA-DR (and associated genes) that they have inherited.

These antibodies may be present for many years prior to the onset of any clinical disease; indeed, a large number of patients with these antibodies may never develop clinically significant disease.

The SS-A and SS-B are proteins that are derived from dying cells, a process called apoptosis. It has been postulated that some virus damages particular cells in the salivary gland, leading to the release of the SS-A and SS-B proteins, and that an immune response against "self-antigens" becomes a self-perpetuating autoimmune response in genetically predisposed individuals. We will

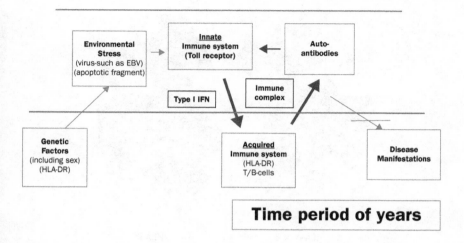

Figure 6.1 Time course of autoimmune response.

Time course of autoimmune response:

1. Environmental stress is interpreted in context of genetic factors

2. Antibodies precede disease

3. Presence of antibody does not mean disease

discuss later in the chapter some of the environmental agents and apoptotic fragments that contribute to the immune process.

The (HLA-DR-Dependent) Acquired Immune System

The genome encodes two types of immune response. The part that involves "immune memory" and is associated with the antibodies characteristic of Sjögren's is called the *acquired or adaptive* immune system. This is the part of the immune system first identified as being important in tissue transplantation. These histocompatibility genes are made of DNA and encode a series of proteins called HLA genes (Figure 6.2). The HLA antigens were named in the order of their discovery: HLA-A, then HLA-B and HLA-C, and finally HLA-D.

The most important of these transplantation genes for the development of Sjögren's or SLE was found to be HLA-D. The genes encoded by HLA-A and

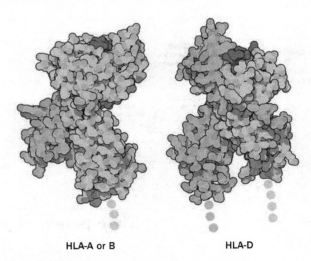

HLA-A or B   HLA-D

Figure 6.2 The histocompatibility antigens bind small peptides.

HLA-B have a slightly different structure than the structure of HLA-D (see Figure 6.2). In recognition of the importance of the HLA-D region and its control of autoantibody production, the acquired (transplantation-like) portion of the immune system is also called the HLA-DR-dependent part of the immune system.

The function of these histocompatibility genes is analogous to a plate that holds food in an orientation that can be recognized by certain immune lymphocytes that "come to the table." This is shown in Figure 6.2, where the histocompatibility molecule holds the small string of about 12 amino acids (called peptides) in a particular conformation (shown by the red molecule held in a groove). The stabilization of the peptide allows efficient recognition of the molecule by other immune cells. If the peptide exhibits a correct fit with the immune receptor (generally on the surface of the T cell or B cell, discussed later), then the lymphocyte will be stimulated to make an immune response. This ability to present (or not present) a peptide to the other immune cells is one of the key regulatory steps of the immune system. Under certain circumstances, particular inherited HLA-D genes allow self-peptides to be "presented" to T cells and B cells, thus enabling an autoimmune response.

Each individual inherits one copy of chromosome 6 from each parent and each contains one copy of HLA-DR. Thus, the patient has two chances to be a responder (i.e., a binder of peptide) or a non-responder if neither one of the histocompatibility antigens efficiently binds the peptide. These histocompatibility genes are different in different individuals (like brown eyes or blue eyes) but involve many more choices (as if we could have a hundred different types of eye color). Further, the distribution of these HLA-D antigens is quite different in distinct ethnic populations, which may help explain the different frequency and clinical manifestations in different countries.

The reason for the diversity of HLA-DR genes in the world's population is the strong Darwinian selection pressure to be able to bind some past or future infectious agent and make an immune response. For example, in Hawaii, the native population was "inbred" (lacking diversity of HLA-DR molecules) and thus could not respond to the measles infection brought by foreign sailors, leading to the decimation of the native population. In a sense, the price we pay for autoimmunity (the excessive response to certain self-genes) is the protection from known and unknown viruses.

One of the surprising findings of the study of immunology is that a key role for the immune system is the disposal of fragments of dead cells that may die of natural causes or after a viral infection. We create about a billion new cells per day, and an equal number die a "normal death." The debris from these dead cells must be removed and digested so the protein and nucleic acid building blocks can be reused to form new cells. Indeed, one of the immune system's most important functions is to be the "garbage collector" for cell debris.

One of the leading theories of autoimmune disease is that a mistake in processing of the fragments from dead cells is a key stimulus to development of autoimmune disease. Rather than simply disposing of the dead cell material, a mistake is made, and the dead cell's material is identified as foreign and the immune system is activated (as if it were a foreign graft or invading virus). For example, in Sjögren's patients, the characteristic antibody is anti-SS-A, and immune responses against the SS-A protein may have a role in perpetuating the damage to the glands and other tissues.

SS-A is a normal nuclear protein found in all cells, and its job is to be the "chaperone" for another protein into the cell's cytoplasm. However, this protein (and its associated RNA molecule) is particularly difficult for the immune system to break down, and thus SS-A may accumulate after a cell dies, and the result is a stimulus to the immune system. Part of that reaction is the formation of antibodies to SS-A, a characteristic laboratory finding in many Sjögren's patients.

To summarize the contribution of the acquired immune system, autoimmunity is caused when self-antigens cannot be properly removed by the "garbage collectors," and the residual protein is inappropriately bound to the HLA-D molecule. This in turn stimulates a cascade of other immune factors that constitute the acquired immune system. This includes production of autoantibodies and the release of inflammatory factors that are measured when we try to assess the activity of the disease, such as the level of anemia, sedimentation rate, or attack of the immune system on organs other than the salivary and lacrimal glands. Many of the medicines used in autoimmune disease were initially developed to prevent organ rejection in the transplant model; these include prednisone, hydroxychloroquine, methotrexate, and many others.

The (HLA-DR-Independent) Innate Immune System

We noted that the acquired (HLA-DR) system was important but could not explain the entire story. In parallel with the search for an understanding of organ transplantation, other scientists were trying to understand the immune system's response to infectious organisms. Why do we get fevers, muscle and joint pains, and even a profound sense of fatigue that we associate with feeling "flu-ish"? This led to recognition of a different part of the immune system that did not involve the HLA-DR system: the "innate" (inborn) or the HLA-DR-independent immune response.

In autoimmune disorders such as Sjögren's or SLE, there is a close mutual stimulation of the innate and the acquired immune system. To assess disease activity and understand symptoms of Sjögren's, we must understand both arms of the immune system.

The acquired immune system is important, but it takes about 2 to 3 weeks after a foreign infection for this system to recognize the invader and make the appropriate T-cell/B-cell and antibody responses. With most infections, we would have succumbed long before, assuming it was not an infection we recognized from a prior encounter and had an acquired immune memory.

Thus, studies of our response to infections such as pneumococcal infection led to recognition of a separate branch of the immune system called the innate (HLA-D-independent) system. The acquired system (defined by HLA-D) and the innate system work closely together to defend us from external infections, but when they function together in excess, the result may be autoimmune disease such as Sjögren's or SLE.

The innate immune system provides our first line of defense against bacteria and viruses. It consists of a different set of cells, such as *macrophages* and *dendritic cells*, that are not dependent on HLA-D proteins for their response. Instead, it has evolutionarily evolved a series of receptors that is more limited but can immediately recognize particular proteins, sugars, or nucleic acids that are common to many pathogens in the environment. Indeed, many of the symptoms such as fever or muscle aches that we feel in response to viruses or bacteria derive from the immediate release of inflammatory hormones (commonly referred to as cytokines) from the cells of the innate immune system. A further consequence of stimulating the innate immune system is the stimulation of the acquired immune system described earlier. It is the perpetual mutual stimulation of the innate (HLA-D-independent) and the acquired (HLA-D-dependent) systems that characterizes autoimmune disorders such as Sjögren's and SLE.

The Relationship Between Sjögren's and SLE

The immunologic and clinical features of Sjögren's and SLE show a great deal of overlap (Figure 6.3; Box 6.1). However, there are distinct differences that are important. Perhaps the easiest way to simplify this overlap is to consider Sjögren's to be an attack of the exocrine (secretory) glands mediated largely by lymphocytes, whereas SLE is a disease where the "organ" damage usually occurs in multiple organ systems and is mediated by autoantibodies. However, the results are similar: glands and organs are damaged either directly by lymphocytes or autoantibodies, and autoantibodies can play a role in both diseases. Autoantibodies can bind with self-antigens, which are mistaken for foreign proteins. The autoantibody may be directed against an antigen (i.e., protein) located on the surface of a red blood cell (leading to hemolytic anemia), a platelet (leading to a condition called thrombocytopenia), or the skin (leading to certain types of rashes).

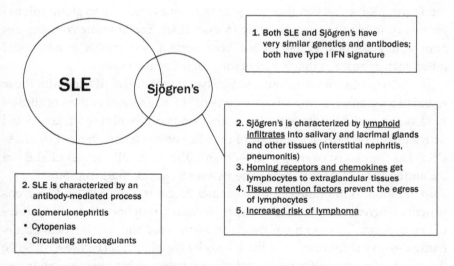

Figure 6.3 What is the relationship between SLE and Sjögren's?

Box 6.1 Sjögren's at a Glance

- An autoimmune disorder characterized by severely dry eyes and dry mouth, due to lymphocytic infiltrates
- Prevalence: 0.1% to 0.3% of adult females
- Female:male ratio is 9:1.
- Two peak ages of onset—in the 30s and in the 50s
- Many older patients diagnosed with "SLE" actually have Sjögren's.
- Patients have a characteristic HLA-DR (extended haplotype): In Caucasians, it is extended DR3.
- The genetic background is different in distinct ethnic groups (Chinese, Japanese, Greeks), but these groups have similar antibody profiles.
- The autoantibody profile is similar to subset of SLE.
- Increases mortality risk, particularly due to lymphoproliferative complications.
- Causes high burden of illness and diminished quality of life
- May lead to disability, especially for those with fatigue and cognitive issues
- Is limiting for basic tasks: for instance, dry eyes cause the patient to have difficulty working on a computer and reading; dry mouth affects talking, eating, and social interaction; both affect sleep

---

Also, autoantibodies may bind to circulating proteins or DNA to form immune complexes that can then lodge in the kidney (leading to glomerulonephritis) or in blood vessels (leading to vasculitis). The immune complex can bind to an additional protein called "complement" and trigger an additional inflammatory cascade that is part of the innate immune system.

The pattern of antibodies found in SLE has a great deal of overlap with those found in Sjögren's. It is important to think of SLE as a series of different clinical syndromes, each with its own characteristic autoantibodies (each associated with a distinct HLA-DR), and one of the SLE subsets (characterized by HLA-DR3) has the closest overlap with Sjögren's. The HLA-DR3 subset of SLE has the antibody to SS-A, and these patients have Sjögren's-like symptoms.

In addition to immune complex features found in both SLE and Sjögren's patients, Sjögren's is also characterized by dryness throughout the body. Features of dry eye and dry mouth are shown in Figures 6.4 and 6.5. Dryness occurs partly due to the infiltration of the glands by lymphocytes (Figure 6.6). Since the glands of most healthy individuals do not have any lymphocytic infiltrates,

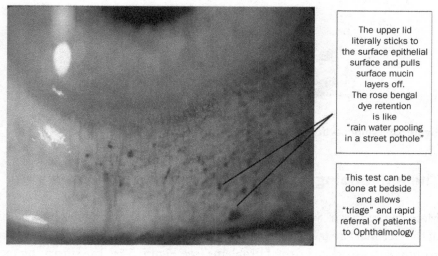

The upper lid literally sticks to the surface epithelial surface and pulls surface mucin layers off.
The rose bengal dye retention is like "rain water pooling in a street pothole"

This test can be done at bedside and allows "triage" and rapid referral of patients to Ophthalmology

Figure 6.4 Dryness results in the clinical appearance of keratoconjunctivitis sicca (KCS) characteristic of Sjögren's.

we must consider Sjögren's a disease of "aggressive" lymphocytes in which they get into tissues where they do not belong. This aggressive tendency can become very pronounced (Figure 6.7), to the point where the salivary glands become massively infiltrated and the patient may develop a lymphoma.

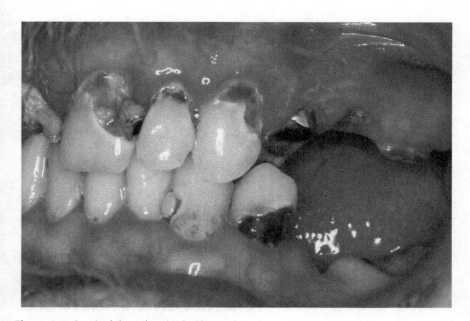

Figure 6.5 Cervical dental caries in Sjögren's

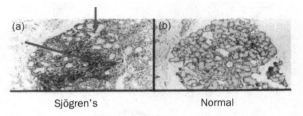

Sjögren's   Normal

Figure 6.6 Lymphocytic infiltrates (*arrows*) in Sjögren's (**a**) versus normal (**b**).

The Immunology of Clinical Symptoms in Sjögren's

More commonly in Sjögren's, we see only the results of glandular infiltration of the lacrimal and tear glands that results in dry eyes (see Figure 6.4) and dry mouth with associated dental problems (see Figure 6.5). The surprising feature of this severe dryness is that the glands are not totally destroyed by the lymphocytic infiltrates (see Figure 6.6).

Although we previously pointed out the lymphocytes that form clusters in the gland, we now emphasize that about 50% of the glands remain viable. So one of the key questions in Sjögren's is: *Why are the residual glands not functioning at a high level?*

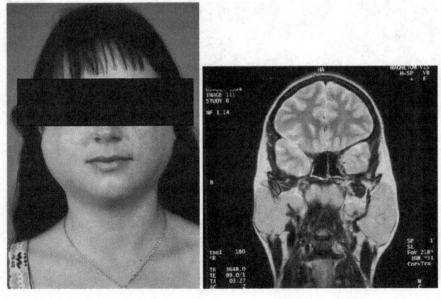

Figure 6.7 Parotid enlargement in Sjögren's.

In other diseases, a kidney continues to secrete fluid until it is over 90% destroyed; similarly, a liver or lung continues to function until it is over 90% damaged. Thus, we must conclude that the local release of inflammatory mediators within the gland causes the residual cells to become "paralyzed." This concept is extremely important, because it suggests that as newer and better treatments are discovered, there is the potential for salivary and lacrimal glands to recover function.

Studies in animal models indicate that the inflammatory mediators (such as type I interferon, tumor necrosis factor [TNF], and interferon gamma) greatly decrease the gland's ability to respond to neural stimulation. An example of a salivary gland biopsy with cells producing type I interferon is shown in Figure 6.8 (where the arrow depicts a few of the cells with red color that is the type I interferon). Also in this figure, the right-hand panel shows the gene expression signature from the lip biopsy from different individuals. The three columns on the left are from "normals," the next three columns are from Sjögren's patients, and the three columns on the right side are from patients with dryness not due to Sjögren's. The pattern of colored bands indicates the strength of gene expression. In the middle columns (from the Sjögren's patients), the dark green bands at the top of each column indicate a very high level of expression and

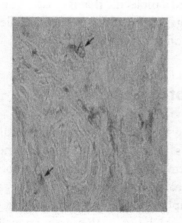

Arrows indicate cells in
Sjögren's SG biopsy with
type I IFN

Normal lip biopsies lack type I interferon
gene signature

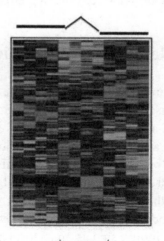

Sjögren's SG biopsy with type I IFN
gene profile

Figure 6.8 Interferon type I in the salivary gland suggests a role in Sjögren's.

show the characteristic pattern associated with response to type I interferon. We see that the lip biopsies from different Sjögren's patients all share a pattern of genes that are upregulated by type I interferon.

To re-emphasize this important point: One of the pivotal inflammatory molecules in both Sjögren's and SLE is type I interferon. This molecule is normally produced by the innate immune system in response to infection. It leads to low-grade fevers, myalgias, arthralgias, cognitive symptoms, and all the symptoms we associate with having the flu. It leads to elevation of the erythrocyte sedimentation rate (ESR) and C-reactive protein (CRP) levels, which we routinely measure in Sjögren's patients to assess activity. When the lymphocytes infiltrate the salivary or lacrimal gland, they paralyze the gland's response to normal stimuli. Thus, the gland may be only 50% destroyed, but the residual glandular tissue cannot secrete adequately due to the presence of inflammatory mediators such as type 1 interferon.

However, most of us get over flu symptoms in a day or two, so the next key question is: *What leads to the persistence of production of the type I interferon signal in the glands and other tissues?* This appears to be the link between the acquired (HLA-DR) and innate (non-HLA-DR) systems.

Perhaps an additional factor in causing Sjögren's is the finding that certain genes appear to increase the sensitivity of type I interferon production and response. Sjögren's patients have an increased frequency of two of these genes called *interferon response factor 5* (IRF5), and a molecule that is closely bound to the type I interferon receptor (Stat 4). In genome-wide screens, IRF5 alleles and Stat 4 are associated with a predisposition to develop Sjögren's.

Extraglandular Manifestations of Sjögren's

In addition to dryness, Sjögren's patients may have other symptoms, including rash, muscle pains (myalgia), joint pains (arthralgia), nerve pain (neuropathy), and fatigue. Lymphocytes that leave their site of origin (the bone marrow) and travel through the bloodstream can settle in various organs that may be involved (Figure 6.9). The lymphocytes are generated with a series of cell surface molecules that tell them which organs they are responsible for patrolling (the molecules on the lymphocyte are called "addressins" since they encode the address of the target organ). Any tissue that has inflammation may induce signals on its local blood vessels to attract those circulating lymphocytes (molecules called vascular adhesive molecules). The combination of addressins and vascular adhesive molecules determines which tissues will be involved by lymphocytic infiltration. The genes that encode these

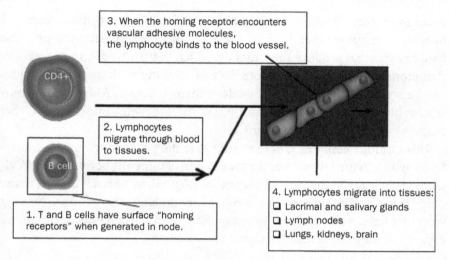

3. When the homing receptor encounters vascular adhesive molecules, the lymphocyte binds to the blood vessel.

CD4+

2. Lymphocytes migrate through blood to tissues.

B cell

4. Lymphocytes migrate into tissues:
☐ Lacrimal and salivary glands
☐ Lymph nodes
☐ Lungs, kidneys, brain

1. T and B cells have surface "homing receptors" when generated in node.

Figure 6.9   Clinical manifestations of Sjögren's reflect lymphocyte homing and retention patterns.

addressins and cell surface adhesion molecules also serve as a risk factor for development of disease and provide a target for future therapy. The type of tissue usually involved in Sjögren's is known as epithelium. Epithelial tissue contains cells that form the lining of organs, glands, and the skin. Why the epithelium is a particular target of autoreactive lymphocytes in Sjögren's is not entirely known but may in part be due to expression of adhesion molecules as well as peptides expressed by the tissue.

In addition to the glands discussed earlier, we mentioned that other tissues such as lung, kidney, skin, and nerves might have lymphocytic infiltration. For this to occur, the lymphocytes must travel through the bloodstream until they reach the target organ. The lymphocytes know when to take the "exit ramp off the highway" of the bloodstream due to addressins on the lymphocyte and vascular adhesion molecules on the local blood vessels. The additional genes that lead to susceptibility to Sjögren's (and its extraglandular manifestations) play a key role in regulating this process of lymphocytes "homing" to the target organs.

Role of Antibodies Against SS-A and SS-B Antigens

The HLA-DR system encodes a tendency to make antibodies against the SS-A antigen, so a person born with the HLA-DR3 gene has a higher tendency to make the autoantibody. In salivary or lacrimal gland tissue that is damaged by a virus or some other process, the SS-A antigen stimulates the immune lymphocytes that produce the antibody, which in turn binds to a normal cell chaperone called hYRNA. A more detailed binding of these two molecules can be predicted by computer models of their structure. Although this molecular biology is esoteric, it is fun to see the probable "smoking gun" that perpetuates the process of Sjögren's.

This immune complex is able to stimulate the production of type I interferon, which in turn stimulates the production of more antibody to SS-A. A vicious cycle leads to the clinical picture of Sjögren's or SLE. Of course, many other genes and hormones play a role in modulating this process. Finding ways to interrupt this cycle without crippling the important infection-fighting capacity of the body is a goal of current research.

Hormonal Influences

Estrogen activity may be involved in developing dryness symptoms because of two factors:

1. Sjögren's affects women much more frequently than men.
2. Symptoms of dry mouth and dry eye are more prevalent in patients who are receiving hormone replacement therapy than those who are not.

Viruses, the Immune System, and Sjögren's

It is thought that some viral infections could have a role in the pathogenesis of Sjögren's by this mechanism: After a virus or bacterium enters the body, an immune reaction is almost always activated. (Parasitic infections are less of a threat to us than they were to our forebears.) Thankfully, the infection is almost always defeated, and the person returns to normal health.

But sometimes this initial response against the virus or bacterium becomes chronic, because the body cannot clear the infection, and sometimes the immune response heads off in the direction of autoimmune disease. Examples of infections that can cause chronic problems include *streptococci* (which can cause rheumatic fever), human immunodeficiency virus (HIV), and hepatitis C virus (chronic hepatitis). Indeed, hepatitis C virus can cause dry eye, dry mouth, and arthritis, all symptoms found in Sjögren's.

Epstein–Barr Virus

Epstein–Barr virus (EBV) has been suggested as a possible activator or co-factor in the development of Sjögren's. Once we are infected with this virus, we remain infected for the rest of our lives, and nearly everyone is infected. Therefore, nearly all of us have antibodies directed against EBV. It is important to note, however, that having EBV antibodies (a positive EBV test) does not mean that a person necessarily has Sjögren's or in fact any autoimmune disease. Evidence that this virus is important in Sjögren's has not yet convinced most scientists, and it remains an idea that is not generally accepted.

Hepatitis C

Chronic hepatitis C can cause symptoms that are similar to Sjögren's (dry mouth, dry eye, and arthritis in association with an enlarged parotid gland with lymphocytic infiltration). Anti-SSA and anti-SSB, which are present in the blood of Sjögren's patients, are typically absent in the blood of the patient with chronic hepatitis C infection. Most Sjögren's experts lean toward including hepatitis C as one of the differential diagnoses, as other features distinguish it. Anti-SSA and anti-SSB are usually absent in hepatitis C patients, as are the usual pathologic findings of autoimmune Sjögren's.

Retroviruses

Two retroviruses, HIV and human T-cell leukemia virus (HTLV-1), are known to cause a syndrome that presents with a clinical picture similar to that seen in Sjögren's. Those viruses affect males more than females, and the auto-antibodies that define Sjögren's have not been found in the patients who carry those viruses. HLTV-1 may cause muscle deterioration and causes a condition with the unattractive name of tropical spastic paraparesis. This virus is endemic in some parts of the world.

The medical literature now has many, many reports describing the dry eye and mouth associated with HIV infection. Both Sjögren's and HIV infection have diffuse lymphocyte infiltration in the affected tissues. However, the kind of lymphocyte that dominates in HIV-infected patients tends to be different than those that dominate in Sjögren's. The characteristic autoantibodies, anti-SSA and anti-SSB, are typically not found in HIV-infected patients. There are other gene-related differences as well. Consequently, HIV-infected patients are not usually considered to have Sjögren's, but there is some disagreement among doctors on this point.

The Microbiome

Much research over the past several years has been directed toward understanding the interaction between the microbiome and our immune system in health and disease. The microbiome refers to the viruses, bacteria, and fungi that live on or within our bodies and comprises approximately 100 trillion microorganisms. There are 10 times more bacterial cells than human cells in our bodies. Most of these microorganisms live in harmony with us; in fact, they play key roles in regulating our nutrition, homeostasis, and, importantly, our immune system. Because there are so many microorganisms in our oral cavities, it is not surprising that the disequilibrium between the oral microbiome and our immune system may be important in the pathogenesis of Sjögren's. Diet and exposure to antibiotics and environmental pollutants all may alter the normal oral microbiome and thus expose our immune systems to unfamiliar bacterial peptides and other molecules. Thus, we can see that alteration in the oral microbiome (a condition called dysbiosis) may be important in Sjögren's pathogenesis. (See more on the microbiome in Chapter 9.)

The Functional Circuit That Links Ocular/Oral Symptoms and Secretory Function

To understand the spectrum of disorders that contribute to dry eye and mouth, it is important to recognize that these symptoms result from an imbalance in a functional circuit that controls lacrimal and salivary function. The functional circuit can be considered to start at the mucosal membrane (either the ocular surface or buccal mucosal surface) where the patient has decreased aqueous secretions (Figures 6.10 and 6.11). These highly innervated surfaces send unmyelinated nerves to specific regions of the midbrain, termed the lacrimatory and salvatory nuclei. This midbrain region sends signals to the brain's cortex, where dryness is sensed, and receives input from cortical centers that reflect input such as depression or stress reactions associated with dryness. The clearest evidence of these cortical inputs is the classical Pavlovian response of salivation in response to other cortical stimuli such as the smell of food.

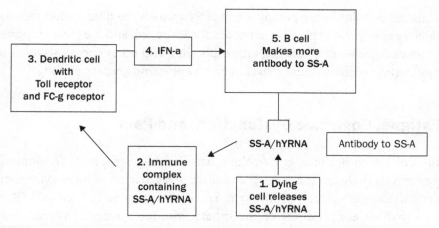

Figure 6.10 The vicious cycle of innate and acquired immunity leads to interferon type I (links genetic and autoantibody response).

After the midbrain receives input from the mucosa and higher cortical centers, efferent (outgoing) nerves that innervate the glands using cholinergic neurotransmitters (especially acetylcholine and vasoactive intestinal peptide) and blood vessels using adrenergic (adrenalin-containing) neurotransmitters are activated. Therefore, the presence of inflammatory infiltrates in the glands contributes to inadequate secretory response not only by destroying glandular elements but also by interfering with effective release of neurotransmitters by the nerves in the end organ and the response of the glandular cells at the level of post-receptor signaling. As a result, there is decreased activation of the receptors that subsequently produce the energy source for water transport.

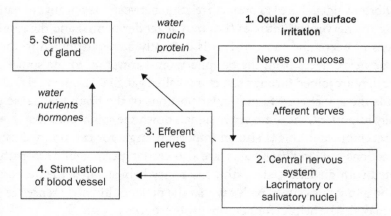

Figure 6.11 Normal tearing or salivation secretion requires a functional unit.

Thus, a key point in the pathogenesis of Sjögren's is the observation that the salivary and lacrimal glands are not totally destroyed, and the local immune-generated release of cytokines, autoantibodies, and other chemicals leads to dysfunction of the residual glands in part by blocking neural signaling.

Fatigue, Cognitive Dysfunction, and Pain

In addition to dryness, one of the most disabling symptoms in Sjögren's patients is fatigue and vague cognitive dysfunction. These symptoms do not correlate closely with our normal laboratory tests such as ESR or CRP (which are products of the innate immune system). Indeed, these symptoms, similarly found in fibromyalgia, are reminiscent of the "flu" or "jet lag," but the patient does not quickly bounce back. We can learn more about Sjögren's from ongoing research in fibromyalgia. Dysautonomia, or the dysfunction of the autonomic nervous system, also is garnering new attention by investigators and clinicians as a potential contributor to the fatigue, cognitive dysfunction, and chronic pain often experienced in Sjögren's, and we will learn more about its role in these symptoms with additional research.

Studies in animal models and using new-generation magnetic resonance imaging techniques have suggested that the subtle interplay of inflammatory products in particular portions of the brain influences the function of nerves responsible for alertness and muscle pain. Since these symptoms are also found in many patients with depression, it is not surprising that many medications useful in depression may be helpful for these symptoms in Sjögren's and fibromyalgia.

In fibromyalgia, there is a poor correlation between the findings of patient's pain in the nerves and muscles (i.e., muscle tender points) and the results of biopsies of nerve and muscle. This is currently being attributed to the fact that the nerve fibers from the periphery must travel up to the spinal cord, where they are joined through structures called ganglia. The nerve signal then ascends the spinal cord to particular portions of the brain that sense pain. Equally important, the brain sends signals down the spinal cord that dampen pain receptors, and this is also an important target for certain medications. Medications used in fibromyalgia are also used in peripheral neuropathy associated with diabetic neuropathy, since they help stabilize the neurotransmission along this critical pathway that the patient ultimately senses as pain. They may also be helpful for neuropathy in Sjögren's.

The concept of fibromyalgia has now been upgraded to "central pain sensitization" to reflect the importance of how pain signals are transmitted. Many therapeutic trials have failed to understand that the patient's quality of life may depend more on how their brain senses the dryness rather than the millimeters of tears that are generated and measured or that overall functional status depends strongly on the muscle pain, nerve pain, or energy level that are not reflected in other measurements of glandular or inflammatory activity. The role of the brain and the immune and neurologic systems and their interactions all may play roles in many of the symptoms and complications of Sjögren's.

Summing Up

Sjögren's results from the interaction of genetic and environmental factors. It is likely that multiple genes interact to predispose an individual to Sjögren's. However, even when all of the genes are present (as in identical twins), it is clear that other (presumed) environmental factors play a role, since less than 20% of identical twins are concordant for the disorder.

No single environmental agent has been identified despite an intensive 50-year search. It is more likely that many different agents can stimulate the innate immune system, which is a primitive immune system, and thus prime the more sophisticated acquired immune system to perpetuate the autoimmune process. The molecules that define the innate immune system and the acquired immune system and that link the two systems are the subjects of intensive research. It is hoped that an understanding of these molecular events will lead to a new generation of therapies for patients.

For Further Reading

Chivasso C, Sarrand J, Perret J, et al. The involvement of innate and adaptive immunity in the initiation and perpetuation of Sjögren's syndrome. *Int J Mol Sci.* 2021;22(2):658.

James JA, Harley JB, Scofield RH. Role of viruses in systemic lupus erythematosus and Sjögren's syndrome. *Curr Opin Rheumatol.* 2000;13:370–376.

Rivière E, Pascaud J, Tchitchek N, et al. Salivary gland epithelial cells from patients with Sjögren's syndrome induce B-lymphocyte survival and activation. *Ann Rheum Dis.* 2020;79(11):1468–1477.

Shimizu T, Nakamura H, Kawakami A. Role of the innate immunity signaling pathway in the pathogenesis of Sjögren's syndrome. *Int J Mol Sci.* 2021;22(6):3090.

Shoenfeld Y, Ryabkova VA, Scheibenbogen C, et al. Complex syndromes of chronic pain, fatigue and cognitive impairment linked to autoimmune dysautonomia and small fiber neuropathy. *Clin Immunol*. 2020;214:108384.

Verstappen GM, Pringle S, Bootsma H, Kroese FGM. Epithelial-immune cell interplay in primary Sjogren syndrome salivary gland pathogenesis. *Nat Rev Rheumatol*. 2021;17(6):333–348.

Weißenberg SY, Szelinski F, Schrezenmeier E, et al. Identification and characterization of post-activated B cells in systemic autoimmune diseases. *Front Immunol*. 2019;10:2136.

7

Environmental Effects

Jeffrey W. Wilson, Peter Olsson, and Thomas Mandl

We know that a combination of genetic susceptibility and an environmental trigger, whether infection or something else in the environment, leads to the development of Sjögren's. Inherited immunogenetics provide a setting for the potential development of autoimmune diseases, and then an environmental event triggers disease development. Infections are well known as likely triggers of these diseases, and studies suggest that other environmental triggers might be responsible as well. Progress is under way to identify genes that lead to susceptibility for Sjögren's (Chapter 8), but no one specific environmental effect has been identified as responsible for Sjögren's. Researchers even raise the question as to whether different environmental exposures might lead to development of Sjögren's in different individuals. This chapter will introduce what is currently known.

Infections

Infections as triggers of autoimmune disease have been recognized since the relationship between streptococcal infection and development of rheumatic fever was identified. In this early example, even when the streptococcal infection is eradicated, the immune system continues to react against the patient's joints, skin, and heart, resulting in the autoimmune reaction of rheumatic fever. This brought forth the important question: Why are only certain individuals susceptible to this reaction, and what was its nature?

Few studies have been done specifically in Sjögren's on environmental factors in development of the disease. A 2019 study from Sweden by Mofors et al. found that a history of infection was associated with nearly double the risk for developing Sjögren's, suggesting that microbial triggers of immunity may be a part of the pathogenesis of Sjögren's. In particular, infection of the lungs, skin, and urogenital tract increased the risk of Sjögren's

Jeffrey W. Wilson, Peter Olsson, and Thomas Mandl, *Environmental Effects* In: *The Sjögren's Book*. Edited by: Daniel J. Wallace, Oxford University Press. © Sjögren's Foundation 2022. DOI: 10.1093/oso/9780197502112.003.0007 and the appearance of the autoantibodies anti-SSA/Ro and anti-SSB/La. Another 2019 study, by Ben-Eli et al., found the association between infection requiring hospitalization and Sjögren's to be nearly five times that of the study's matched controls. This research looked at Sjögren's patients in addition to those who did not have Sjögren's but did have complications related to Sjögren's: dry eye patients and those with B-cell non-Hodgkin's lymphoma (NHL). All three conditions were independently associated with previous infection requiring hospitalization.

Other research into a link between specific viral and bacterial infections has taken place without finding a clear connection. The most studied virus in relation to Sjögren's is Epstein–Barr virus (EBV), which has been detected in the salivary glands and blood and tissue samples of patients with Sjögren's. However, EBV is one of the most common viruses found in humans throughout the world, and no direct link with Sjögren's has been proven, leading to caution in declaring a causal relationship. Studies on *Helicobacter pylori*, a bacterial infection, have also shown an association with development of Sjögren's; however, results have been deemed controversial, and like many other aspects of Sjögren's, more well-designed studies are needed. Nevertheless, it is important to note that a definitive link between *H. pylori* and the development of stomach cancer in Sjögren's has been found. Other infections that have been studied in relation to Sjögren's are listed in Table 7.1.

While infections are believed to play a role in the pathogenesis of Sjögren's, researchers have not yet found a definitive link between specific infections and development of Sjögren's.

Table 7.1 Infections Studied in Sjögren's

Cytomegalovirus (CMV)	Associated with autoimmune disease but no clear connection specifically to Sjögren's is apparent at this time
Hepatitis B (HBV)	No association identified
Hepatitis C (HCV)	Some conjecture that an association with Sjögren's exists; this virus currently is considered an exclusion factor for a Sjögren's diagnosis.
Human T-cell leukemia virus type 1 (HTLV-1)	Some evidence of reducing the frequency of ectopic germinal centers in lip biopsies (associated with increased development of NHL in Sjögren's) of HTLV-1-positive Sjögren's patients (Takatani, 2021). This study found that the virus inhibited BAFF and CXCL13 expressions of established follicular dendritic cells.
Coxsackie	Potential association with Sjögren's

Other Environmental Factors

Infections are well-accepted triggers of disease, but could there be other triggers based on environmental exposures? Investigators have pursued potential links between environmental factors and disease development and found clear or probable associations, so it would not take a great leap of faith that we will one day identify clear links with Sjögren's. Only one study to date has found a direct link between development of Sjögren's and an environmental trigger. But first, we will cite instances of links between environmental factors and development of diseases other than Sjögren's to illustrate the concept that some as-yet-unidentified environmental exposure could also be found to lead to Sjögren's. It is possible that a multitude of potential environmental exposures may have a pathogenic role in the development of Sjögren's, as a clear association has been identified between environmental factors and development of other diseases, including related autoimmune disorders.

One of the clearest and most interesting examples demonstrating a link between environment and disease is the lymphatic vessel disease podoconiosis, which was shown to be triggered by walking barefoot on red clay (in Ethiopia, in a 2012 article in the *New England Journal of Medicine*) and on volcanic soil (in Uganda, in a 2017 article in the *American Journal of Tropical Medicine and Hygiene*). In these cases, disease developed from absorbing mineral particles through the feet, which caused an inflammatory reaction and scarring of the lymphatics and led to the diagnosis of podoconiosis, a disease that mimics elephantiasis, an infection brought by mosquitoes. The lesson? An environmental trigger may cause a disease that mimics an infection. Could an environmental trigger bring on autoimmune disease?

Agent Orange, an herbicide used during the Vietnam War, has been linked to development of diseases of the endocrine, nervous, circulatory, respiratory, and digestive systems. It has also been linked to lymphoma. Links to autoimmune diseases include Graves disease (Antonelli, 2020), rheumatoid arthritis (Ebel, 2021), and autoimmune thyroiditis and diabetes mellitus (Yi, 2014). Disease development has been seen not just in veterans exposed to the herbicide but in their progeny as well. This finding has led experts to speculate that Agent Orange might provide an example of the role of epigenetics in disease development, in which the environmental trigger causes a change in the DNA of the person exposed to the agent, and then the DNA changes are passed on to the person's children.

The only study connecting environmental factors specifically with Sjögren's is a 2019 study by Lee et al. that found a significantly higher prevalence of

Sjögren's in Taiwanese populations exposed to large amounts of chromium in farm soil, leading the authors to suggest that chromium exposure could be a risk factor for development of Sjögren's. Other studies have found links between environmental exposures and related autoimmune diseases, including an increased risk of lupus related to higher levels of air pollution with nitrous dioxide and carbon monoxide as well as with exposure to UVA and UVB light. In addition, an increased risk of lupus and rheumatoid arthritis has been found with occupational exposure to silicone. While an association between silicone breast implants and autoimmune rheumatic diseases remains controversial, studies have identified such connections, including one study that found Sjögren's to be the most closely associated, followed by systemic sclerosis and sarcoidosis (Watad, 2018). Symptoms found in Sjögren's such as dysautonomia, small-fiber neuropathy, and myopathies also have been linked with silicone implants.

Tobacco smoking is one of the greatest health problems worldwide. The well-known negative effects include increased risk of myocardial infarction, stroke, chronic obstructive pulmonary disease (COPD), several forms of cancer, impaired wound healing, and many more. Tobacco smoke consists of thousands of different chemical compounds, many of which are carcinogenic. The effect of smoking on the immune system is both pro-inflammatory and anti-inflammatory. One of the reasons for the higher risk of cancers among smokers can be its effect on the immune system.

Smoking has been associated with the development of rheumatoid arthritis and systemic lupus erythematosus. However, studies have led to confusion by showing both negative and protective effects on disease. For example, there are reports that smoking ameliorates autoimmune diseases such as ulcerative colitis and Behçet's disease, which may be due to different mechanisms in those diseases and the above-mentioned dual effect of smoking.

Few Sjögren's patients, once diagnosed, have been found to smoke. Epidemiologic studies have demonstrated that smoking is less prevalent among Sjögren's patients compared to controls. One study that gathered smoking data from a health survey analyzed patients' smoking habits years before they were diagnosed with Sjögren's. In the group of individuals who were later diagnosed with Sjögren's, a lower prevalence of current smokers compared to controls was found; there was also a higher prevalence of former smokers among patients.

Did exposure to smoking contribute to the development of Sjögren's? We do not know. It is much easier to make guesses as to why Sjögren's patients no longer smoke following diagnosis. Dryness in the oral cavity, nose, and airways probably increases the irritation caused by the smoke, making patients more prone to quit smoking. In addition, smoke might irritate the parotid glands and cause increased pain and/or swelling. Interestingly, a large study from the United States compared Sjögren's patients with a control group of patients with dry eyes and dry mouth who did not fulfill criteria for Sjögren's and still found a lower prevalence of smoking among patients diagnosed with Sjögren's. The same study also confirmed previous findings of a lower prevalence of anti-SSA/Ro autoantibodies and positive minor salivary gland biopsy among current smokers. Could this contradictory information indicate a protective effect of smoking on Sjögren's, or could it simply mean that those who have signs of potential Sjögren's intuitively quit smoking? Again, we do not know. However, these questions do not affect the longstanding recommendation to Sjögren's patients not to smoke, as there is overwhelming scientific evidence of the harmful effects of smoking on everyone.

In addition to direct environmental effects, such as those cited earlier, we might expand our considerations to include indirect environmental effects as well. An example of an indirect environmental effect might be global warming, which is bringing an expansion in the habitat of mosquitoes and subsequent geographic distribution of certain mosquito-borne viruses. Ticks, likewise, are expanding their range and associated diseases (such as Lyme and alpha-gal). These infections cause symptoms found in autoimmune diseases, including skin rashes, acute and chronic inflammatory arthritis and paresthesias, as well as asthma, allergies (to mammalian meat with alpha-gal infection), and diarrhea.

Summing Up

Our environment contributes to our overall health and, at times, is believed to provide triggers for autoimmune disease. We still have much to learn about environmental factors as they relate to Sjögren's, but consider this proposed mechanism of disease: A patient in the setting of inherited immunogenetics (and perhaps additional factors such as vitamin D deficiency) is exposed to an infectious or environmental trigger that initiates the development of an autoimmune disease.

The ultimate hope in understanding these factors is to gain knowledge that may allow us to prevent or decrease the likelihood of these disorders. What could the future hold? Imagine at birth the individual's genomic mapping identifies inherited disease tendencies. Infectious triggers for the individual's particular genetic makeup determine specific vaccines for those infections. Direct environmental triggers once identified can be avoided, but indirect environmental triggers may be more difficult to manage.

With scientific advances progressing at a rapid pace, causal relationships will become more clear. Further research into environmental contributors is needed to elucidate the role of environmental factors in Sjögren's and to better help patients, practitioners, and researchers to best prevent, manage, and treat this complex disease.

For Further Reading

Antonelli A, Ferrari SM, Ragusa F, et al. Graves' disease: Epidemiology, genetic and environmental risk factors and viruses. *Best Pract Res Clin Endocrinol Metab.* 2020 Jan;34(1):101387.

Arnson Y, Shoenfeld Y, Amital H. Effects of tobacco smoke on immunity, inflammation and autoimmunity. *J Autoimmun.* 2010;34(3):J258–J265.

Ben-Eli H, Aframian DJ, Ben-Chetrit E, et al. Shared medical and environmental risk factors in dry eye syndrome, Sjogren's syndrome, and B-cell non-hodgkin lymphoma: A case-control study. *J Immunol Res.* 2019 Jan 21;2019:9060842.

Björk A, Mofors J, Wahren-Herlenius M. Environmental factors in the pathogenesis of primary Sjögren's syndrome. *J Intern Med.* 2020;287:475–492. https://doi.org/10.1111/joim.13032

Ebel AV, Lutt G, Poole JA, et al. Association of agricultural, occupational, and military inhalants with autoantibodies and disease features in US veterans with rheumatoid arthritis. *Arthritis Rheumatol.* 2021 Mar;73(3):392–400.

Igoe A, Scofield RH. Autoimmunity and infection in Sjögren's syndrome. *Curr Opin Rheumatol.* 2013;25(4):480–487.

Karabulut G, Kitapcioglu G, Inal V, et al. Cigarette smoking in primary Sjögren's syndrome: Positive association only with ANA positivity. *Mod Rheumatol.* 2011;21(6):602–607.

Kihembo C, Masiira B, Lali WZ, et al. Risk factors for podoconiosis: Kamwenge district, western Uganda, September 2015. *Am J Trop Med Hyg.* 2017 Jun;96(6):1490–1496.

Lee C, Hsu P, Su C. Increased prevalence of Sjögren's syndrome where soils contain high levels of chromium. *Sci Total Environ.* 2019;637:1121–1126.

Lemery J, Auerbach P. *Enviromedics: The Impact of Climate Change on Human Health.* Rowman & Littlefield; 2017.

Mofors J, Arkema EV, Björk A, et al. Infections increase the risk of developing Sjögren's syndrome. *J Intern Med.* 2019;285:670–680.

Nielsen PR, Kragstrup TW, Deleuran BW, Benros ME. Infections as risk factor for autoimmune diseases: A nationwide study. *J Autoimmun.* 2016;74:176–181.

Olsson P, Turesson C, Mandl T, et al. Cigarette smoking and the risk of primary Sjögren's syndrome: A nested case control study. *Arthritis Res Ther.* 2017;19(1):50.

Takatani A, Nakamura H, Furukawa K, et al. Inhibitory effect of HTLV-1 infection on the production of B-cell activating factors in established follicular dendritic cell-like cells. *Immun Inflamm Dis.* 2021 Sep;9(3):777–791.

Tekola Ayele F, Adeyemo A, Finan C, et al. HLA class II locus and susceptibility to podoconiosis. *N Engl J Med.* 2012 Mar 29;366(13):1200–1208.

Watad A, Rosenberg V, Tiosano S, et al. Silicone breast implants and the risk of autoimmune/rheumatic disorders: A real-world analysis. *Int J Epidemiol.* 2018 Dec 1;47(6):1846–1854.

Yi SW, Hong JS, Ohrr H, et al. Agent Orange exposure and disease prevalence in Korean Vietnam veterans: The Korean veterans health study. *Environ Res.* 2014 Aug;133:56–65.

8

Genetics and Sjögren's

Kathy L. Sivils

Genetics broadly refers to the study of genes, which control the physical traits that are passed from parents to their offspring. Genes determine observable features such as hair and eye color. They also determine how our bodies will metabolize medications, what hormones we produce, and, perhaps most importantly, our innate predisposition to develop certain diseases. Indeed, all of the genetic information required to govern functions of the human body is contained in approximately 22,000 genes. Furthermore, the expression of all diseases is influenced to some degree by the genetic makeup of each individual.

Genes determine physical traits by essentially serving as an instruction manual that guides how cells function. Other cellular components (primarily proteins) are produced that carry out the work of a cell based on the information provided by genes. Differences in traits such as hair or eye color result from changes or variants in the information contained within the relevant gene. Some variants are like typos in the instruction manual, where mistakes can cause significant problems. Other variants have very little, if any, consequence. Humans naturally carry millions of variants across all 22,000 genes, and not only are these variants what make each human unique (except in the case of identical twins), but they also hold the key to understanding why some individuals are more vulnerable to developing autoimmune diseases such as Sjögren's. Thus, the goals of genetic research are to identify which specific genes cause a disease and to understand how the variation in those genes leads to clinical manifestations.

Simple Versus Complex Genetic Diseases

Family studies can be helpful in genetic research. Many diseases that are obviously "genetic," such as cystic fibrosis, Huntington's disease, sickle cell anemia, and hundreds more that are typically rare in human populations,

Kathy L. Sivils, *Genetics and Sjögren's* In: *The Sjögren's Book*. Edited by: Daniel J. Wallace, Oxford University Press.
© Sjögren's Foundation 2022. DOI: 10.1093/oso/9780197502112.003.0008

follow inheritance patterns in families that are predictable and reflect very basic principles of genetic inheritance. In these cases, the cause can be traced to a single gene with alterations in the genetic code that lead to disease. In such cases, the disease is considered genetically "simple." In contrast, for at least a third of Sjögren's patients, a look at their own family history provides some evidence to support a role for inherited factors as a root cause, but the patterns are not so obvious. Clues from families of Sjögren's patients may include the presence of other members with Sjögren's, or more commonly, other members with either another autoimmune disease or immunologic problems that suggest an underlying genetic link. The patterns of how Sjögren's-related disease manifestations are inherited usually vary from one family to the next and often appear to be random.

The differences in patterns of inheritance between Sjögren's and genetically simple diseases such as cystic fibrosis can be largely explained by how complex the underlying genetic causes are that contribute to the risk of developing disease. We know with certainty that multiple genes are important in Sjögren's. How they work together to cause disease is undeniably complex. However, there are many details we do not yet understand. How many of the approximately 22,000 genes in humans play a role in Sjögren's? Do certain combinations of risk genes result in more severe disease or a specific feature of disease such as lymphoma? How do other factors, such as diet, exposure to UV light, infections, age, race, and gender, interact with susceptible genetic backgrounds to influence the disease risk? Furthermore, we expect that the set of genes that increase risk of developing Sjögren's will not always be the same for every individual.

Recent progress in understanding basic human genetics, coupled with powerful laboratory tools to tackle these questions for complex diseases, has been nothing short of revolutionary. Many common diseases, such as diabetes, many cancers, and most autoimmune diseases, are genetically complex. For many of these diseases, dozens of disease genes have now been identified and extensive efforts are under way to understand more precisely how the variations in those genes lead to disease.

The importance of genetics and understanding how genes work can also be seen in many other aspects of our society. We have modified the genes of livestock and crops to make them heartier and more resistant to diseases, spliced genes into bacteria to produce life-saving medicines, revolutionized the science of criminal forensics, and developed new methods of diagnosing and treating complicated illnesses. Current research in Sjögren's uses cutting-edge technology to investigate the genetic and environmental triggers that lead to the development of Sjögren's. While research into this disease has lagged behind when compared with other autoimmune diseases, we have begun to identify genetic associations that are revealing new insights and changing our understanding of Sjögren's. An accurate and detailed understanding of what causes Sjögren's will most certainly lead to the development of better tools for diagnosis and treatment for patients afflicted with this disease.

Early Genetic Discoveries

In the 1850s, Gregor Mendel, an Augustinian priest and scientist, undertook experiments to study the heritability of the physical characteristics of pea plants and unknowingly laid the foundation for modern human genetics. As he painstakingly documented the physical traits, or phenotypes, of successive generations of pea plants, he established that some unknown element conveying physical characteristics was passed from the parent plants to their offspring in mathematically predictable ratios. His observations led to the establishment of the Mendel's laws of inheritance, rules that accurately predicted how physical traits would manifest in subsequent generations, and paved the way for the discovery of that unknown heritable element: the gene. Genetic counseling for families with single-gene disorders is heavily based on the laws of inheritance established by Mendel.

Mendel's work remained largely unknown for more than three decades, until it was rediscovered at the turn of the 20th century by botanists Hugo de Vries and Carl Correns, who were studying plant hybridization. By this time, scientists had identified a variety of cellular components and hypothesized that structures called chromosomes were the key to understanding the patterns of trait heritability that Mendel described. It was not until 1915, however, that scientist Thomas Hunt Morgan proved definitively that chromosomes carried genetic information from parents to their offspring. We now know there are 23 human chromosomes. Each individual inherits one set of 23 chromosomes from the father and another set from the mother such that the offspring essentially receives two copies of the full set of genetic information. This is important in cases where a carrier of a detrimental gene located on one chromosome may be "rescued" by the second normal copy inherited from the other parent. Expression of some traits may be obviously derived from one parent, while other traits may show influences from both parents.

In 1944, Oswald Avery, Colin MacLeod, and Maclyn McCarty determined that deoxyribonucleic acid (DNA) is the molecule responsible for inheritance. Landmark studies in 1953 by scientists James Watson, Francis Crick, and Rosalind Franklin defined the molecular structure of DNA, at last giving scientists the ability to explain precisely how DNA carries genetic information.

From Genetics to Cellular Functions

DNA is normally present inside a cell as a double-stranded, helical-shaped molecule (Figure 8.1). DNA strands contain four chemical building blocks, called nucleotides: adenosine (A), cytosine (C), guanine (G), and thymine (T). Like a winding staircase, pairs of the four nucleotides form the "steps" and are linked in tandem along two phosphate/sugar backbones. The order of these nucleotides along a stretch of DNA is critically important and acts much like letters in an alphabet to form the basis of how information is conveyed. The full genetic code, or DNA sequence, along all 23 chromosomes in humans consists of about 3 billion A, T, C, or G nucleotides. Abnormalities or changes in the order of any of the 3 billion nucleotides can range from having no effect on cellular function to having devastating effects on health or even life.

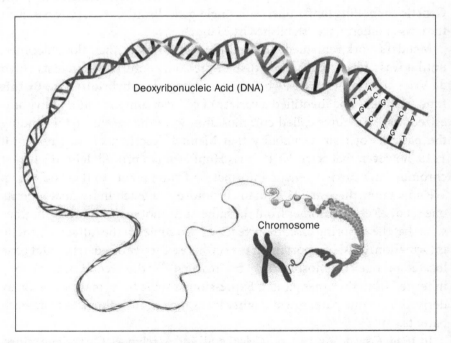

Deoxyribonucleic Acid (DNA)

Chromosome

Figure 8.1 DNA exists in a condensed state within the chromosome when not undergoing replication or gene expression. Note the pairing of A-T and C-G nucleotides on the double-stranded DNA molecule.

A gene is defined as a specific segment of a DNA strand that carries the instructions for producing a certain protein. Examples include genes that code for insulin, hemoglobin, collagen, antibodies, blood-clotting factors, interferons, hormone receptors, and thousands more proteins used by the body to carry out needed functions. A gene may range in size from about 500 nucleotides to about 2.5 million nucleotides.

It is important to note that there are large segments of DNA that are in between genes and do not directly contain the genetic code for proteins. These regions were once called "junk" DNA, but scientists are now learning that many of the secrets of how genes work, such as when to produce a protein, or how much of a protein should be produced, lies in the sequences found in these intergenic regions.

If a protein is needed, the corresponding gene becomes active and the DNA will be used as a template for cellular machinery that copies the gene sequence into a sister molecule called ribonucleic acid (RNA). Hundreds to thousands of copies of the active gene may be produced in a given cell. The RNA strands then serve as messengers that carry the code, or sequence copied off of the DNA, from the nucleus of the cell where the chromosomes are housed to the location of the cell where proteins are then made.

Understanding regulation of gene activity is a major component of genetics research. How much RNA is made from a gene, how long the RNA molecule survives inside a cell before degradation occurs, how fast a protein is produced from the messenger RNA, and other complex processes occur that serve to regulate when and how much of a protein is made. Furthermore, certain genes are active only in certain cell types, at certain times in development, or in response to certain environmental conditions. The regulation of RNA function is determined to a great extent by the specific sequences of DNA between genes. These regions are called "non-coding" and are extremely important to normal cellular functions. Overall, the DNA sequences between genes contain the majority of all genetic variation present in humans. Interestingly, one theme that has emerged from genetic research in many complex diseases is that the majority of genetic associations with diseases are due to sequence variants in these regulatory regions and not directly in the gene coding segments.

Following production of RNA molecules when a gene becomes active, proteins are produced in a process called translation. Scientists have deciphered the code that is used in translation between the molecular language of genes and amino acids. This has led to many important discoveries about protein structure and function. Proteins are also linear molecules made of chains built from 20 possible amino acids. The order of amino acids in a protein chain is derived directly from the coding sequence of nucleotides in the DNA for the relevant gene via the messenger RNA molecules. Short sequences of three nucleotides, referred to as codons, correspond to any of 20 specific amino acid, somewhat analogous to translating a set of instructions from one language to another (Figures 8.2 and 8.3). During translation, chains of amino acids are linked together into a protein molecule based on the order of the codons. For example, insulin and hemoglobin are both composed of amino acid chains, but the order in which the amino acids are linked together is different. Once a protein is made, the amino acid composition determines how the protein may fold or take on a non-linear shape, where the protein

RNA codon table

1st position	2nd position				3rd position	Amino Acids
	U	C	A	G		
U	Phe	Ser	Tyr	Cys	U	Ala: Alamine
	Phe	Ser	Tyr	Cys	C	Arg: Arginine
	Leu	Ser	Stop	Stop	A	Asn: Asparagine
	Leu	Ser	Stop	Trp	G	Asp: Aspartic acid
						Cys: Cysteine
C	Leu	Pro	His	Arg	U	Gln: Glutamine
	Leu	Pro	His	Arg	C	Glu: Glutamic acid
	Leu	Pro	Gln	Arg	A	Gly: Glycine
	Leu	Pro	Gln	Arg	G	His: Histidine
						Ile: Isoleucine
A	Ile	Thr	Asn	Ser	U	Leu: Leucine
	Ile	Thr	Asn	Ser	C	Lys: Lysine
	Ile	Thr	Lys	Arg	A	Met: Methionine
	Met	Thr	Lys	Arg	G	Phe: Phenylalanine
						Pro: Proline
G	Val	Ala	Asp	Gly	U	Ser: Serine
	Val	Ala	Asp	Gly	C	Thr: Threonine
	Val	Ala	Glu	Gly	A	Trp: Tryptophane
	Val	Ala	Glu	Gly	G	Tyr: Tyrosisne
						Val: Valine

Figure 8.2 The molecular language of genes is based on sequences of three nucleotides, known as a codon, corresponding to an amino acid. When DNA is copied into RNA, T nucleotides are substituted for a uracil, or U. In this table, the codon UUU corresponds to the amino acid phenylalanine, while the codon CCG corresponds to the amino acid proline. The codon UAA does not code for an amino acid but rather generates a stop signal that ends further addition of amino acids to the growing protein molecule.

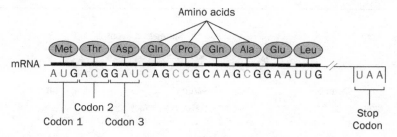

Figure 8.3 Example of a nucleotide sequence and the translation of each codon of the molecular language into a string of amino acids that will make the final protein.

goes inside the cell, if the protein should be secreted out of the cell, and many other functional capabilities such as binding to DNA or other proteins.

Genetic Effects on Disease

Important genetic variants have now been identified for over 2,600 human disorders. There are numerous ways in which the structure and function of DNA can contribute to disease. Most changes to DNA sequence occur as DNA is being replicated when cells grow and divide, or as a result of exposure to damaging elements, such as UV radiation, oxidative stress, or carcinogenic chemicals. In either case, complex cellular mechanisms exist to help prevent or repair detrimental changes. However, the proteins involved in DNA repair or replication may mistakenly add or insert an extra nucleotide, or inappropriately delete a nucleotide (Figure 8.4). By far the most common type of DNA sequence variation is a single nucleotide substitution, commonly called a single nucleotide polymorphism (SNP, pronounced "snip"). Each individual carries about 4 million to 5 million SNPs. These types of variants are the ones most often associated with complex diseases.

Sometimes DNA sequence variations occur on a larger scale, where portions of chromosomes might be deleted, duplicated, inverted (flipflopped), or translocated (swapped), possibly leading to losses, gains, or disruption of genetic information that have widely varying effects (see Figure 8.4). Sometimes during cellular division, entire chromosomes are either added or lost, leading to odd numbers of chromosomes. These chromosomal deletions or additions typically result in massive losses or gains of genetic information and most are incompatible with life. One addition that is compatible with life is trisomy 21, where three copies of chromosome 21 lead to the condition known as Down's syndrome.

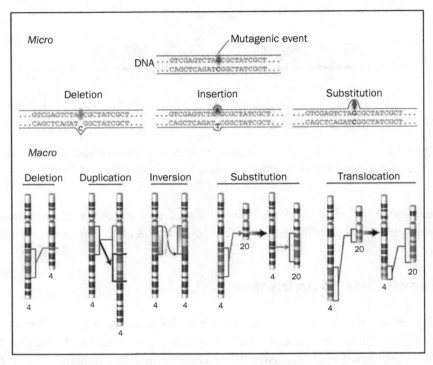

Figure 8.4 Examples of the types of variants that can occur in DNA sequences.

Changes, or variants, in the DNA sequence can sometimes have profound effects on the order of amino acids and may lead to significant problems. Such changes can cause a protein strand to be truncated if an abnormal "stop" codon is introduced by mutated DNA sequence, a faulty protein may no longer be able to bind to other proteins or receptors properly, or other normal protein modifications may be interrupted, such as the attachment of other molecules necessary for normal function. Many variants simply change the amount of protein that is produced.

A classic example of a DNA variant that changes the structure, and hence function, of a protein in a dramatic way is in sickle cell anemia. In this case, a single nucleotide in the DNA sequence is switched from an A to a T. This leads to an amino acid substitution during production of the hemoglobin protein. The resulting protein structure is altered, which causes red blood cells to manifest a "sickle" shape that is stiff, does not move easily through blood vessels, and leads to shorter lifespan of the cells causing anemia. This single gene disorder is present in individuals who have inherited two copies of the abnormal hemoglobin gene. Individuals who inherit one normal copy and one abnormal copy carry the sickle cell "trait" but do not exhibit full-blown disease.

Sometimes changes in the DNA sequence are beneficial. For example, individuals who carry the sickle cell trait are more resistant to malaria infections. This happens because the parasite that causes malaria cannot infect those cells that carry the abnormal hemoglobin protein. This balance between the advantages or disadvantages to the health of human populations derived from DNA sequence variations has developed over thousands of years. For many of the autoimmune diseases, one theory for why they develop is in part based on the idea that "selection" for immune response genes that were once strongly protective for infections and other environmental assaults have persisted in humans and may now be detrimental under circumstances where such robust responses are not required.

In addition to the basic nucleotide sequence, DNA and the proteins it interacts with can undergo permanent chemical and structural modifications that have an effect on when and under what circumstances a gene is expressed or silenced. This adds an additional layer of complexity for understanding how genes contribute to disease. Epigenetics is an emerging field that studies how these heritable modifications, which do not involve changes in the nucleotide sequence, lead to altered gene expression. This area of research is revealing that epigenetic processes are important in many disorders, including autoimmune diseases.

Tools of Genetics Research

With over 100 million SNPs and over 12,000 other sites along the human DNA sequence that are known to vary across human populations, identifying those that are relevant to disease is a significant challenge in complex diseases such as Sjögren's. For SNPs, the essence of identifying the variants that are most likely to contribute to disease often involves comparing the frequency of a specific nucleotide at a specific site between patients (cases) and healthy individuals (controls). For example, one individual may have a base pair of C-G at a particular location on a particular chromosome, where another individual may have a base pair of T-A at the exact same chromosomal location (Figure 8.5). If the C nucleotide is present at that site 58% of the time in cases, compared to 42% of the time in controls, the C variant in the DNA sequence may be associated with disease. Further studies can then test if the associated variant that is more common in patients causes altered expression or structure of

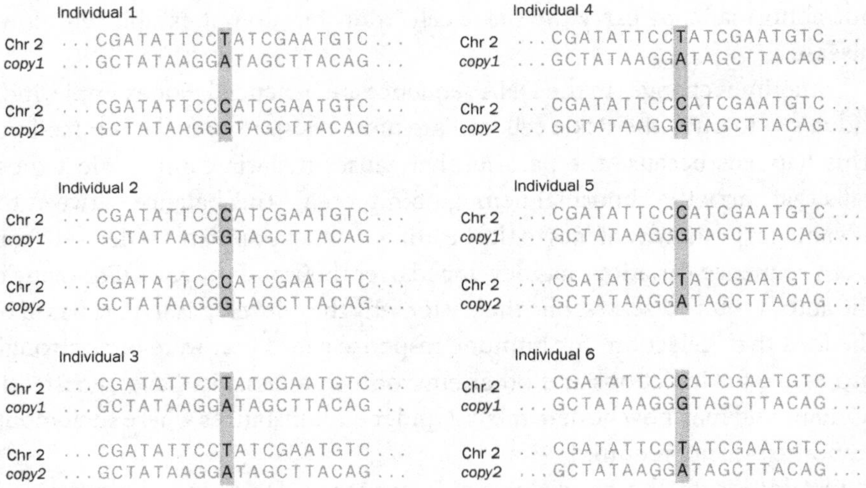

Individual 1

Chr 2   ...CGATATTCCTATCGAATGTC...
copy1   ...GCTATAAGGATAGCTTACAG...

Chr 2   ...CGATATTCCCATCGAATGTC...
copy2   ...GCTATAAGGGTAGCTTACAG...

Individual 2

Chr 2   ...CGATATTCCCATCGAATGTC...
copy1   ...GCTATAAGGGTAGCTTACAG...

Chr 2   ...CGATATTCCCATCGAATGTC...
copy2   ...GCTATAAGGGTAGCTTACAG...

Individual 3

Chr 2   ...CGATATTCCTATCGAATGTC...
copy1   ...GCTATAAGGATAGCTTACAG...

Chr 2   ...CGATATTCCTATCGAATGTC...
copy2   ...GCTATAAGGATAGCTTACAG...

Individual 4

Chr 2   ...CGATATTCCTATCGAATGTC...
copy1   ...GCTATAAGGATAGCTTACAG...

Chr 2   ...CGATATTCCCATCGAATGTC...
copy2   ...GCTATAAGGGTAGCTTACAG...

Individual 5

Chr 2   ...CGATATTCCCATCGAATGTC...
copy1   ...GCTATAAGGGTAGCTTACAG...

Chr 2   ...CGATATTCCTATCGAATGTC...
copy2   ...GCTATAAGGATAGCTTACAG...

Individual 6

Chr 2   ...CGATATTCCCATCGAATGTC...
copy1   ...GCTATAAGGGTAGCTTACAG...

Chr 2   ...CGATATTCCTATCGAATGTC...
copy2   ...GCTATAAGGATAGCTTACAG...

Figure 8.5 Example of single nucleotide polymorphisms (SNPs). Note the variations at the same location on the two copies of the same chromosome (chr) among various individuals.

the relevant protein, which then could lead to important changes in biological function of the cell. Likewise, differences in the frequency of other types of variants (insertions, deletions, etc.) between cases and controls may also indicate an association with disease.

Up until 2013, a small number of studies in Sjögren's focused on testing approximately 20 of the estimated 22,000 genes for genetic associations, largely due to limitations in the technologies used to generate genetic data. Fortunately, extraordinarily powerful tools to perform far more comprehensive studies have been developed and applied to numerous diseases, including Sjögren's. These new tools were developed at a rapid pace over the past two decades and allow us to quickly collect and analyze genetic data. For example, genotyping refers to the genetic typing that must be done in individuals in order to determine which nucleotide is present at a given site in the DNA. The current technology for genotyping allows data for over 4 million known SNPs to be determined in a single experiment. These studies are generally focused on identifying variants that are common in most human populations.

This technology has allowed scientists to perform much more informative genetic studies. Numerous large-scale genetic studies have been completed for autoimmune diseases, including systemic lupus erythematosus (SLE), rheumatoid arthritis (RA), type 1 diabetes, Crohn's disease, psoriasis, and celiac disease. Dozens of new genetic associations have been established, opening up exciting new avenues for further research and providing fundamental new insights into the causes of these diseases. Interestingly, genes that are indisputably associated with multiple autoimmune diseases are common and may eventually help explain why various autoimmune traits or different autoimmune diseases can be found within families.

For sites in the DNA sequence that vary but are present in a population at low frequency and are thus considered rare (i.e., occur in <1% of individuals), determining the entire genetic code for a gene or gene region is often necessary and done through a process known as DNA sequencing. Advances in this technology are also under rapid development, and fully sequencing an individual's entire DNA sequence is possible. Thus, the rate at which we can accumulate and study genetic information is changing dramatically.

Another important tool that has helped advance genetic research is gene expression microarrays and RNA sequencing. Using RNA extracted from blood or other cell types, scientists are able to identify which genes are active by measuring the levels of RNA being produced for each gene. The key to these experiments is that essentially every gene is tested at the same time. This serves scientists in many ways, including one important type of study that compares gene expression between patients and healthy controls. Surprising results are common in these types of studies because new genes or biological pathways are often implicated that had not been previously considered relevant to disease. Hundreds to thousands of genes can be differentially expressed between comparison groups, providing important clues for potential genetic associations, possible new diagnostic markers, or new therapeutic targets that should be developed. The importance of innate immune responses that involve interferons and other proteins that provide antiviral protection in Sjögren's patients has been a common finding in several studies using these tools.

Genetics of Sjögren's

Since the 1970s, scientists have noted a clear association between Sjögren's and genes involved in the human leukocyte antigen (HLA) system. HLA genes, which are located on chromosome 6, code for proteins that reside on the surface of cells and are essential to proper immune function. They play a major role in recognition of "self" proteins in humans. The strongest associations between HLA and Sjögren's have been found in the HLA class II molecules, HLA-DQ and HLA-DR. These particular molecules are highly variable in humans, which reflects the wide variety of nucleotide sequences that are present in these genes. In Sjögren's patients, certain variants in HLA-DR and HLA-DQ are more frequent that may alter functions such as how these molecules bind to foreign antigens presented to T cells.

In 2013, the first large-scale genetic studies in Sjögren's were completed, and several additional studies since that time have added to our current understanding of genetic associations with this complex disease. These studies have revealed about a dozen very convincing genetic associations to date. In addition to genes in the HLA regions, two genes, STAT4 and IRF5, have been consistently found that are associated with Sjögren's as well as RA and SLE. Both genes code for proteins that play an important role in innate immune responses that happen early upon infection. Some genes play major roles in the function of adaptive immune responses, which typically occur after innate immune responses are well under way and involve specific responses by T and B cells. Several genes have now been associated with T and B cells and are thought to play a role in promoting inflammatory and autoimmune reactions. Many of the genes associated with Sjögren's have multiple functions and operate in multiple cell types. In some genes, multiple SNPs are independently associated with Sjögren's, further adding to the complexity. While most genetic studies have been conducted in European-derived populations, studies in Asian populations have been conducted as well, and these show that some genetic associations are shared while others appear to be enriched in a specific racial group. For all of the genes identified thus far, much work remains to develop a detailed explanation for how the variants contribute to altering immune function and result in disease. Once the details are understood, researchers may then be able to use this information to develop therapeutics that correct the problem.

The Future of Sjögren's Research

Ongoing studies are focused on identifying additional genetic associations in Sjögren's to more fully define the genetic contributions to the disease. Genes that play a role in development and control of autoimmune responses, such as cytokines, interferons, antibodies, and receptors on T cells or B cells, are all good candidates. Other genes, such as those involved in production and secretion of saliva or other exocrine gland functions, are also possible candidate genes. Genes with variants that cause lymphomas to develop, neurologic dysfunction, or many of the other possible disease manifestations described throughout this book may also be discovered. We expect that Sjögren's will be similar to many of the related autoimmune diseases such as

SLE or RA, and more than 100 genes will be important in contributing to disease manifestations. Single variants (SNPs) will probably account for most of the genetic effects, but insertions, deletions, and other types of variants could possibly be involved. Once the catalog of genetic variants associated with Sjögren's is developed, researchers will focus on how those genetic changes lead to altered biological functions.

To successfully apply the powerful genetic tools that have been developed over the last few years, researchers will need thousands of samples and comprehensive clinical information from Sjögren's patients for comparison with healthy controls. Over 20 research sites around the world have joined together as the Sjögren's Genetics Network (SGENE) and are conducting larger genetic studies in Sjögren's. As witnessed in so many other complex diseases, we have the tools and are on the path toward many new discoveries that will provide insight into the genetic causes of Sjögren's in the very near future.

For Further Reading

Feero WG, Guttmacher AE, Collins FS. Genomic medicine—an updated primer. *N Engl J Med.* 2010;362(21):2001–2011.

Harris VM, Scofield RH, Sivils KL. Genetics in Sjögren's syndrome: Where we are and where we go. *Clin Exp Rheumatol Suppl.* 2019;118(3):234–239.

Hur K, Kim SH, Kim JM. Potential implications of long noncoding RNAs in autoimmune diseases. *Immune Netw.* 2019;19(1):e4.

Inshaw JRJ, Cutler AJ, Burren OS, et al. Approaches and advances in the genetic causes of autoimmune disease and their implications. *Nat Immunol.* 2018;19(7):674–684.

9

The Gut Microbiome and Sjögren's

Anat Galor, Kara M. Cavuoto, and Santanu Banerjee

There has been a recent interest in the interaction between gut bacteria and mucosal immunity in a number of diseases, including Sjögren's. This is because commensal bacteria that live in our gut can have both positive and negative effects on our health. For example, gut bacteria help us extract nutrients from food. Many plant polysaccharides cannot be digested by our bodies and are thus transformed by gut bacteria into short-chain fatty acids (SCFAs), such as acetic acid and butyric acid. Interestingly, some SCFAs, like butyric acid, have been found to suppress inflammation by enhancing the death of effector T cells (cells that mediate inflammation) and promoting proliferation of regulatory T cells (T_{reg}). T_{regs} help control inflammation and prevent the development of autoimmune disease.

However, the association between gut bacterial and autoimmune disease is likely a two-way street. Gut microbiome abnormalities can lead to systemic inflammation in our bodies, and, conversely, systemic inflammation can preferentially deplete beneficial gut bacteria and promotes the growth of commensal bacteria with potential pathogenic properties.

The Microbiome and Sjögren's

Stool from individuals with Sjögren's has been found to have greater relative abundances of pathogenic bacteria (*Pseudobutyrivibrio*, *Escherichia/Shigella*, and *Streptococcus*) and reduced relative abundance of commensal bacteria (*Bacteroides*, *Parabacteroides*, *Faecalibacterium*, and *Prevotella*) compared to controls. Decreased abundances of commensal species can result in lower production of anti-inflammatory SCFAs. Furthermore, reduced gut microbiome diversity has been correlated with more severe ocular and systemic disease.

Gut Dysbiosis in Autoimmune Diseases in Humans

Individuals with autoimmune diseases other than Sjögren's have also been found to have gut microbiome alterations compared to controls. This includes

Anat Galor, Kara M. Cavuoto, and Santanu Banerjee, *The Gut Microbiome and Sjögren's* In: *The Sjögren's Book*. Edited by: Daniel J. Wallace, Oxford University Press. © Sjögren's Foundation 2022. DOI: 10.1093/oso/9780197502112.003.0009 individuals with rheumatoid arthritis (RA), Behçet's disease (BD), and spondyloarthritis (SpA). For example, individuals with RA have decreased gut microbial diversity compared with controls, with a lower abundance of common commensals such as *Bifidobacteria* and *Bacteroides*. On the other hand, *Prevotella copri* has been found to be abundant in stool samples of patients with RA. The immune relevance of this bacteria was demonstrated by identifying a T-cell epitope (Pc-p27) from *P. copri* in the blood of a patient with chronic RA and then testing for immune responses to this epitope in individuals with RA, other rheumatic diseases, and healthy controls. When combined with peripheral blood from patients, this 27-kd protein of *P. copri* stimulated effector T-cell responses (mostly T_H1) in 17 of 40 RA patients. In addition, 41 of 127 RA patients had IgG or IgA antibody reactivity with *P. copri*, yet this response was rarely found in patients with other types of arthritis and controls.

Individuals with BD were found to have a decreased abundance of *Roseburia* and *Subdoligranulum* and their gut microbiome produced less butyric acid than cohabitating controls. In another study, individuals with BD were found to have a greater abundance of the *Bifidobacterium* and *Eggerthella* and reduced abundance of the *Megamonas* and *Prevotella* when compared with controls. Interestingly, in this study, there was no significant difference in annotated species numbers (as numbers of operational taxonomic unit [OTU]) or bacterial diversity (alpha) between the groups.

Individuals with SpA have a higher abundance of *Ruminococcus gnavus* as compared with both RA and controls that positively correlated with disease activity in patients with inflammatory bowel disease (IBD). *R. gnavus* uses glycans from the intestinal mucous layer as energy, which affects the equilibrium of mucus and thus gut barrier integrity with resultant increased permeability. Also, this bacterium produces a peptide that inhibits colonization by other species and thus offers a competitive advantage to its survival.

Other authors have also found gut alterations in ankylosing spondylitis (AS), particularly higher abundances of *Prevotellaceae* and *Lachnospiraceae* compared to controls. Interestingly, in healthy controls, significant differences in gut microbiome composition were detected between HLA-B27-positive and HLA-B27-negative siblings. Therefore, we can conclude that the correlation between genetics and disease status is at least partially mediated through effects on the gut microbiome.

Gut Dysbiosis in Animal Models of Autoimmune Diseases

While several epidemiologic studies have shown that individuals with various autoimmune diseases have specific microbiome signatures compared to controls, animal models have more elegantly demonstrated that these signatures can impact disease pathogenesis. The importance of commensal bacteria in modulating ocular surface health was demonstrated in mice raised in a germ-free versus conventional environment. In one study, mice (C57BL/6J) who were raised in a germ-free environment, and who did not have any gut bacteria, spontaneously developed a dry eye phenotype. This included corneal epithelial staining, goblet cell loss, and T-cell infiltration into the lacrimal gland. These features are similar to the dry eye phenotype seen in individuals with Sjögren's. Just as in humans, female mice displayed a more severe disease phenotype than male mice. Interestingly, restoring the gut microbiome (via fecal microbiome transplant from conventional mice) improved dry eye in these germ-free mice.

A similar finding was seen in a mouse model of Sjögren's (CD25 knockout [KO]) that spontaneously develops dry eye. CD25KO mice raised in a germ-free environment had a worse dry eye phenotype (greater corneal barrier dysfunction, lower goblet cell density) and higher levels of ocular surface inflammation (increased lymphocytic infiltration score and increased expression of IFN-γ, a protein made by T_H1 effector cells) compared to CD25KO mice housed in a conventional environment. Fecal transplant in these germ-free CD25KO mice reversed the spontaneous dry eye phenotype and decreased the generation of pathogenic CD4-positive, IFN-γ-positive cells.

The exclusive role of the microbiome in driving disease has also been demonstrated in RA. In one study, gut bacteria from patients with RA and healthy controls were inoculated into germ-free arthritis-prone mice. The inoculation of RA-derived gut bacteria let to an increase in intestinal T_H17 effector cells and the development of more severe arthritis as compared to inoculation of control stool. In another model of RA (collagen-induced arthritis), partial depletion of natural gut flora with an oral administration of the antibiotic enrofloxacin worsened disease severity when compared to control mice. These experiments highlight the important role of commensal bacteria in systemic immune regulation.

Rats were used to examine the exclusive role of the HLA-B27 gene (the strongest risk factor for SpA) on shaping the gut microbiome. In this experiment, gut microbiome composition was compared between rats transgenic for HLA-B27 and human β2-microglobulin and wild-type rats. This study found an increased abundance of *Prevotella* spp. and *Bacteroides vulgatus* and a decreased abundance of *Rikenellaceae* in transgenic versus wild-type animals.

As noted earlier, this demonstrates how genetic background can influence gut microbiome composition. Interestingly, raising HLA-B27/human β2-microglobulin transgenic rats in a germ-free environment prevented the development of disease. This is in contrast to the Sjögren's-like dry eye model where germ-free mice developed worse disease.

In a model of experimental autoimmune uveitis (EAU) (induced with interphotoreceptor binding protein [IBP] peptide), mice treated with oral antibiotics (specifically, metronidazole and vancomycin) had reduced ocular inflammation compared to water-treated animals. These clinical findings were linked to an increase in T_{regs} in the gastrointestinal lamina propria and extraintestinal lymphoid tissues and a decrease in T-effector cells and inflammatory cytokines. Interestingly, 16S sequencing of the gut microbiome demonstrated that mice immunized with IBP had a different gut microbiome from mice not immunized (and thus mice that did not develop disease). Not surprisingly, microbial differences were also found in mice treated with uveitis-protective antibiotics compared to those not treated with antibiotics. A similar effect was found when EAU induction was attempted in germ-free mice. Not only was the clinical severity of inflammation reduced, but germ-free mice also had lower numbers of infiltrating macrophages and T cells in the retina. At the same time, germ-free mice had reduced numbers of IFN-γ and IL-17-producing T-effector cells and increased numbers of T_{regs} in the eye-draining lymph nodes. Interestingly, initial activation of retina-specific T cells that were involved in uveitis was found to occur in the intestine and was dependent on commensal bacteria.

Potential Pathophysiologic Explanation Linking the Microbiome to Ocular Autoimmune Disease

A growing body of literature suggests that the gut microbiome may provide a common link to understanding ocular and systemic autoimmune diseases. This is primarily a result of the host immune system responding to compositional changes in the microbiome.

The host immune system and the gut microbiota constantly interact and maintain a state of homeostasis. Over the lifespan of the host, sudden changes in microbial composition (e.g., antibiotic treatment) or host immune apparatus (e.g., chemotherapy) have been shown to profoundly affect each other. Any perturbation in the composition of gut microbiota is instantly detected by the immune-surveillance cells (macrophages and dendritic cells) within the intestinal mucosa, which constitutes the innate (or native) immune response, largely mediated by pattern recognition receptors known as the Toll-like receptors (TLRs). Depending on the predominant bacterial species in the altered microbiota interacting with the innate immune cells, TLR2 (which respond to gram-positive bacteria) or TLR4 (which respond to gram-negative bacteria) are activated. This results in local and systemic inflammation, immune cell chemotaxis, and eventual tutoring and activation of adaptive (or acquired) immune response, mediated by T lymphocytes (T cells).

T cells respond to direct stimulation from the innate immune system to mobilize and initiate a second phase of immune response by activation and proliferation of effector cell phenotypes. Primarily, these are type 1 (T_H1), type 2 (T_H2), and type 17 (T_H17) effector cells, which have different functions. T_H1 cells predominantly secrete IFN-γ, a pro-inflammatory molecule whose main function is to fight infection. After the infection is cleared, T_H2 cells secrete IL-4 to dampen the T_H1 response. T_H17 cells produce IL-17 and IL-22, which are pro-inflammatory cytokines that are triggered in response to predominantly gram-positive pathogens. By way of checks and balances, a fourth T-cell phenotype, the T_{reg}, maintains the relative levels of the pro-inflammatory effector T cells with reported plasticity between the cell types, among other mechanisms.

Commensal microbiota influence the whole cascade of innate immune activation building up to an adaptive response and effector-T-cell differentiation. For example, commensals, such as *Clostridia* and *Bacteroides*, have been shown to promote the differentiation of T_{regs} in the colon. On the other hand, *Erysipelotrichaceae*, *Prevotellaceae*, and *Alcaligenaceae* have been shown to negatively affect the ability of effector T cells to differentiate, thus decreasing the body's ability to clear infection. Overall, in the setting of dysbiosis, one frequently sees a non-resolving T_H2 and T_H17 response, which has been implicated in autoimmune diseases.

Microbiome Modulation: A Future Therapeutic Avenue in Sjögren's?

Given the potential role of the gut microbiome on autoimmune eye diseases, changing the microbiome through diet, probiotics, orally administered immunoglobulins, or fecal microbial transplant may be a potential therapeutic avenue. Data on microbiome manipulation with diet have not been encouraging. A meta-analysis of 15 studies involving 837 individuals with RA did not find conclusive evidence for a favorable disease response by various changes in diet (vegetarian, Mediterranean, elemental).

The data on probiotics is slightly more encouraging. In an animal model of RA (type II collagen immunization), mice that were given *Prevotella histicola* (a bacterium native to the human gut) by oral lavage had decreased incidence and severity of arthritis compared to controls when treated either prophylactically (before immunization) or therapeutically (after immunization). This therapeutic effect was accompanied by generation of T_{regs} in the gut and suppression of T_H17-effector-cell responses. In a similar manner, oral ingestion of a polysaccharide of *Bacteroides fragilis* protected against central nervous system demyelinating disease in a mouse model. When mice were given a probiotic containing wild-type *B. fragilis*, they maintained resistance to inflammation and thus were protected against disease, whereas those given *B. fragilis* deficient in polysaccharide A were susceptible to disease.

These findings do not translate as cleanly into human disease. In a meta-analysis of nine rheumatoid arthritis studies involving 361 patients, individuals receiving probiotics had a lower pro-inflammatory cytokine IL-6 level compared to those receiving placebo. However, there was no difference in clinical disease activity between groups. Similarly, probiotics were not found to improve clinical manifestations in juvenile idiopathic arthritis (JIA). One problem with probiotics is that, as summarized earlier, there are likely unique bacterial signatures in different autoimmune diseases, and it is not known which commercially available probiotics are best for which diseases. Perhaps the development of disease-specific probiotics will result in clinical improvements that were not seen using commercially available products.

Immunoglobulin A (IgA) is the main antibody type secreted into the intestine and plays an important role in the defense against pathogens. One group identified an IgA subtype (W27) that binds to multiple pathogenic but not beneficial bacteria. They gave mice that spontaneously develop colitis an oral preparation of IgA. This resulted in a change in the microbiome by decreasing dysbiosis, which resulted in a less severe disease phenotype when compared to placebo-treated animals. The relative abundance of *Lachnospiraceae* and *Ruminococcaceae* was increased, which is important as these families are considered inducers of beneficial immune regulatory cells. The authors postulate the reason for the selective enhancement of beneficial bacteria and decrease in pathogenic bacteria is that nearly 90% of IgA derived from the small intestine of mice recognizes a key sequence of four amino acids that are important for W27 binding. This sequence is found in the majority of pathogenic bacteria in the *Gammaproteobacteria* and *Betaproteobacteria* classes. In contrast, this sequence is lacking in many beneficial bacteria, thus allowing the beneficial bacteria to flourish. Given the specificity for binding in their mouse model, they recommend seeking and testing a corresponding sequence in humans.

Fecal microbial transplantation (FMT) is another method used to change the composition of the gut microbiome. In FMT, a fecal preparation of bacteria from carefully screened, healthy donors is transplanted into the colon of a patient, most often via enema or colonoscopy. FMT is an approved treatment for recalcitrant *Clostridium difficile* infections and has also been used to remove multidrug-resistant organisms from the gut. More recently, FMT has been studied as a treatment for immune-mediated diseases. In graft-versus-host disease, a condition that also results in severe dry eye, four patients underwent FMT derived from a spouse or relative and delivered once or twice via naso-duodenal tube. Some patients showed improvements in gastrointestinal symptoms and peripheral regulatory T cells.

In ulcerative colitis, FMT or placebo was given by colonoscopic infusion, followed by self-administered enemas 5 days per week for 8 weeks. FMT enemas were each derived from between three and seven unrelated donors. At 8 weeks, 27% of patients in the FMT group achieved steroid-free clinical and endoscopic remission compared to 8% of patients not receiving FMT. Furthermore, microbial diversity increased with and persisted after FMT.

Summing Up

There is ample evidence that gut microbiome alterations are found in individuals with autoimmune diseases, including Sjögren's. Animal models have clarified that these are not just associations but that the gut microbiome affects disease phenotype. There are several methods by which the gut microbiome can be changed, and this avenue may be a potential future treatment in Sjögren's. More research is needed, however, to identify the specific microbiome signature in Sjögren's that can be used to guide preventive and therapeutic strategies.

For Further Reading

Banerjee S, Sindberg G, Wang F, et al. Opioid-induced gut microbial disruption and bile dysregulation leads to gut barrier compromise and sustained systemic inflammation. *Mucosal Immunol.* 2016;9:1418–1428.

Breban M. Gut microbiota and inflammatory joint diseases. *Joint Bone Spine.* 2016;83:645–649.

Breban M, Tap J, Leboime A, et al. Faecal microbiota study reveals specific dysbiosis in spondyloarthritis. *Ann Rheum Dis.* 2017;76:1614–1622.

Chen J, Wright K, Davis JM, et al. An expansion of rare lineage intestinal microbes characterizes rheumatoid arthritis. *Genome Med.* 2016;8:43.

de Paiva CS, Jones DB, Stern ME, et al. Altered mucosal microbiome diversity and disease severity in Sjogren syndrome. *Sci Rep.* 2016;6:23561.

Ferreira CM, Vieira AT, Vinolo MA, et al. The central role of the gut microbiota in chronic inflammatory diseases. *J Immunol Res.* 2014;2014:689492.

Heissigerova J, Seidler Stangova P, Klimova A, et al. The microbiota determines susceptibility to experimental autoimmune uveoretinitis. *J Immunol Res.* 2016;2016:5065703.

Honda K, Littman DR. The microbiome in infectious disease and inflammation. *Annu Rev Immunol.* 2012;30:759–795.

Iwasaki A, Medzhitov R. Control of adaptive immunity by the innate immune system. *Nat Immunol.* 2015;16:343–353.

Jacobs JP, Braun J. Immune and genetic gardening of the intestinal microbiome. *FEBS Lett.* 2014;588:4102–4111.

Kamada N, Chen GY, Inohara N, Nunez G. Control of pathogens and pathobionts by the gut microbiota. *Nat Immunol.* 2013;14:685–690.

Kelly CJ, Colgan SP, Frank DN. Of microbes and meals: The health consequences of dietary endotoxemia. *Nutr Clin Pract.* 2012;27:215–225.

Maeda Y, Kurakawa T, Umemoto E, et al. Dysbiosis contributes to arthritis development via activation of autoreactive T cells in the intestine. *Arthritis Rheumatol.* 2016;68:2646–2661.

Marietta EV, Murray JA, Luckey DH, et al. Suppression of inflammatory arthritis by human gut-derived *Prevotella histicola* in humanized mice. *Arthritis Rheumatol.* 2016;68:2878–2888.

McHardy IH, Goudarzi M, Tong M, et al. Integrative analysis of the microbiome and metabolome of the human intestinal mucosal surface reveals exquisite inter-relationships. *Microbiome.* 2013;1:17.

Mohammed AT, Khattab M, Ahmed AM, et al. The therapeutic effect of probiotics on rheumatoid arthritis: A systematic review and meta-analysis of randomized control trials. *Clin Rheumatol.* 2017;36:2697–2707.

Nakamura YK, Metea C, Karstens L, et al. Gut microbial alterations associated with protection from autoimmune uveitis. *Invest Ophthalmol Vis Sci.* 2016;57:3747–3758.

Paramsothy S, Kamm MA, Kaakoush NO, et al. Multidonor intensive faecal microbiota transplantation for active ulcerative colitis: A randomised placebo-controlled trial. *Lancet.* 2017;389:1218–1228.

Power SE, O'Toole PW, Stanton C, et al. Intestinal microbiota, diet and health. *Br J Nutr.* 2014;111:387–402.

Scher JU, Sczesnak A, Longman RS, et al. Expansion of intestinal *Prevotella copri* correlates with enhanced susceptibility to arthritis. *Elife.* 2013;2:e01202.

Vaahtovuo J, Munukka E, Korkeamaki M, et al. Fecal microbiota in early rheumatoid arthritis. *J Rheumatol.* 2008;35:1500–1505.

Yiu JH, Dorweiler B, Woo CW. Interaction between gut microbiota and Toll-like receptor: From immunity to metabolism. *J Mol Med.* 2017;95:13–20.

Zaheer M, Wang C, Bian F, et al. Protective role of commensal bacteria in Sjogren syndrome. *J Autoimmun.* 2018;93:45–56.

10

Causes of Exocrine Gland Dysfunction in Sjögren's

Efstathia K. Kapsogeorgou, Michael Voulgarelis, and Athanasios G. Tzioufas

Exocrine glands are the organs producing and secreting the fluids that are required for the hydration and lubrication of the cavities/organs where they reside, which are usually easily accessible or in direct contact with exogenous factors, such as skin, eyes, oral cavity, gastrointestinal tract, bronchi, and so forth. The composition of the exocrine gland secretions varies according to the body tissue/cavity where they reside; generally, they contain aqueous (water), mucous, and/or lipid components and various antimicrobial factors. They are vital for the proper function of the cavities/organs, as well as the first line of defense against pathogens, since they prevent the attachment of pathogens in tissues or kill them by the antimicrobial factors.

Sjögren's is characterized by the dysfunction of the exocrine glands resulting in insufficient moisture and a feeling of dryness, the so-called sicca symptoms. In the vast majority of patients with Sjögren's, the exocrine glands affected are the lacrimal and salivary glands (95% and 90% of patients, respectively). Their dysfunction has been associated with both reduced production and altered quality of tears and saliva, resulting in eye and mouth dryness (keratoconjunctivitis sicca and xerostomia, respectively). Other sites commonly affected in Sjögren's are the upper respiratory system, vagina, and skin.

The desiccation of the upper respiratory tract may lead to dry, crusted secretions in the nose, sinusitis, nose bleeding, hoarseness, and bronchial hyperresponsiveness manifested as persistent dry cough and shortness of breath, whereas vagina dryness is associated with pain during sexual intercourse s (dyspareunia). The causes of the exocrine gland dysfunction in Sjögren's remain elusive; however, it seems that several factors contribute. To date, flawed nerve signaling, destruction of the glands by inflammatory infiltrates, and defective function of the secretory epithelial cells have been incriminated. The normal function of the major glands affected in Sjögren's

Efstathia K. Kapsogeorgou, Michael Voulgarelis, and Athanasios G. Tzioufas, *Causes of Exocrine Gland Dysfunction in Sjögren's* In: *The Sjögren's Book*. Edited by: Daniel J. Wallace, Oxford University Press. © Sjögren's Foundation 2022.
DOI: 10.1093/oso/9780197502112.003.0010

(namely the lacrimal and salivary glands), their hypofunction, and possible causes will be discussed in this chapter.

Exocrine Glands and Secretions in the Eye and Oral Cavity

Eyes

The ocular surface is covered by a tear film consisting of three layers: (1) the mucus adjacent to the ocular surface, (2) the aqueous, and (3) the outer lipid layer, which prevents the evaporation of the watery tear phase. This film protects the eye, provides a smooth optical surface at the air–cornea interface, and facilitates the removal of debris and pathogens. The tear film is produced by the lacrimal and meibomian exocrine glands as well as small goblet cells in the conjunctiva. The lacrimal glands, one for each eye, are bilobed, almond-shaped glands located at the upper lateral corner of the orbit formed by the frontal bone. They produce the aqueous phase of the tear film consisting of water, salts, and antimicrobial components enabling protection from pathogens. These are called basal tears and serve in keeping the eye moist and nourished.

In addition to basal tears, lacrimal glands secrete the reflex tears in response to irritation that lubricate and clean the eyes, as well as tears produced in response to strong emotions, stress, or pain. The oily layer of the tear film is produced by the meibomian glands that reside along the rims of the eyelids, whereas goblet cells in the conjunctiva produce the mucins, which form the inner mucous layer of the tear film that increases its velocity and facilitates the attachment in the ocular surface. Dry eye may result from lacrimal and/ or meibomian gland dysfunction, resulting in decreased production of the aqueous and/or the oily layer of the tear film, respectively. Both conditions are associated with higher evaporation rates and inadequate lubrication of the eye. In some cases, eye dryness presents with excess tears due to irritation of the dry eye and production of the reflex tears, a situation that might be confused with excess tearing. In Sjögren's, both reduced quantity and altered quality of tears have been reported. During focusing on reading, working on a computer, or watching TV, eyes blink less, resulting in increased evaporation of the tear film. Thus, in patients with Sjögren's who have defective tear film, such activities may worsen the feeling of dryness and lead to difficulty achieving relief.

Oral Cavity

The oral cavity is covered by the aqueous saliva that coats the teeth and oral mucosa. The saliva is secreted by the salivary glands, which include three pairs of major salivary glands, located outside the oral cavity but draining into it, and numerous minor salivary glands in the mucosal tissues lining the oral cavity. The major salivary glands are (1) the parotid glands located between the ear and the jaw, (2) the submandibular glands under the jawbone, and (3) the sublingual glands beneath the tongue. The minor salivary glands are classified according to their location in the oral cavity as the labial, buccal, glossopalatine, palatine, and lingual glands.

Salivary glands consist of the secretory structures called acini, which empty into the intercalated ducts, which in turn drain into the striated ducts and these into the interlobular, excretory ducts. Acini are composed of secreting epithelial cells that secrete a watery fluid, or mucous acinar cells, which produce a viscous secretion rich in mucins. The secretion of serous or mucous acini drains into the ducts, where the fluid is further enriched with lysozymes, various proteins, and growth factors until it drains into the oral cavity. According to the type of acinar cells, these can be classified as serous, mucous, or mixed (containing both serous and mucous acini; Figure 10.1). The parotid, submandibular, and sublingual glands produce the major proportion of saliva, whereas minor salivary glands produce mainly mucous secretions that have a major role in the coating of the oral cavity with saliva, enabling the lubrication and protection of the mucous surfaces of the mouth.

The secretions of all types of salivary glands drain into the oral cavity and constitute the saliva. Approximately 0.5 to 1 liter of saliva is produced per day under physiologic conditions, and this production is controlled by sympathetic and parasympathetic stimulation. The saliva is mainly composed of water, whereas electrolytes, enzymes, mucins, immunoglobulins, cytokines/chemokines, growth factors, and other proteins, as well as lipids, amino acids, and antimicrobial components, constitute only 1%. Saliva also contains desquamated epithelial cells, a few inflammatory cells, debris, and microorganisms and their products. In addition to hydration/lubrication of the oral mucosa, saliva has many other important physiologic functions, including the following:

1. *Protection of mucosae*: Hydration, lubrication, and protection of the oral structures, including teeth, from friction during mastication. Tooth hygiene is also mediated by the provision of inorganic ions that maintain tooth integrity and repair enamel and mucins that participate in

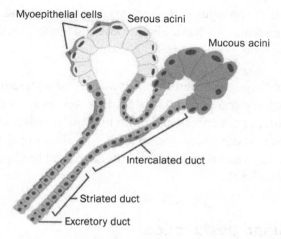

Myoepithelial cells   Serous acini

Mucous acini

Intercalated duct

Striated duct

Excretory duct

Figure 10.1 A schematic presentation of a salivary gland unit. Acinar cells producing the saliva components are organized in structures called acini. Depending on the type of secretion, watery or viscous and rich in glycoproteins called mucins, acini are classified as serous or mucous, respectively. Salivary glands consist of only serous, only mucous, or both serous and mucous acini, and they are respectively characterized as serous, mucous, or mixed salivary glands. The secretions of acini drain into the intercalated ducts, followed by striated ducts and then by interlobular, excretory ducts. Acinar secretions are further modified during their passage in the ducts, resulting in saliva that is excreted into the oral cavity.

thermal and chemical insulation. The constant flow of saliva floats away the accumulated food debris and microorganisms. In addition, saliva contains several growth factors, such as epithelial growth factor, that facilitate tissue repair.

2. *Antimicrobial activity*: The oral cavity abounds with bacteria, fungi, and other microorganisms. Saliva mucins prevent the attachment of microorganisms to teeth and mucosae, providing a physical barrier to infections. In addition, saliva contains a plethora of antimicrobial factors, such as lysozyme, peroxidase, lactoferrin, histatin, agglutinin, and defensins that directly kill or neutralize the microorganisms. Moreover, immune defense is mediated by immunoglobulins that are secreted in the saliva.

3. *Taste and digestion of food*: In order to taste dry food, the food must be solubilized (broken down by liquid). The molecules of the masticated food are diluted in the watery phase of saliva and only then can be tasted. Furthermore, saliva, through both the aqueous and mucous content, aids in binding masticated food into a slippery bolus that slides easily

through the esophagus without damaging the mucosae. Finally, saliva contains enzymes, such as alpha amylase and lipase, that initialize digestion of the food.

In patients with Sjögren's, xerostomia is associated with reduced flow rates in which the watery component is reduced, as well as altered quality of saliva. These result in poor mouth and tooth hygiene as reflected by infections, plaque formation, tooth decay, and so forth, as well as difficulties with food consumption and swallowing; often patients cannot eat hard, dry food and/or need water to swallow it.

Exocrine Gland Dysfunction

Although the exact causes of exocrine gland dysfunction in Sjögren's have not been identified, it is considered to be a complex phenomenon owing to the reduction and/or inhibition of water transport machinery and altered quality of epithelial secretions. This exocrinopathy is associated with dense lymphocytic infiltration of the glands, located mainly around ducts, and destruction of the glandular epithelial structures (Figure 10.2). The injurious effects of chronic inflammation and its byproducts, such as function-modulating cytokines and cytotoxic and apoptotic signals, are considered capable of driving exocrine gland hypofunction by destroying glandular innervation and nerve signaling and by promoting defective epithelial secretory function and destruction of epithelial glandular structures. On the other hand, studies of the affected minor salivary glands in Sjögren's have shown that more than autoimmune responses affect the epithelial cells. Factors unrelated to inflammatory infiltrates, such as endogenous defects, may contribute to epithelial secretory hypofunction. Moreover, numerous studies have shown that salivary gland epithelial cells in Sjögren's are endogenously activated and act as the major orchestrators of autoimmune responses by recruiting, activating, and promoting the differentiation of inflammatory cells and the organization of the infiltrates. We will discuss all of these aspects contributing to salivary gland dysfunction in more detail.

Altered Epithelial Secretory Function in Sjögren's

As mentioned before, the secretion process in salivary glands is controlled by sympathetic and parasympathetic nerve fibers, and the differential

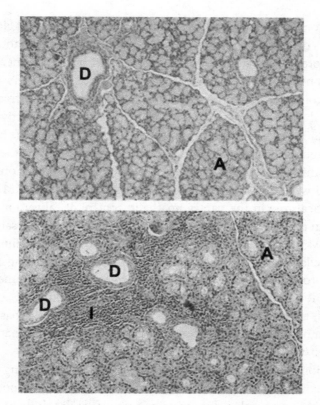

Figure 10.2 Histopathologic images of labial minor salivary gland sections obtained from an individual who does not suffer from Sjögren's (control; upper panel) and a patient with Sjögren's (lower panel). In the minor salivary gland of the patient with Sjögren's, lymphoid infiltrates (I, small round cells) are developed around the ducts (D) and are associated with significant destruction of acini (A) compared to the nonaffected tissue from the control individual. Tissue sections are stained with hematoxylin and eosin.

stimulation of epithelial cholinergic and adrenergic receptors determines the quantity and quality of secreted saliva. Thus, acetylcholine stimulation of cholinergic receptors results in saliva rich in water and electrolytes but low in proteins and glycoproteins, whereas adrenergic stimulation results in saliva rich in proteins and glycoproteins but with a low water and electrolyte content. Thus, it has been hypothesized that defective innervation, nerve signaling, and/or stimulation may contribute to altered epithelial secretions in Sjögren's.

Indeed, initial observations supporting the concept that vasoactive intestinal peptide (VIP)-containing nerve fibers are reduced in the areas of high inflammation at the minor salivary gland lesions suggested that glandular innervation is defective in Sjögren's patients. However, this was not confirmed by later, more elegant studies, which showed that both the innervation and consequent nerve stimulation are, indeed, not altered in Sjögren's.

On the contrary, altered neural signal transmission, water transport machinery, and protein synthesis seem to participate in the defective saliva secretion in Sjögren's. Thus, studies in mouse models of Sjögren's have shown that cytokines released in the inflammatory lesions reduce the release of neurotransmitters, leading to salivary hypofunction. Furthermore, autoantibodies against the muscarinic type 3 acetylcholine receptor (M3R), which plays a critical role in the parasympathetic control of salivation, have been identified in patients with Sjögren's and implicated in reduced salivary function. Anti-M3R autoantibodies have been shown to reduce the fluid secretion by acinar cells, possibly by disrupting the intracellular trafficking of the water transport protein aquaporin-5 (AQP5), whereas cellular immune responses against M3R have been linked to the destruction of epithelial cells. On the other hand, altered AQP5 distribution in acini, consisting of basal, and not apical, membrane localization, further supports the concept that water machinery transportation is also defective in Sjögren's.

In addition, altered production, modification, and trafficking of mucins, another significant component of saliva, seem to malfunction in the disease. Mucins are complex glycoproteins acting as hydrophilic polymers that bind water on the epithelial surface and thereby preserve mucosa humidity. Reduced expression of mucins, accumulation in the cytoplasm of acini, and ectopic secretion in the extracellular matrix instead of lumen, possibly mediated by inflammation, have been described in Sjögren's and in relation to the altered saliva quality of patients.

Apoptotic Cell Death of Epithelial Cells in Sjögren's

As already mentioned, the dysfunction of exocrine glands is associated with destruction of epithelial glandular structures, which is considered to be mediated by apoptotic cell death. Apoptosis is a tightly regulated form of programmed cell death that occurs after danger signals drive the cell to self-destruction. Although it is a physiologic process occurring during various physiologic conditions, it is considered extremely significant for the development of autoimmune disorders and particularly for the development of humoral autoimmune responses, namely the production of autoantibodies, since intracellular antigens are presented to the immune system in an immunogenic fashion through this pathway. In Sjögren's, epithelia have been described to elevate apoptotic cell death in the minor salivary glands, and these cells, containing the Ro/SSA and La/SSB autoantigens, probably mediate the development of the autoantibody responses that characterize the disease. Multiple causes are considered to underlie the increased apoptosis of the glandular epithelia in Sjögren's, including the inflammatory microenvironment, pathogen infections, autoantibodies, and sex hormones. Inflammation seems to be an important inducer of epithelial cell apoptosis. The pro-apoptotic signals are delivered either directly by the interaction with inflammatory cells, such as cytotoxic or other T cells, or indirectly by the cytokines produced by them, such as IFN-γ and TNF-α. Viral infections may contribute to the destruction of epithelial cells either directly by killing them or through the induction of apoptosis mediated by the stimulation of sensing receptors on epithelia that recognize viral components, such as the Toll-like receptor 3 (TLR3), which has been shown to induce apoptotic cell death of salivary gland epithelial cells.

In addition, autoantibodies against the Ro/SSA and La/SSB autoantigens that are abundant in Sjögren's have been shown to induce epithelial apoptosis, whereas sex hormones have been implicated in the regulation of epithelial survival. Sjögren's usually affects women after menopause, during which estrogen levels are significantly reduced. Indeed, estrogen deprivation has been shown to induce apoptosis of salivary gland epithelial cells, thereby implicating estrogen withdrawal in glandular destruction. The significance of epithelial apoptosis in the pathogenesis of Sjögren's has been further verified in an experimental mouse model, in which lacrimal epithelial apoptosis resulted in dacryoadenitis and development of serum anti-Ro/SSA and anti-La/SSB autoantibodies.

Epithelial Cells as the Orchestrators of the Autoimmune Lesions in Sjögren's

The aforementioned defects of the glandular epithelia are more or less dictated by the tissues' inflammatory microenvironment, suggesting that epithelial cells are innocent bystanders suffering from the influence of autoimmune responses. However, studies during the last two decades have proved that this is not the case. Although the survival and the function of the salivary gland epithelial cells are significantly harmed by their interaction with immune cells and their products, they are also involved with the lymphocytic infiltration of tissue and autoimmune lesions. Histopathologic and in vitro studies, analyzing salivary gland epithelial cells from patients and controls both in situ in tissues and in vitro in long-term cultures, shed light on the role of epithelia in Sjögren's. Histopathologic analyses indicate that infiltrating mononuclear cells (particularly T and B lymphocytes and dendritic cells) are often found to invade ducts or to be in close proximity with ductal epithelial cells, suggesting that glandular epithelia communicate and interact with immune cells. Indeed, salivary gland epithelial cells in patients with Sjögren's have been found to express constitutively a plethora of immune-competent molecules implicated in innate and acquired immune responses, suggesting that they are able to mediate the recruitment, homing, activation, differentiation, and proliferation of lymphoid cells as well as the expansion and organization of lymphoid infiltrates. Furthermore, salivary gland epithelial cells from patients with Sjögren's have been shown to fruitfully interact with T and B cells and to drive their activation and differentiation in a manner similar to that observed in the affected tissue. Finally, epithelial cells are probably implicated in the development of autoantibody responses against Ro/SSA and La/SSB autoantigens by introducing them into the immune system through apoptosis or the release of autoantigen-loaded vesicles, called exosomes.

These immune-modulating features of the salivary gland epithelial cells from patients with Sjögren's are constitutive, evident in long-term cultures devoid of immune cells and their products, and remain stable after several months of culture, suggesting that they are intrinsically activated. The offending factor(s) of the epithelial activation are not known. Epigenetic changes or latent viral infections, which have long been suspected to participate in disease pathogenesis, may be causally implicated by altering epithelial biological properties and initiating an aberrant immune response. Indeed, infection by hepatitis C (HCV) or human immunodeficiency (HIV) viruses is associated with chronic sialadenitis that mimics Sjögren's, whereas several viruses or viral elements, such as cytomegalovirus (CMV), Epstein–Barr virus (EBV), human herpes virus type 6 (HHV6), human T-lymphotropic virus type I (HTLV-1), human herpes virus type 8 (HHV-8), and retroviral and coxsackie viral elements, have been described to reside in the salivary gland tissues of patients.

Summing Up

The secretory function of the exocrine glands is a perplexing and tightly regulated process that needs to readily respond to internal and external stimuli or environmental changes to facilitate the hydration, lubrication, and protection of tissues, organs, or cavities that are easily accessible or in direct contact with exogenous factors and pathogens. For this reason, besides internal regulatory mechanisms, secretorty functions are also controlled by various systems, the foremost being the autonomic nervous system. The perplexities of the regulation of exocrine gland function hinder the identification of their hypofunction causatives. Especially in Sjögren's, identification of the cause is exacerbated by the complexity of the disease, the variety of the pathogenetic mechanisms underlying disease pathogenesis, and our inability to identify the offending factors. However, according to the data presented in this chapter, the following hypothesis outlines our current knowledge about the causes of exocrine gland dysfunction in Sjögren's. The glandular epithelial cells in patients become permanently activated, possibly by an exogenous factor, and begin to express a variety of immunomodulatory molecules and

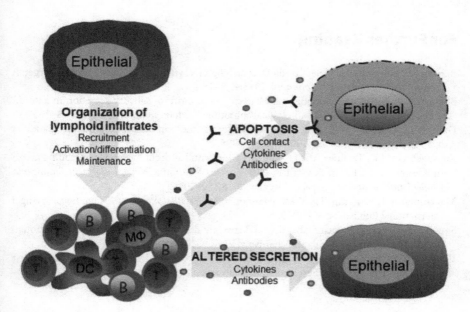

Figure 10.3 A hypothetical schematic representing the causes of exocrine dysfunction in Sjögren's. The glandular epithelial cells of patients with Sjögren's express a variety of immunomodulatory molecules and seem able to mediate the recruitment, activation, and/or differentiation of T and B lymphocytes, macrophages (MΦ) and dendritic cells (DC) as well as the organization of infiltrates in the minor salivary glands through the production of cytokines/chemokines. On the other hand, immune cells and their products (cytokines, antibodies, etc.), constituting the inflammatory tissue microenvironment, induce the reduction of the secretory function by (a) inducing the apoptotic cell death of glandular epithelia or (b) directly affecting the secretory function of epithelial cells by disrupting the signaling of neurotransmitters stimulating saliva secretion, water transport machinery, and/or the quality of the secreted components.

act as regulators of local immune responses. They recruit immune cells to the glands and then interact with them by promoting their activation, proliferation, and differentiation, ultimately resulting in organized infiltrates. On the other hand, the immune cells and the inflammatory microenvironment affect the secretory function of epithelial cells by reducing both the quantity and quality of secretions as well as epithelial survival by promoting their apoptotic death. Thus, the final result is altered secretion along with destruction of epithelial structures of the glands (Figure 10.3). The identification of the offending factors of epithelial activation, and the role of the latter in the observed epithelial secretory dysfunction, is of great importance for the understanding of disease pathogenesis and the development of effective therapeutic interventions.

For Further Reading

Barrera MJ, Bahamondes V, Sepúlveda D, et al. Sjögren's syndrome and the epithelial target: A comprehensive review. *J Autoimmun*. 2013;42:7–18.

Bhattarai KR, Junjappa R, Handigund M, et al. The imprint of salivary secretion in autoimmune disorders and related pathological conditions. *Autoimmun Rev*. 2018;17:376–390.

Dawson LJ, Fox PC, Smith PM. Sjögren's syndrome: the non-apoptotic model of glandular hypofunction. *Rheumatology*. 2006;45:792–798.

Kapsogeorgou EK, Tzioufas AG. Glandular epithelium: Innocent bystander or leading actor? In Alunno A, Bartoloni E, Gerli R, eds. *Sjögren's Syndrome: Novel Insights in Pathogenic, Clinical and Therapeutic Aspects*. Elsevier; 2016:189–204.

Moutsopoulos HM, Zampeli E, Vlachoyiannopoulos PG. *Rheumatology in Questions*. Springer International Publishing AG; 2018.

Smatti MK, Cyprian FS, Nasrallah GK, et al. Viruses and autoimmunity: A review on the potential interaction and molecular mechanisms. *Viruses*. 2019;11:762.

Vivino FB, Bunya VY, Massaro-Giordano G, et al. Sjogren's syndrome: An update on disease pathogenesis, clinical manifestations and treatment. *Clin Immunol*. 2019;203:81–121.

PART III

HOW IS THE BODY AFFECTED?

11

Diagnosis of Fatigue

Daniel J. Wallace, Richa Mishra, and Frederick B. Vivino

What Is Fatigue, and How Do We Define It?

Fatigue is a common and disabling symptom for patients with Sjögren's and is best defined as a low-energy state characterized by physical or mental weariness. This typically results in an inability to sustain normal activities or, in a worst-case scenario, any activity whatsoever. In some cases, the fatigue is severe enough to lead to misdiagnosis of Sjögren's as chronic fatigue syndrome; the latter diagnosis, however, is always considered a diagnosis of exclusion. Fatigue may take a variety of forms and have a variety of causes. Although constantly present, fatigue is also a dynamic state with waxing and waning intensity that responds to various physiologic and situational influences, including emotional state, recent activities, disease activity, weather patterns, medication use, sleep patterns, and diurnal variation.

How Often Does Fatigue Occur in Sjögren's, and What Is Its Impact?

Fatigue is found in the majority of patients with Sjögren's, and the prevalence varies according to the method of assessment used in different studies. The 2016 "Living with Sjögren's" survey conducted by the Harris Poll on behalf of the Sjögren's Foundation listed fatigue as the third most troubling symptom (prevalence 80%), after dry eyes (92%) and dry mouth (92%). Numerous studies before and after have documented similar findings as well as significantly diminished quality of life among people with Sjögren's compared to normal individuals. These results parallel the diminished quality of life found in other patient groups, including people with rheumatoid arthritis (RA) and fibromyalgia. In 2009 Segal et al. reported that fatigue and pain are two of the most important factors that affect quality of life (i.e., physical and emotional well-being) in Sjögren's. Additionally, when compared to healthy people of

Daniel J. Wallace, Richa Mishra, and Frederick B. Vivino, *Diagnosis of Fatigue* In: *The Sjögren's Book*. Edited by: Daniel J. Wallace, Oxford University Press. © Sjögren's Foundation 2022. DOI: 10.1093/oso/9780197502112.003.0011 the same age and background, Sjögren's patients have lower rates of employment and higher rates of disability.

No specific biomarkers are available to distinguish most fatigued from non-fatigued individuals. However, Sjögren's patients in a phase 2 clinical trial recently demonstrated changes in blood cell gene expression as well as reduced inflammation, both of which might be associated with fatigue. Significant improvement in fatigue was attained in the trial, and phase 3 trials were planned for 2021 during which we should learn more about the therapy targets and fatigue. In addition, our hope is that specific biomarkers for the fatigue in Sjögren's will be identified during the Foundation for the National Institutes of Health Biomarkers Consortium and related National Institutes of Health Accelerating Medicines Parternship*-Autoimmune and Immune-Mediated Diseases (NIH AMP*-AIM) initiative (see Chapter 49 for more information on these). Recent research has shown that the vagus nerve might play a role in the regulation of fatigue. Several initial studies across multiple sites have shown that stimulation of the vagus nerve can modulate immune response, thereby reducing fatigue. Additional, larger, studies are needed for this novel approach to treating fatigue.

What Do You Feel, and What Is Causing Your Fatigue?

The majority of patients with connective tissue disorders, including lupus, RA, and Sjögren's, suffer from fatigue. Fatigue has many forms and descriptions. Basic fatigue is always present but worsens during periods of peak disease activity (disease flares). It is most common in individuals with involvement of the internal organs and sometimes is associated with flu-like symptoms. The exact cause is unknown but may be related to the release of cytokines (chemical mediators of inflammation) in the blood—a sign of systemic inflammation. Another possible cause of fatigue is neuroendocrine dysfunction, a type of hormonal imbalance.

Many Sjögren's patients are notoriously poor sleepers and wake up frequently at night or complain of "nonrestorative" sleep. This causes a sensation of fatigue immediately upon awakening (i.e., waking up tired) and can occur for multiple reasons, including restless leg syndrome, periodic limb movement disorder of sleep, sleep apnea, medication side effects, or discomfort from dry eyes and mouth. This kind of fatigue is sometimes associated with impaired concentration and memory, termed "brain fog."

Some of the most important causes of fatigue in Sjögren's are listed in Table 11.1. Inflammation and tissue damage (e.g., interstitial lung disease impairing oxygen exchange) are the most common disease-related causes.

Immobilizing or "rebound" fatigue sometimes occurs during periods of disease quiescence due to a sudden increase in activity levels (i.e., overdoing it the preceding day) beyond what the body can tolerate. Sudden fatigue or the "crumple and fold" phenomenon that is not related to a change in activity levels raises the possibility of infection, especially when a fever is present. Weather-related fatigue that feels like a sweeping wave and is associated with muscle aches suggests fibromyalgia.

Fibromyalgia is commonly associated with Sjögren's (prevalence up to 47%) and is characterized by diffuse body pain, chronic fatigue, nonrestorative sleep, morning stiffness, a subjective feeling of swelling, and modulation of the symptoms by the weather. It is often associated with other disorders, including depression, irritable bowel syndrome, temporomandibular joint dysfunction, migraine headaches, pelvic urethral (spastic bladder) syndrome, and costochondritis (inflammation of a rib and adjoining cartilage, causing chest pain).

Fatigue with the "molten lead phenomenon," like someone has poured molten lead into the limbs during sleep or like walking with a heavy weight, suggests an inflammatory process (especially with morning stiffness for >1 hour), and arthritis should be excluded. A similar phenomenon can also occur due to proximal muscle weakness; the latter is suspected when a patient has difficulty lifting the limbs (e.g., getting out of a chair or raising the arms to comb one's hair). It can be caused by myositis (muscle inflammation), steroid myopathy, hypothyroidism, or vitamin D deficiency. Vitamin D deficiency is common in the general population, especially among autoimmune disease patients. It has been implicated as a cause of not only fatigue and weakness but also generalized muscle and bone pain. Fatigue related to other physical

Table 11.1 Some Causes of Fatigue in Sjögren's

Systemic inflammation	Severe anemia
Disturbed sleep	Infection
Anxiety and depression	Celiac disease
Fibromyalgia	Lymphoma
Medication side effects	Malnutrition
Vitamin B_{12} deficiency	Tissue damage
Hypothyroidism	Autonomic nerve dysfunction
Vitamin D deficiency	Anemia

causes such as thyroid problems or anemia makes people feel as if they are climbing a steep hill while walking on level ground.

A "tired-wired" feeling can result from use of certain medications such as prednisone or too much caffeine. With this type of fatigue, the body feels tired but the mind wants to keep going and can't let the body rest. Prednisone typically causes insomnia and is therefore best taken in the morning. Some medications, such as painkillers (for example, tramadol [Ultram], oxycodone [OxyContin], or gabapentin [Neurontin]), may cause drowsiness and increased dryness and therefore are best taken at night. The use of narcotics (oxycodone, hydrocodone, tramadol) should be minimized due to their addictive potential.

People who suffer from chronic illnesses frequently develop psychosocial problems. Prevalence rates for depression and anxiety as high as 48% have been reported in individuals with Sjögren's. In some cases, the energy spent fighting these illnesses causes severe emotional fatigue that at times can seem overwhelming. Anxiety and depression also may interfere with restful sleep and exacerbate the fatigue; these disorders also may worsen chronic pain, headaches, and other symptoms.

How Is Fatigue Assessed?

Generally used fatigue scales are not specific for Sjögren's, with the exception of the Patient Reported Outcome Measurement Information System (PROMIS) methodology currently being developed by the National Institutes of Health and the Sjögren's Foundation and the three-question ESSPRI used in clinical trials (ESSPRI stands for European Alliance of Associations for Rheumatology (EULAR) Sjögren's Syndrome Patient Reported Index). Nonspecific measures that have been used include the Multidimensional Fatigue Inventory, Fatigue Severity Scale, Fatigue Impact Scale, Chalder Fatigue Scale, and the Functional Assessment of Cancer Therapy Scale—Fatigue (FACIT), the latter of which is commonly employed in autoimmune clinical trials. Since fatigue is inversely correlated with health-related quality of life, both physical and mental components of the Short Form-36 (SF-36) have been used as well.

Summing Up

Fatigue is pervasive in patients with Sjögren's and one of the main aspects that account for an altered quality of life. Primary factors such as inflammation can be reversible and should be ruled out first. Associated factors such as medication and thyroid dysfunction (present in 20% of Sjögren's patients) deserve attention as well. Environmental and psychosocial factor adjustments can often ameliorate fatigue. The management of fatigue is reviewed in Chapter 32.

For Further Reading

Dias LH, Miyamoto ST, Giovelli RA, et al. Pain and fatigue are predictors of quality of life in primary Sjögren's syndrome. *Adv Rheumatol.* 2021;61(1):28. doi:10.1186/s42358-021-00181-9

Karageorgas T, Fragioudaki S, Nezos A, et al. Fatigue in primary Sjogren's syndrome: Clinical, laboratory, psychometric and biologic Associations. *Arthritis Care Res.* 2016;68:123–131.

Miyamoto ST, Lenmdrem DW, Ng WF, et al. Managing fatigue in patients with primary Sjögren's syndrome: Challenges and solutions. *Open Access Rheumatol Res Rev.* 2019;11:77–88.

Ng W-F, Bowman SJ. Primary Sjögren's syndrome: Too dry and too tired. *Rheumatology.* 2010;49(5):844–853.

Pinto ACPN, Piva SR, da Silva Vieira AG, et al. Transcranial direct current stimulation for fatigue in patients with Sjögren's syndrome. *Brain Stimul.* 2021;14(1):141–151. doi:10.1016/j.brs.2020.12.004

Segal B, Bowman S, Fox P, et al. Primary Sjögren's syndrome; health experiences and predictors of health quality among patients in the United States. *Health and Quality of Life Outcomes.* 2009;7:46.

Strombeck B, Ekdahl C, Manthorpe R, et al. Health-related quality of life in primary Sjögren's syndrome, rheumatoid arthritis and fibromyalgia compared to normal population data using the SF-36. *Scand J Rheumatol.* 2000;29:20–28.

Tarn J, Legg S, Mitchell S, Simon B, Ng WF. The effects of noninvasive vagus nerve stimulation on fatigue and immune responses in patients with primary Sjögren's syndrome. *Neuromodulation.* 2019;22(5):580–585.

12

Musculoskeletal Manifestations of Sjögren's

Donald E. Thomas Jr.

> Conjunctivitis associated with rheumatoid or arthritic conditions (which) occurred chiefly, if not invariably in women, one of whom had peliosis rheumatica, and there was no tear secretion.
>
> **Dr. J. Gray Clegg**

This quotation from 1927 is the first description of what we today call Sjögren's associated with rheumatoid arthritis (RA). Dr. Clegg of Manchester, England, wrote this in response to a Dutch ophthalmologist named A.W. Mulock Houwer. Dr. Houwer had cared for 10 patients with keratitis filamentosa, six of whom had chronic polyarthritis that he thought may have been gout. Since gout was much more common in England than in the Netherlands, Dr. Houwer traveled to London to present and discuss his patients with his English peers of the esteemed Ophthalmological Society of the United Kingdom.

> It was difficult, however, to get more facts regarding the nature of the arthritis as most patients did not like to submit to a clinical examination. We imagined that possibly we were dealing with cases of irregular gout. This possibility occurred to us on examining patient No. 9 (a woman of 60), where the x-ray examination of the hands revealed some changes suggesting gout.

Dr. Houwer ended his paper with:

> As in England gout seems to be far more prevalent than in the Netherlands, I am very curious to learn whether any of you have come across similar cases.

Three years later, in January 1930, Dr. Henrik Sjögren, an ophthalmologist practicing in the Eye Clinic at the Seraphim Hospital (also known as the Serafen

Donald E. Thomas Jr., *Musculoskeletal Manifestations of Sjögren's* In: *The Sjögren's Book*. Edited by: Daniel J. Wallace, Oxford University Press. © Sjögren's Foundation 2022. DOI: 10.1093/oso/9780197502112.003.0012 or "Serafim" Military Hospital) in Stockholm, Sweden, encountered E.Ö., a 49-year-old woman with extreme dryness of the mouth and eyes. Her dryness problems began 6 years earlier when she concomitantly developed very painful, swollen joints. She was seen in the medical polyclinic of the hospital at that time and was diagnosed with "chronic rheumatism." Dr. Sjögren suspected that this was an unusual combination of medical problems and presented the case to his local Swedish ophthalmological society. His older colleagues said that this disease was unknown to them. These events led to Dr. Sjögren—with the aid of his wife Maria, also an ophthalmologist—to document the 19 patients with sicca syndrome and present them in his now-famous 1933 doctoral thesis. It is noteworthy that 13 of his original 19 patients also had chronic arthritis. So, from the very beginning, arthritis was identified as one of the primary associations with sicca complex. Dr. Sjögren's 158-page manuscript (in the English translation) describing these patients was extremely detailed and laid the foundation for the recognition and study of patients suffering from what we now know is a systemic autoimmune disease. This analysis was recognized by the best ophthalmologists of the time, leading to the eponym "Sjögren's syndrome" (even though it could just as correctly have been named "Clegg syndrome" or "Houwer syndrome").

The Joints

Henrik Sjögren went on to accumulate a total of 80 patients with keratoconjunctivitis sicca (KCS). In a 1951 paper, he described 62% of them as having a concurrent polyarthritis. Between 1947 and 1956, five articles were published in the medical literature, each of which included RA patients and their association with KCS. Among a total of 1,213 RA patients in these studies, 153 (13%) had KCS, demonstrating a high prevalence of KCS among patients who had RA. Joseph J. Bunim, MD, in the 1960 Heberden Oration of the American Rheumatism Association (the predecessor of the American College of Rheumatology), described 40 patients with Sjögren's cared for at the Arthritis Branch of the National Institutes of Arthritis and Metabolic Diseases of the National Institutes of Health (NIH) in Bethesda, Maryland. He described in great detail many of the extraglandular aspects of Sjögren's. Of the 40 patients, 15 appeared to have Sjögren's alone, while the remaining 25 were classified as other "clinical subgroups," including 17 with definite RA, two with possible RA, two with scleroderma, and two with myositis.

Today we describe joint involvement as either arthralgia or arthritis. By arthritis, we mean that there is inflammation or damage of any of the structures making up the joint, including the articular cartilage, synovial membrane, joint capsule, periosteum, adjacent bony structures, and the intervening synovial fluid (Figure 12.1). In ascribing arthritis in a Sjögren's patient to the disease itself, it is implied that we are focusing on inflammatory arthritis that is due to the pathogenic mechanisms related to the autoimmune disorder. It is essential to distinguish non-autoimmune causes of arthritis—such as traumatic arthritis and the primary osteoarthritis of aging—from the inflammatory arthritis of Sjögren's. Osteoarthritis has the hallmarks of osteophytes, subchondral sclerosis, and bony cysts on imaging studies; the presence of non-inflammatory synovial fluid in the joints; and the presence of bony swellings on physical examination. Inflammatory arthritis causes soft tissue swelling of the joint. The medical history can also be of help in that the inflammatory arthritis of an autoimmune disease typically causes prolonged, more severe morning stiffness (often lasting 30 minutes or longer) compared to the briefer and less severe stiffness of degenerative osteoarthritis. However, it is important to point out that the duration and severity of morning stiffness are not so specific as to be diagnostic of the type of arthritis (that is, the arthritis of Sjögren's can potentially cause brief morning stiffness). Crepitus (grating or feeling of friction in the joint), either by history or on physical examination, can also be a clue that points more toward degenerative arthritis. This point of differentiating inflammatory arthritis due to the autoimmune mechanisms associated with Sjögren's versus the possibility of unrelated degenerative arthritis is vital because osteoarthritis begins to become more prevalent in

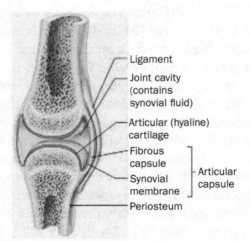

Figure 12.1 Schematic view of synovial joint [adapted from studyblue.com/notes/ lecture 5 joints and articulations]

Source: Prekasan, D. & Saju, K.K. (2016). Review of the Tribological Characteristics of Synovial Fluid. Procedia Technology. 25. 1170-1174. 10.1016/j.protcy.2016.08.235.

people in their mid-30s and is almost universal after the age of 50. This age range includes most patients who have Sjögren's. Therefore, osteoarthritis is a common coexisting condition in people who have Sjögren's.

Synovitis is an even more specific term when referring to inflammatory arthritis. It refers to actual inflammation of the synovial membrane of the joint. Although its occurrence in a patient with Sjögren's is usually assumed to be due to inflammation from the autoimmune process, synovitis may also occur in osteoarthritic joints, though to a lesser degree. The use of "synovitis" is considered to be more specific than that of "arthritis" when referring to inflammation of the joints in autoimmune diseases such as Sjögren's.

Arthralgia is the term we use to mean joint pain. A person can have objective evidence of arthritis (for example, evidence of joint damage on X-ray) yet not have accompanying arthralgia of that joint. Conversely, people can have arthralgias of joints that may or may not have evidence of actual arthritis. Sjögren's research studies demonstrate that many Sjögren's patients may have arthralgia (or polyarthralgia when referring to joint pain in many joints) in the absence of demonstrable arthritis on physical examination. The mechanism for this occurrence is not entirely understood. However, with the increasing use of musculoskeletal ultrasound (MSK-US), we are beginning to better understand that many of these patients have an anatomic explanation for their pain, such as synovitis or other causes such as tenosynovitis (inflammation of the tendon sheath on top of the joint; see the ultrasound section of this chapter).

Sjögren's patients may have joint involvement in the form of arthralgias (plus or minus actual arthritis) attributed to the Sjögren's disease process itself or due to an accompanying systemic autoimmune disease. When Sjögren's occurs with RA, it is a given that the inflammatory arthritis is presumably due to the RA component of the autoimmune disease. However, when Sjögren's occurs with other systemic autoimmune disorders—such as systemic lupus erythematosus (SLE), systemic sclerosis (a.k.a. scleroderma), polymyositis, or dermatomyositis—it is much more difficult, and usually impossible, to determine if the arthralgias or arthritis is due to the Sjögren's or the other autoimmune disorder. The remainder of this section of the chapter will only deal with joint involvement in patients who have Sjögren's, to remove any ambiguity as to the actual cause of the joint problems.

The prevalence of arthralgias in Sjögren's ranges from 36% to 84%, while the frequency of actual arthritis or synovitis is 15% to 77% in studies that do not utilize more advanced imaging such as ultrasound (US) or magnetic resonance imaging (MRI). These wide ranges of prevalence are explained by the various ways each study was performed, the authors' definitions of "arthralgia" and "arthritis," the demographics of the patient population studied, and the primary reasons the study was performed in the first place. For example, some of the studies directed at evaluating the use of therapeutic agents to treat Sjögren's—for instance, the Kruize et al. study with 74% arthralgia and the Carubbi et al. study with 49% arthritis—may overestimate the frequencies because they are studies looking for patients who have potentially treatable symptoms. Studies—such as those by Ramos-Casals et al., who studied 1,010 Sjögren's patients, and Fauchais et al., who evaluated 499 patients—may underestimate arthritis (15% and 16% respectively) as their retrospective studies may not have been as stringent in recording arthritis or synovitis in the chart records. The 1983 study by Castro-Poltronieri and Alarcón-Segovia is an outlier, identifying 84% of their Sjögren's cohort as having arthralgia while 77% had arthritis. Because this study only had 31 patients, this higher frequency may be an overestimation related to the small sample size.

Patients with Sjögren's exhibit a type of arthritis similar to that found in SLE patients: a non-erosive, symmetrical, polyarticular arthritis most commonly affecting the small joints of the hands. "Non-erosive" refers to the absence of bony erosions on plain-film X-rays. "Symmetrical" refers to the involvement of the same joint area on both sides of the body (such as involving some of the metacarpophalangeal [MCP] joints, or knuckles, in both hands). Having synovitis of the left second MCP joint and the right thumb MCP joint would be considered symmetrical even though they do not involve precisely the same digits. "Polyarticular" means that more than three or four joints are affected. Some patients with Sjögren's can have an oligoarthritis (two to four joints involved), while having a monoarthritis (one joint affected) is most unusual but can occur. Patients with Sjögren's do not typically develop deforming arthritis. If reversible deforming arthritis occurs (Jaccoud's arthropathy), where joints can be straightened by the examiner on physical examination, then a diagnosis of SLE should be strongly considered along with Sjögren's. If there are permanent, nonreversible joint deformities on physical examination that are related to inflammatory arthritis, then RA with Sjögren's should be suspected by the clinician.

Another lupus-like attribute of Sjögren's arthritis is that there is typically not much synovial swelling present on physical examination. Joint tenderness along with a loss of passive range of motion on physical examination and prolonged morning stiffness (that is, inflammatory symptomatology) is more prevalent than having notable boggy synovial swelling of the joints (as is more typical of RA). This phenomenon of little synovial swelling seen on physical examination is even more recognized today with the use of US by rheumatologists in the examination room. Studies that did not utilize US (those referred to in the preceding paragraphs) often show a large number of Sjögren's patients having arthralgia without actually having apparent arthritis. For example, the studies by Haga and Peen, Fauchais et al., and Ramos-Casals et al. showed an "arthralgia" prevalence of 74%, 45%, and 48% respectively, while only finding "arthritis" in 18%, 16%, and 15% respectively. The studies that utilize US to assess for synovitis show significantly higher rates of actual joint synovitis. For example, the 2013 US study by Amezcua-Guerra showed that more than three-quarters of their patients with Sjögren's had synovitis of the joints.

The distribution of the joints affected by Sjögren's also appears to be similar to that of SLE patients, with small to medium joints being affected more frequently than large joints. However, the studies differed as to which joints were most affected. Haga and Peen found the ankles to be the most affected joints by arthritis in Sjögren's, followed by MCP joints, shoulders, metatarsophalangeal (MTP) joints, then wrists. Haga and Peen's findings contrast with those from the Fauchais et al. study, where the MCP joints, upper extremity proximal interphalangeal (PIP) joints, and the wrists were more commonly involved, followed by the knees. The MTP joints, distal interphalangeal (DIP) joints, and shoulders were least affected (while no patients had hip arthritis from Sjögren's). The US study by Amezcua-Guerra et al. showed that the wrists, followed by the elbows and knees, were most commonly affected by synovitis in Sjögren's without an accompanying autoimmune disease, while MCP involvement was much more common in patients who had Sjögren's and RA.

Interestingly, several studies point to the occurrence of sacroiliitis in patients who have Sjögren's. Sacroiliitis is classically felt to be part of the seronegative spondyloarthritides, such as ankylosing spondylitis, psoriatic arthritis, inflammatory bowel disease, and reactive arthritis. However, Fauchais et al. found radiographic sacroiliitis and inflammatory back pain in 1% of their Sjögren's patients, but they lacked the enthesitis (painful inflammation where tendons and ligaments attach to the bone) that is more typical of the spondyloarthritides. A more recent study by Eren et al. in 2018 found a 10.5% prevalence of radiographic sacroiliitis in 85 patients with Sjögren's (compared to only 2% of the control patients). Both Whaley et al. in 1971 and Collins et al. in 1992 showed an increased association of Sjögren's in patients with psoriatic arthritis and ankylosing spondylitis. Then, when Kobak et al. found that 10% of their ankylosing spondylitis patients had Sjögren's as proven by a biopsy of a minor salivary gland, they proposed a possible pathogenic association between Sjögren's and the spondyloarthritides.

Rare arthritis patterns in Sjögren's include one case of cricoarytenoid arthritis (affecting the pair of small joints in the back of the larynx) described by Sève et al. in 2005; this patient, who was diagnosed by indirect laryngoscopy, had dysphonia that resolved with prednisone therapy. One patient in Fauchais et al.'s series had small hand-joint polyarthritis associated with distal extremity edema reminiscent of remitting seronegative symmetrical synovitis with pitting edema (RS_3PE).

The articular manifestations of Sjögren's can occur before sicca symptoms. This delay in noting dryness is not too surprising, because we know that it takes a certain threshold of decreased saliva and tear production before many patients notice it. As expected, the numbers vary quite a bit in the studies, with as many as 30% of patients developing arthritis before the onset of sicca in the Castro-Poltronieri et al. paper but in only 7% of all Sjögren's patients in the study by Fauchais et al. Most patients appear to present with arthritis and dryness problems simultaneously and at the time of their Sjögren's diagnosis. Some patients develop arthritis after their diagnosis. Among the entire Sjögren's group who had inflammatory arthritis in Fauchais et al.'s cohort, 31% of the patients (14% of the whole Sjögren's cohort) developed their arthritis after their sicca symptoms occurred.

Having inflammatory arthritis with Sjögren's appears to predict more severe disease in several studies. Fernandez Castro et al. in 2018 showed a higher rate of severe to very severe dry eye—as measured by the Tear Film and Ocular Surface Society Dry Eye Workshop 2007 classification—in patients who had arthritis with Sjögren's. Mirouse et al. found a six-fold higher rate of lymphadenopathy in Sjögren's patients who had synovitis as well as a four-fold higher European Union League Against Rheumatism (EULAR) Sjögren's Syndrome Disease Activity Index (ESSDAI). Over 60% of Fauchais et al.'s Sjögren's patients who had inflammatory arthritis at the time of their Sjögren's diagnosis had other extraglandular manifestations. These patients especially had an increased chance of having Raynaud's phenomenon, cutaneous vasculitis, cryoglobulinemia, peripheral neuropathy, and interstitial nephritis compared to patients who did not have arthritis. Their patients had most of their flares of arthritis during the early years of their Sjögren's diagnosis, and the flares often coincided with flares of parotid gland enlargement, cutaneous vasculitis, and neurologic disease. Since previous studies had also shown an association between Sjögren's arthritis and enlargement of the salivary glands, Raynaud's, and cutaneous vasculitis, Fauchais et al. recommend close follow-up of Sjögren's patients who have inflammatory arthritis and suggest being on the lookout for multisystemic involvement, especially vasculitis.

Tendonitis and Tenosynovitis

Most Sjögren's studies have overlooked the possibility of tendon involvement. For example, tenosynovitis was noted in only 2% of Stevens et al.'s 2005 Sjögren's patients. However, Riente et al.'s 2009 US study found, upon a thorough evaluation of a group of Sjögren's patients, that 21% had flexor tenosynovitis of the hands. This high rate of tenosynovial involvement is again in line with the pattern of the similarity of Sjögren's and SLE, where US studies have also shown a high rate of tenosynovitis among SLE patients. One must also wonder whether tenosynovitis could explain such a high ratio of arthralgia to inflammatory arthritis in many pre-US Sjögren's studies. If these studies had actively looked for tenosynovitis, could the occurrence of tenosynovitis explain why some of the arthralgia patients did not have clinical arthritis? Future studies should investigate the prevalence of inflammatory tendosynovitis by physical examination and MSK-US in Sjögren's patients.

Myalgia and Myositis

Actual inflammatory myositis appears to be uncommon in patients with Sjögren's outside of those patients who have polymyositis or dermatomyositis in addition to Sjögren's. Interestingly, Bloch et al. showed in their 1965 study of Sjögren's patients that 72% of the muscle biopsies performed in 36 patients showed a perivascular myositis, even in some asymptomatic patients. In 1994, Kraus et al. described three cases of myositis in 104 patients with Sjögren's. However, one must ask if these may have represented instances of polymyositis with Sjögren's rather than Sjögren's with inflammatory myositis. Given the high frequency of asymptomatic myositis in Bloch et al.'s cohort of Sjögren's patients, this matter deserves further investigation.

The occurrence of muscle discomforts or muscle pain (myalgia) is common in Sjögren's. The Kruize et al. hydroxychloroquine study listed a 74% prevalence of myalgia among their Sjögren's patients, Markusse et al. found about a 50% prevalence after a 9-year average follow-up of 50 patients, and the 2012 "cutting-edge" paper by Tincani et al. stated that "myalgias are frequent." The high frequency of muscle pain in these studies is in contrast to Fauchais et al.'s study, which listed "muscular manifestations" in only 5% of their 419 Sjögren's patients. However, this was a retrospective study, and the physicians caring for this group of patients may not have been diligent in noting all symptoms such as myalgia in the clinical records. Interestingly, the Meijer et al. study from the Netherlands of rituximab stated that "tendomyalgia" occurred in 83% of their patients. I have never seen this term used before, so I am not confident as to what this precisely refers. Of note, these studies mentioning myalgia in Sjögren's did not discuss what percentage of these patients may have had fibromyalgia (presented later in this section) as the cause of their myalgia.

Arthritis Referrals to Rheumatologists

Fauchais et al. stated that 11% of their Sjögren's patients were referred to them based upon the occurrence of articular symptoms. They mention that previous investigators had noted that 10% of arthritis workups result in a diagnosis of Sjögren's as the cause of arthritis and that another undifferentiated arthritis study demonstrated that 5% of cases evolve into Sjögren's within 1 year of initial evaluation. Therefore, physicians must keep in mind the possibility of Sjögren's as one of the possible causes of inflammatory arthritis of uncertain etiology.

Evolution of Sjögren's Patients Developing Additional Autoimmune/Rheumatic Diseases

How can the clinician predict which Sjögren's patients will evolve to an overlap syndrome (that is, develop another major, related rheumatic disease)? Researchers have not studied this question very well thus far. In Fauchais et al.'s cohort, it was uncommon for patients to develop another related disease after diagnosis of Sjögren's alone: Only 4% of their patients who had Sjögren's and articular symptoms eventually progressed to develop an additional systemic autoimmune disorder. However, this was three-fold more often than those patients who did not have articular manifestations. Those patients who had hypergammaglobulinemia or who were positive for rheumatoid factor (RF), anti-SSA/Ro, or anti-SSB/La antibodies were more likely to develop an additional connective tissue disease (three patients developed SLE and four developed polymyositis in the articular group). Other studies have suggested that having antibodies to cyclic citrullinated peptide (CCP) may increase the chances of evolution to RA in addition to a patient's Sjögren's (discussed later in this chapter).

Fibromyalgia

Fibromyalgia is a syndrome characterized by chronic, widespread pain felt to be related to central sensitization mechanisms. Other symptoms often associated with it are fatigue that does not improve with rest, nonrestorative sleep, cognitive difficulties, and oversensitivity to physical touch. Other problems, such as irritable bowel syndrome, migraine, chronic pelvic pain disorders, and interstitial cystitis, often occur with fibromyalgia. While fibromyalgia is present in approximately 2% of the population, numerous studies show that there is a much higher rate among patients who have systemic autoimmune disorders such as Sjögren's. The prevalence of fibromyalgia in patients who have Sjögren's varies from 12% to 55%, depending on the research study, patient demographics, and the criteria used to make the diagnosis. Iannuccelli et al. found in their 2012 Italian cohort that although 90% of their Sjögren's patients reported having widespread pain, only 18% of them satisfied criteria for fibromyalgia. These researchers suggested that there must be an underlying mechanism other than fibromyalgia for many patients with Sjögren's to have widespread pain.

Torrente-Segarra et al. reviewed the literature to assess the prevalence of fibromyalgia in patients who have SLE. Having concomitant Sjögren's increased the chances of having fibromyalgia by 2.4-fold compared to SLE patients who did not have Sjögren's.

Looking at this from another direction, Bonafede et al. examined 72 patients with fibromyalgia to assess if any of them might have Sjögren's. Thirty-five percent of the patients had a positive Schirmer's test for dry eye (used as a screening test for possible Sjögren's), and these patients then underwent a minor salivary gland biopsy. Those with a positive biopsy result for Sjögren's were also found to be positive for antinuclear antibody (ANA), anti-SSA/Ro, anti-SSB/La, and/or RF. A total of 14% of the 72 patients with fibromyalgia were found to have Sjögren's (half were definite Sjögren's, while the other half were "probable" Sjögren's). The results of this study should alert clinicians to ensure that fibromyalgia patients are screened for possible Sjögren's by asking about sicca symptoms, performing a Schirmer's test, and ordering autoantibody testing.

Medications That Cause Pain

Of course, it is essential to consider other causes of MSK pain, such as medications, in patients who have Sjögren's. Some of the most common drugs include the fluoroquinolones (e.g., ciprofloxacin and levofloxacin), statins used for cholesterol, and the bisphosphonates (e.g., alendronate, ibandronate) used to treat osteoporosis. All of these are commonly used in patients who have Sjögren's and can be potential causes of pain.

The aromatase inhibitors (e.g., anastrozole, letrozole, and exemestane), commonly used as adjuvant therapy for breast cancer, deserve special mention. Approximately 40% to 50% of women who take these medications develop significant pain, described as disabling in 5% to 10% of patients. A knockout mouse model showed that aromatase inhibitors could cause a Sjögren-like condition. Laroche et al. then studied 24 women who had joint pain while taking aromatase inhibitors and found that 29% had "probable" Sjögren's and one had definite Sjögren's.

Checkpoint inhibitors, a type of immunotherapy used to treat many types of cancers, have revolutionized the management of some tumors that until recently had little to no good treatments. As their use has become more common, they have shown the ability to induce immune-related adverse events, causing medical problems that closely mimic systemic autoimmune diseases, including inflammatory synovitis and severe salivary and ocular gland hypofunction (causing severe dry mouth and dry eyes) in some patients. Therefore, it is essential to recognize these medications as possible causes when a patient presents with new-onset sicca complex along with MSK pain.

Laboratory Tests in Sjögren's and Arthritis

Anti-CCP antibodies are relatively specific for diagnosing RA. However, they are also found in other systemic autoimmune diseases, including Sjögren's. Depending upon the laboratory method used, the prevalence in Sjögren's ranges from 3% to 10%. Most of these studies show a clear association with an increased risk of having non-erosive arthritis with Sjögren's and an increased risk of evolution to RA with Sjögren's. One of the more extensive and well-done studies, by Atzeni et al., concluded that anti-CCP in Sjögren's may be a predictor of future progression to RA or at least synovitis. Other abnormal lab results such as RF, anti-SSA/Ro, anti-SSB/La, and hypergammaglobulinemia are common in patients who have Sjögren's but do not appear to predict the occurrence of articular manifestations in most studies.

Imaging Studies

Plain-film X-rays tend to either be normal or show mild joint space loss without erosions in Sjögren's studies. Radiographic erosions are unusual and more common in those patients who evolve to RA with Sjögren's. Tsampoulas and the highly respected MSK radiologist Donald Resnick suggested in their

1986 study that plain-film X-rays could help differentiate between patients who have Sjögren's alone and those who have RA with Sjögren's. Patients with Sjögren's and inflammatory arthritis (without RA) had less joint space narrowing and did not have erosive disease. Interestingly, having Sjögren's appeared to have a relatively protective effect on joints in RA patients in that they tended to have fewer erosions and less joint space loss than RA patients who did not have Sjögren's.

As previously mentioned, sacroiliitis appears in some patients who have Sjögren's. Therefore, clinicians should make sure to ask about inflammatory back pain in Sjögren's patients, and, if present, obtain an anteroposterior pelvic X-ray along with consideration of special sacroiliac joint views such as the modified Ferguson view. If the diagnosis is uncertain on plain-film X-rays, then semicoronal MRI images of the sacroiliac joints may be needed to look for signs of bone marrow edema in subchondral bone as a sign of early sacroiliitis. However, caution should be used to ensure that an experienced radiologist reads the films, because healthy individuals can occasionally have findings such as the bone marrow edema abnormalities found in sacroiliitis. Although Fauchais et al. did not find enthesitis in their patients with sacroiliitis, an US study in these patients would be interesting to see if there is sonographic evidence for enthesitis as is found in the spondyloarthritides.

MSK-US has shed much additional light on the articular manifestations of Sjögren's. The first study to assess the use of MSK-US in Sjögren's was published in 2002 by Iagnocco et al. and showed an increased prevalence of knee synovitis and effusions. She and her group went on to find in their 2010 follow-up study that 37.5% of their patients with Sjögren's had US evidence of inflammatory synovitis in the wrists, especially synovial proliferation. Although the synovitis was often "silent," its presence did correlate with increased disease activity as measured by the ESSDAI. Riente et al. in 2009 examined the MCP and upper extremity PIP joints in anti-CCP-negative Sjögren's patients and showed that 19% of the patients had inflammatory arthritis involving these joints. Two-thirds of those had erosions present on US. Flexor tenosynovitis was also present in 21% of all their Sjögren's patients. The finding of erosions and flexor tenosynovitis were surprising to the group. Amezcua-Guerra et al. performed an even more exhaustive study in 2013 and found that synovial hypertrophy was present in over three-quarters of their Sjögren's patients—especially in the MCPs, wrists, and knee joints. Eighteen percent of their Sjögren's patients had US evidence for carpal joint erosions, while the presence of MCP erosions was found to be 100% specific for RA with Sjögren's. The finding of erosions on MSK-US, but not on plain-film radiographs, has caused some investigators to wonder if the pathophysiology of Sjögren's erosions may differ from that of RA erosions. Rather than being due to osteoclastic bone resorption (as is hypothesized for RA), they may be due to a different mechanism, such as from tendon traction on demineralized bone with subsequent ischemic bone resorption (as has been hypothesized in scleroderma patients).

The high prevalence of synovitis in these studies led Lei et al. to compare the use of MSK-US to physical examination and laboratory testing. They showed that MSK-US was superior for diagnosing synovitis and erosive disease. More importantly, the use of MSK-US led to necessary management changes, such as optimizing immunosuppressive therapy in 35% of the patients who otherwise would not have had important adjustments in treatment.

These MSK-US studies suggest that clinical evaluation of inflammatory joint involvement by medical history and physical examination is not adequate in our patients who have Sjögren's. Rheumatologists have increased their usage of MSK-US during the past 10 to 15 years, but many practices still do not utilize it to help with diagnostic and management decisions. If future studies replicate these findings by Lei et al.'s group, and I suspect they will, then MSK-US should become an essential tool in all rheumatology practices and should be strongly considered in future clinical trials involving Sjögren's patients. Currently, EULAR offers excellent MSK-US courses for beginners up to advanced students and even provides an exceptional "Teach the Teachers" course. The American College of Rheumatology has also been expanding its teaching of MSK-US and offers formal certification in ultrasonography, where those who prove their proficiency can use the title RhMSUS (Rheumatology MSK-US certification) after their name.

Summing Up

Inflammatory arthritis is common in Sjögren's. It most often presents as non-deforming, non-erosive, symmetrical polyarthritis affecting most commonly the wrists and MCP joints, followed by the upper extremity PIP joints and knees. MSK-US shows us that the prevalence of synovitis is much higher than can be appreciated by physical examination and can potentially improve diagnoses and the management of Sjögren's patients. US also demonstrates a high prevalence of small erosions that are absent on plain-film X-rays as well as the occurrence of tenosynovitis of the hands. These findings suggest that MSK-US should be used more often in both the clinical setting and in research studies of Sjögren's patients.

When inflammatory arthritis occurs in a Sjögren's patient, it is essential to keep in mind that there is an increased risk for other problems such as cutaneous vasculitis, parotitis, and other extraglandular manifestations. The Sjögren's patient who is positive for anti-CCP antibodies may have an increased risk of developing inflammatory arthritis or evolve to an overlap syndrome with concomitant RA. The finding of increased sacroiliitis in some studies is a fascinating phenomenon and should alert the clinician to consider sacroiliac joint imaging in the patient who may have inflammatory back pain.

Overt myositis is rare outside of patients who have polymyositis or dermatomyositis with Sjögren's, but the possibility of subclinical, biopsy-proven myositis may be a common finding that needs further investigation. Myalgia appears to be common. Fibromyalgia occurs much more commonly than in the general population, but fibromyalgia may not explain the high rate of widespread pain in Sjögren's patients. Conversely, it is also important to have due diligence in including Sjögren's in the differential diagnosis when evaluating patients who present with fibromyalgia or inflammatory arthritis.

For Further Reading

Amezcua-Guerra LM, et al. Joint involvement in primary Sjögren's syndrome: An ultrasound "target area approach to arthritis." *BioMed Res Int.* 2013;2013:640265.

Atzeni F, et al. Anti-cyclic citrullinated peptide antibodies in primary Sjögren syndrome may be associated with non-erosive synovitis. *Arthritis Res Ther.* 2008;10(3):R51.

Bloch KJ, Buchanan WW, Wohl MJ, Bunnim JJ. Sjögren's syndrome: A clinical, pathological and serological study of sixty-two cases. *Medicine.* 1992;71(6):386–403.

Bonafede RP, Downey DC, Bennett RM. An association of fibromyalgia with primary Sjögren's syndrome: A prospective study of 72 patients. *J Rheumatol.* 1995 Jan;22(1):133–136.

Bournia VK, Vlachoyiannopoulos PG. Subgroups of Sjögren syndrome patients according to serological profiles. *J Autoimmun.* 2012;39(1–2):15.

Boutry N, et al. MR imaging findings in hands in early RA: Comparison with those in systemic lupus erythematosus and primary Sjögren's syndrome. *Radiology.* 2005;236(2):593.

Bunim JJ. Heberden Oration: A broader spectrum of Sjögren's syndrome and its pathogenetic implications. *Ann Rheum Dis.* 1961;20:1.

Cappelli L, et al. Inflammatory arthritis and sicca syndrome induced by nivolumab and ipilimumab. *Annals Rheum Dis.* 2017;76:43.

Carubbi F, et al. Efficacy and safety of rituximab treatment in early primary Sjögren's syndrome: A prospective, multi-center, follow-up study. *Arthritis Res Ther.* 2013;15(5):R172.

Castro-Poltronieri A, Alarcón-Segovia D. Articular manifestations of primary Sjögren's syndrome. *J Rheumatol.* 1983;10(3):485.

Collins P, et al. Psoriasis, psoriatic arthritis and the possible association with Sjögren's syndrome. *Brit J Dermatol.* 1992;126(3):242.

Eren R, et al. Prevalence of inflammatory back pain and radiologic sacroiliitis is increased in patients with pSS. *Pan-African Med J.* 2018;30:98.

Fauchais A-L, et al. Articular manifestations in primary Sjögren's syndrome: Clinical significance and prognosis of 188 patients. *Rheumatology*. 2010;49(6):1164–1172.

Fernandez Castro M, et al. Inflammatory joint involvement is associated with severe dry eye in patients with primary Sjögren's syndrome. *Ann Rheum Dis*. 2018;77:724.

Haga HJ, Peen E. A study of the arthritis pattern in primary Sjögren's syndrome. *Clin Exp Rheumatol*. 2007;25(1):88.

Iagnocco A, et al. Subclinical synovitis in primary Sjögren's syndrome: An ultrasonographic study. *Rheumatology*. 2010;49(6):1153.

Iannuccelli C, et al. Fatigue and widespread pain in SLE and Sjögren's syndrome: Symptoms of the inflammatory disease or associated fibromyalgia? *Clin Exp Rheumatol*. 2012;30:S117.

Iwamoto N, et al. Determination of the subset of SS with articular manifestations by anticyclic citrullinated peptide antibodies. *J Rheumatol*. 2009;36(1):113.

Kobak S, Kobak AC, Kabasakal Y, et al. Sjögren's syndrome in patients with ankylosing spondylitis. *Clin Rheumatol*. 2007 Feb;26(2):173–175.

Kruize AA, et al. Hydroxychloroquine treatment for primary Sjögren's syndrome: A two-year double-blind crossover trial. *Ann Rheum Dis*. 1993;52(5):360.

Laroche M, et al. Joint pain with aromatase inhibitors: abnormal frequency of Sjögren's syndrome. *J Rheumatol*. 2007;34(11):2259.

Lei L, et al. Hand US-guided therapeutic decisions in inflammatory arthritis associated with SLE and SS. *Lupus Science Med*. 2018;5(Suppl 1). https://lupus.bmj.com/content/5/Suppl_1/A94.2

Lindvall B, et al. Subclinical myositis is common in primary Sjögren's syndrome and is not related to muscle pain. *J Rheumatol*. 2002;29:717.

Kraus A, Cifuentes M, Villa AR, Jakez J, et al. Myositis in primary Sjögren's syndrome. Report of 3 cases. *J Rheumatol*. 1994 Apr;21(4):649–653.

Markusse HM, Oudkerk M, Vroom TM, et al. Primary Sjögren's syndrome: Clinical spectrum and mode of presentation based on an analysis of 50 patients selected from a department of rheumatology. *Neth J Med*. 1992 Apr;40(3-4):125–134.

Meijer JM, et al. Effectiveness of rituximab treatment in primary Sjögren's syndrome: A randomized, double-blind, placebo-controlled trial. *Arthritis Rheum*. 2010;62(4):960.

Mirouse A, et al. Arthritis in primary Sjögren's syndrome: Characteristics, outcome and treatment from French multicenter retrospective study. *Ann Rheum Dis*. 2018;77:693.

Mohammed K, et al. Association of severe inflammatory polyarthritis in primary Sjögren's syndrome: Clinical, serologic, and HLA analysis. *J Rheumatol*. 2009;36(9):1937.

Ramos-Casals M, Solans R, Rosas J, et al. Primary Sjögren syndrome in Spain: Clinical and immunologic expression in 1010 patients. *Medicine* (Baltimore). 2008 Jul;87(4):210–219.

Riente L, et al. US imaging for the rheumatologist. XXIII. Sonographic evaluation of hand joint involvement in primary Sjögren's syndrome. *Clin Exp Rheumatol*. 2009;27(5):747.

Sève P, et al. Cricoarytenoid arthritis in SS. *Rheumatol Int*. 2005;25(4):301.

Sjögren H. *A New Conception of Keratoconjunctivitis Sicca (Keratitis Filiformis in Hypofunction of the Lacrimal Glands)*. (Translated by J. Bruce Hamilton.) Australasian Medical Publishing Company, Ltd.; 1943.

Solans-Laque R, et al. Arthritis prevalence and biological markers in primary Sjögren's syndrome. *Ann Rheum Dis*. 2013;71:679.

Stevens RJ, Hamburger J, Ainsworth JR, et al. Flares of systemic disease in primary Sjögren's syndrome. *Rheumatology* (Oxford). 2005 Mar;44(3):402–403.

Tincani A, Andreoli L, Cavazzana I, et al. Novel aspects of Sjögren's syndrome in 2012. *BMC Med*. 2013 Apr 4;11:93. doi:10.1186/1741-7015-11-93.

Torrente-Segarra V, Salman-Monte TC, Rúa-Figueroa Í, et al Fibromyalgia prevalence and related factors in a large registry of patients with systemic lupus erythematosus. *Clin Exp Rheumatol*. 2016 Mar-Apr;34(2 Suppl 96):S40–47. Epub 2015 Nov 17.

Tsampoulas CG, Skopouli FN, Sartoris DJ, et al. Hand radiographic changes in patients with primary and secondary Sjögren's syndrome. *Scand J Rheumatol*. 1986;15(3):333–339.

Whaley K, et al. Sjögren's syndrome in psoriatic arthritis, ankylosing spondylitis and Reiter's syndrome. *Acta Rheumatol Scand*. 1971;17:105.

13

Sjögren's and Central Nervous System Disorders

Arun Varadhachary

The concept of central nervous system (CNS) manifestations of rheumatologic disease is a well-recognized clinical phenomenon. Discussions regarding the association between rheumatologic disorders and neurologic involvement, however, require understanding of the difference between how rheumatologists and neurologists view disease definitions and classifications for conditions that fall under their respective domains.

As a group, rheumatologists rely upon disease definitions based upon polythetic criteria. In contrast, neurologists use a neuro-anatomic localization method to identify dysfunction of the nervous system and avoid etiologic diagnoses until a neuroanatomic substrate has been defined. Once the site of neurologic dysfunction has been "localized," then the clinical neurologist considers potential syndromic formulations until a pathologic or etiologic diagnosis can be reached. The neurologist attempts to avoid the cognitive error of ascribing prematurely an etiology to a sign that could be the result of any number of etiologies. Whenever reasonable and safe, the neurologist attempts to obtain tissue for examination, as this adds the certainty of histopathology to the clinical study.

Most of the rheumatic diseases lack a single distinguishing feature; however, each disease is usually identified by the presence of a combination of clinical and laboratory manifestations. Therefore, the clinical observation of an expert clinician may be considered the only available "gold standard" to define a rheumatologic diagnosis.

Classification of diseases is to think of them in groups, these groups being in such an order as best leads to the ascertainment and remembrance of their laws. According to the view of Flier and Robbe, the *definiens* of a diagnostic term consists of one or more essential characteristics, which are chosen prior to empirical investigation. Research may reveal accidental or nonessential characteristics that are empirically correlated to the initial disease definition. The term "nosological classification" is often used in connection with medical

Arun Varadhachary, *Sjögren's and Central Nervous System Disorders* In: *The Sjögren's Book*. Edited by: Daniel J. Wallace, Oxford University Press. © Sjögren's Foundation 2022. DOI: 10.1093/oso/9780197502112.003.0013 classification systems, and the tendency is to equate it with "diagnosis" and "validity." However, particularly in the case of rheumatologic diagnoses, this is far from always being the case.

Thus, use of polythetic disease definitions serves to group conditions until underlying mechanisms can be discovered. Thereafter, the definition of any given disease will be changed to align with the biological underpinning. The classification criteria for Sjögren's constituting ocular and oral symptoms, ocular signs, salivary gland pathology and dysfunction, and autoantibodies represents a standard approach to defining rheumatologic disorders.

New biomarkers are actively being sought to help classify subpopulations of patients with neurologic involvement. Some antibodies described as potential serologic markers of neurologic involvement in Sjögren's include IgA and/or IgG anti-alpha-fodrin antibodies, which appear to be more common in Sjögren's with putative neurologic involvement. Another potential marker of Sjögren's with neurologic manifestations are the anti-GW182 antibodies directed against cytoplasmic structures called GW bodies. The anti-type 3 muscarinic receptor antibodies have been described in Sjögren's and may be involved in the pathogenesis of autonomic neuropathic dysfunction.

Other serologic markers have been described in neurologic involvement of Sjögren's. Among these, patients with sensorimotor neuropathy have been reported to have higher rates of mixed cryoglobulin compared to Sjögren's without neurologic manifestations. On the other hand, Sjögren's patients with sensory neuropathy may have lower prevalence of the anti-SSA/Ro and anti-SSB/La antibodies.

Interpretation of any serologic data from patients with rheumatic disorders is problematic as rheumatologic disorders are often associated with polyclonal B-cell activation, which results in nonspecific assay detection. Therefore, studies evaluating the utility of serum biomarkers for the presence of neurologic signs and symptoms in association with Sjögren's without including rheumatologic disease controls when evaluating assay specificity need to be interpreted with caution.

The sensitivity and specificity data of every assay must be interpreted in terms of clinically relevant predictive value. In clinical laboratories where the prevalence of anti-SSA/Ro may be high, excellent sensitivity would translate into a poor positive predictive value. Moreover, it is important to search for the Ro/La antibodies only in selected patients, and the clinician should not consider serologic testing as a routine analysis in the same vein as a complete blood count or a complete metabolic panel. Serologic testing is best limited to patients with significant symptoms. The unintended consequences of inappropriately selecting patients for testing leads to a high proportion of false positives compared to true positives and the attendant risks from follow-up investigation or unnecessary treatment.

Attempts at discerning whether Sjögren's had specific CNS involvement began in the 1980s with retrospective observations of the range of neurologic symptoms experienced by Sjögren's patients. Those observations added to the literature by creating epidemiologic estimations of frequencies between neurologic symptoms, signs, and disorders and Sjögren's disease. Ranges of neurologic and Sjögren's co-involvement ranged from 0% to 70%. Early work used a range of neurologic diagnostic baskets defined variably by neuro-anatomic localization, symptomatology, and presumed pathology. Limitations in interpretation of these studies stemmed from variable methodologies and case definitions, the absence of CNS tissue histopathology to correlate with accepted Sjögren's pathology, and the lack of disease-specific control groups.

Most authors conducting the observational retrospective cross-sectional studies collected patients from either academic neurology departments or rheumatology or immunology clinics, leading to potential selection biases as milder cases of both rheumatologic and neurologic symptoms may have gone unnoticed. As highlighted earlier, the challenge in ascertaining the prevalence of neurologic involvement of Sjögren's is the lack of specific neurologic case definitions and varying diagnostic categories.

However, broadly speaking, numerous authors have divided CNS symptoms into four categories: focal neurologic signs, diffuse/non-localizing symptoms, spinal cord disorders, and demyelinating diseases. Examples of the disorders that can be grouped under these categories include stroke, seizures, movement disorders, encephalopathy, meningoencephalitis, neuropsychiatric symptoms, inflammatory spinal cord disease, optic neuropathy and multiple sclerosis (MS)-like conditions. Such classification schemes, to the mind of a neurologist, are problematic as they mix neuro-anatomic and symptom-based schemes with pathophysiologic criteria that may or may not be overlapping or exclusive from one another.

It is certainly easier to investigate the peripheral nervous system compared to the CNS due to the differential accessibility of tissue for both physiologic and pathologic testing; nonetheless, the pathogenic mechanisms accounting for neurologic symptoms associated with Sjögren's are unclear. The target antigens of the defining Ro/La antibodies are intracellular and thus are unlikely to be directly pathogenic. Similarly, the Sjögren's-defining pathologic feature of the autoimmune exocrinopathy has not been found to be a constant feature of peripheral nerve disease. Mechanisms suggested in the development of peripheral nerve disease in Sjögren's patients include vascular or peripheral inflammatory infiltrates and vasculitis of the nerve's vasa vasorum.

Even less is known about mechanisms of how Sjögren's may contribute to CNS symptoms. Hypotheses include direct infiltration of the CNS by mononuclear cells, vascular injury related to autoantibodies, and microvascular ischemia from small vessel vasculitis. The difficulty in ascertaining disease mechanisms stems from the challenges of being able to obtain CNS tissue.

Tools commonly used to investigate disease processes of the CNS include brain and spinal cord imaging with magnetic resonance imaging, analysis of cerebrospinal fluid obtained via lumbar puncture, evaluation of large vessel pathology through catheter-based and imaging-based angiograms, and cortical neuron electrical activity through the use of electroencephalography. Less frequently used techniques include metabolic activity measured through the use of positron emission tomography scans and brain biopsy. This listing is not exhaustive, and these techniques are not available at all centers. Each technique has risks and benefits, and each must be used with a particular hypothesis in mind. One of the pitfalls of clinical neurology is to perform a test without a clear sense of what information is being sought, as then an unexpected result becomes particularly challenging to interpret.

Recent interest has focused on the relationship between Sjögren's and neuromyelitis optica (NMO; Devic's disease). NMO was considered a severe subcategory of MS up until the discovery of the aquaporin-4 antibody in 2004. The antibody, NMO-IgG or AQP4-Ab, was found almost exclusively in patients with NMO but not in patients with classic MS. Discovery of the antibody coupled with evidence from histopathologic and immunologic studies supported the concept of NMO as a humorally mediated autoimmune disease distinct from MS.

NMO is considered to be an antibody-mediated astrocytopathy with complement-mediated injury to the blood–brain barrier in areas of higher AQP4 expression. NMO features are typically discernable on MRI affecting the optic nerves, brainstem, and spinal cord. The possible relationship between NMO and Sjögren's relates to the concept of abnormal humoral immune mechanisms. However, it is uncertain whether the relationship between Sjögren's and NMO is specific, as other rheumatologic disorders, including lupus and rheumatoid arthritis, have also been described as frequently comorbid with NMO. The strong association of NMO-IgG/AQP4-Ab-positive NMO with connective tissue disorders suggests that the two conditions might arise from the same general autoimmune predisposition.

Summing Up

Considering CNS manifestations of Sjögren's is an exciting area of multidisciplinary investigation, but also highlights the difficulties inherent with biomedical research in an era of changing definitions of disease. Sjögren's was initially defined by a constellation of symptoms that were recognizable to the expert clinician. As underlying autoimmune disease mechanisms are uncovered, it is our challenge to continuously consider how we categorize disease such that groupings remain clinically relevant and allow us to take care of our patients. See Chapters 29, 30, and 31 for additional discussions on peripheral and central nervous system disorders as well as management and treatment options.

For Further Reading

Bougea A, Anagnostou E, Konstantinos G, et al. A systematic review of peripheral and central nervous system involvement of rheumatoid arthritis, systemic lupus erythematosus, primary Sjögren's syndrome and associated immunological profiles. *Int J Chronic Dis.* 2015;2015:910352.

Margaratten M. Neurologic manifestations of primary Sjögren's syndrome. *Rheum Dis Clin North Am.* 2017;43:519–529.

Moreira I, Teixeira F, Martins Silva A, et al. Frequent involvement of central nervous system in primary Sjögren's. *Rheumatol Int.* 2015;35:289–294.

Tobon GJ, Pers J-O, Devauchelle-Pensec V, Youinou P. Neurological disorders in primary Sjögren's syndrome. *Autoimmune Dis.* 2012; Article ID 645967.

14

The Internal Organs in Sjögren's

R. Hal Scofield, Fotini C. Soliotis, Stuart S. Kassan,
and Haralampos M. Moutsopoulos

In Sjögren's, the immune system typically targets the salivary and lacrimal glands. In addition, the disease can manifest in other organs, including the lungs, heart, gut, liver, kidney, and nervous system. Major organ disease is seen in about half of Sjögren's patients. Some patients are affected early with so-called extraglandular (that is, outside the lacrimal and salivary glands) disease at about the same time that the symptoms of dry mouth and dry eye begin. On the other hand, in some patients, major organ involvement has its onset months or even years after the diagnosis of Sjögren's.

Manifestations of lung and liver disease as well as one type of kidney disease (interstitial nephritis) usually occur early, around the time of diagnosis of Sjögren's, and are unlikely to occur later on. These diseases are characterized by a common immune process: infiltration of the affected organ by a group of white blood cells called lymphocytes.

Conversely, the less common type of kidney disease, glomerulonephritis, and the involvement of the peripheral nerves often occur later in the disease process and are not usually present at the time of the onset of sicca or the diagnosis of Sjögren's. These two diseases also are characterized by a common immune process: inflammation of blood vessels, known as vasculitis, caused by the deposition of immune complexes (structures made up of antibodies) on the vessel walls.

Although disease of the major body organs (Table 14.1) is rarely severe or life-threatening in Sjögren's, these manifestations should be diagnosed promptly so that effective treatment is given. This is one of the reasons why Sjögren's patients should be monitored by their physician on a regular basis.

Respiratory Tract

The entire respiratory tract can be affected in Sjögren's. Starting with the nose, thinning of the mucous membrane of the nose, or atrophic rhinitis, can

R. Hal Scofield, Fotini C. Soliotis, Stuart S. Kassan, and Haralampos M. Moutsopoulos, *The Internal Organs in Sjögren's* In: *The Sjögren's Book*. Edited by: Daniel J. Wallace, Oxford University Press. © Sjögren's Foundation 2022. DOI: 10.1093/oso/9780197502112.003.0014

Table 14.1 Examples of Major Organ Involvement in Sjögren's

Respiratory Tract	Atrophic rhinitis
	Laryngotracheobronchitis & Traceobronchitis
	Atelectasis
	Interstitial lung disease
	Pleurisy & Pleural effusion
	Pulmonary hypertension
Kidneys & Bladder	Interstitial nephritis
	Renal tubular acidosis
	Nephrogenic diabetes inspidus
	Glomerulonephritis
	Interstitial cystitis
Gastrointestinal Tract	Difficulty swallowing
	Esophageal dysmotility
	Gastroesophageal reflux disease (GERD)
	Chronic atrophic gastritis
	Dyspepsia
	Diarrhea & Steatorrhea
	Pancreatitis
Liver	Chronic autoimmune hepatitis
	Primary biliary cholangitis
Heart	Pericardial effusion
	Pericarditis
	Congenital heart block
Nervous System	Sensory neuropathy
	Mononeuritis
	Trigeminal neuropathy
	Carpal tunnel syndrome
	Neuromyelitis optica
	Anxiety & Depression
	Brain fog
Blood Vessels	Vasculitis
	Palpable purpura

occur, giving rise to nasal dryness. Moving down the airway, the voice box (larynx), windpipe (trachea), and bronchial tubes can become inflamed; this is known as laryngotracheobronchitis. The main symptoms of this condition are hoarseness, dry cough, wheezing, and shortness of breath.

Because there is less mucus produced in the airway, Sjögren's patients have difficulty clearing foreign material that has been inhaled into the respiratory tract. This can also contribute to the chronic inflammation of the bronchi and can predispose the patient to bacterial infections. Also, mucus can become stuck in the small bronchi, blocking the ventilation of a small segment of the lung. This can lead to the collapse of that lung segment (atelectasis).

Inflammation of the trachea and bronchi (tracheobronchitis) can be diagnosed by performing breathing tests known as pulmonary function tests. The patient blows into a tube connected to a machine that measures the flow of air in the bronchi. In this way the reduced flow of air in the bronchial tubes can be detected. In tracheobronchitis, a standard chest X-ray can be normal.

The use of room humidifiers can help relieve symptoms of mild tracheobronchitis. Also, prescribed nebulizers, which can deliver tiny water droplets into the small airways, can help. If the patient is wheezing or if the pulmonary function tests confirm blockage of airflow in the bronchi, then inhalers containing medications that dilate the bronchi can be prescribed. However, these are only partially effective, as they cannot clear the mucus blocking the bronchi; in this respect, drugs that break down mucus (mucolytics) may be of some benefit. This chronic obstructive lung disease, or emphysema, was once thought to be rare among patients with Sjögren's, but recent studies have shown obstructive lung disease to be more common than previously known, even among patients who did not smoke (smoking tobacco causes obstructive lung disease) or did not have symptoms of shortness of breath.

The lung itself can also become inflamed in Sjögren's (interstitial lung disease [ILD]). As the bronchi branch out, they end in small air sacs known as the alveoli, where carbon dioxide is exchanged for oxygen. Around the alveoli there is supporting tissue known as the interstitium. This contains small blood vessels that take up the oxygen from the alveoli. If there is inflammation or scarring within the interstitium, then less oxygen can enter the blood within the lungs.

The symptoms of interstitial lung disease vary depending on the severity of the disease. In the early stages patients may have no symptoms or may complain of a dry cough and mild shortness of breath on exertion. In the late stages of severe ILD, which is rare, patients may have disabling breathlessness on exertion.

The chest X-ray may show a lacy or honeycomb type of shadowing within the lungs. Pulmonary function tests show impairment of gas exchange from the alveoli into the blood vessels and a reduced volume of air in the lungs. High-resolution computed tomography (HRCT) scans of the lungs are very useful in confirming the diagnosis. When looking at HRCT films, areas of inflammation appear as patches of white "ground glass" within the dark lungs. However, other lung conditions can mimic ILD associated with Sjögren's, so further investigations are sometimes necessary to confirm the diagnosis. In a procedure known as bronchoscopy, a lighted, flexible tube can be inserted from the mouth inside the lungs with the patient undergoing what is called conscious sedation. Then a sample of bronchial secretions can be obtained and examined under the microscope. In ILD associated with Sjögren's, fluid from bronchial secretions typically contains numerous lymphocytes, which are cells involved in inflammation. Sometimes a lung biopsy, done either during bronchoscopy or through a chest incision under local anesthetic (open-lung biopsy), is needed to make the diagnosis.

The standard treatment for ILD is corticosteroids given either by mouth or intravenously. (Corticosteroids, also known as glucocorticoids, are commonly referred to as simply "steroids," but corticosteroids are one of several types of steroids. Other steroids include estrogen, testosterone, vitamin D, and aldosterone. Throughout the chapter I will use the word "corticosteroid" to refer to the anti-inflammatory hormones, usually prescribed in the form of prednisone or prednisolone.) Depending on the response and on the severity of the disease, it may be necessary to add other immunosuppressive drugs, such as azathioprine (Imuran, Azasan), cyclophosphamide (Cytoxan), or rituximab (Rituxan). If treated early, ILD does not cause any long-term disability. Recently a new class of drugs known as biologics, which are antibodies directed against inflammatory mediators produced as part of ILD, have proven useful among patients with ILD, including patients with Sjögren's.

Inflammation of the lining around the lung (pleurisy) can occur in Sjögren's. This condition is usually seen in patients with Sjögren's, particularly in those with systemic lupus erythematosus (SLE) or rheumatoid arthritis (RA). Pleurisy usually causes chest pain on breathing. Fluid can sometimes accumulate in the pleural space (pleural effusion), causing shortness of breath. Pleurisy is treated with nonsteroidal anti-inflammatory drugs or corticosteroids. Drainage of the pleural effusion may sometimes be necessary.

Very rarely, Sjögren's patients develop an abnormally high pressure in the pulmonary arteries, the vessels that carry blood from the heart to the lungs. This is known as pulmonary hypertension. The main symptom of pulmonary hypertension is shortness of breath on exertion. In Sjögren's, pulmonary hypertension can develop in isolation or as a result of ILD and lung scarring (fibrosis). Pulmonary hypertension can be diagnosed on a routine cardiac echocardiogram. To obtain an accurate measurement of the pulmonary artery pressure, the patient undergoes cardiac catheterization. Under local anesthesia, a thin wire is guided from the main artery in the leg into the aorta (artery that takes blood directly from the heart) and then into the heart so that pressure can be measured. If left untreated, severe pulmonary hypertension can cause heart failure. Treatment of any underlying ILD can help improve the degree of pulmonary hypertension. Current treatment of moderate to severe pulmonary hypertension in Sjögren's includes the use of anticoagulants such as warfarin (Coumadin), endothelin receptor antagonists such as bosentan (Tracleer), and phosphodiesterase-5 inhibitors such as sildenafil (Revatio).

In severe cases, a continuous infusion of intravenous epoprostenol (Flolan, Veletri) may be used.

An expert committee of rheumatologists and pulmonologists has prepared guidelines for the management of pulmonary disease in Sjögren's, which were published in 2020.

Kidneys

The kidneys remove waste products from the blood and form urine. The most common kidney problem in patients with Sjögren's is inflammation of the tissue around the kidney filters, known as interstitial nephritis. Interstitial nephritis is found early in the disease and has a benign course. This problem generally causes only mild deterioration in kidney function, manifested as a slight elevation in the plasma creatinine concentration. This usually requires no treatment. Progression to end-stage renal disease is rare.

When there is a progressive deterioration of kidney function in a patient with Sjögren's, a kidney biopsy is often done. This involves removing a small piece of kidney tissue with a needle while the patient is awake but under local anesthesia. The tissue is examined under the microscope, and if the diagnosis of interstitial nephritis is made, a course of corticosteroids is given as treatment. Kidney function usually improves within a few weeks unless irreversible scarring in the kidneys has already occurred.

Interstitial nephritis can cause abnormalities in the kidney tubules, which are part of the kidney filtering mechanism. One such abnormality is renal tubular acidosis (RTA). In RTA the kidney tubules cannot excrete acid in the urine. This can occur in up to 25% of patients with Sjögren's. As a result, the urine becomes more alkaline (high urine pH) and the blood becomes more acidic (low blood pH). This can lead to low levels of potassium in the blood and can give rise to kidney stones. Patients with RTA usually have no symptoms. Rarely, when the blood potassium level is very low, muscle weakness or even paralysis can occur. Rarely, the initial presentation of a Sjögren's patient is severe muscle weakness from low blood potassium. Also, recurrent pain in the loin area from kidney stones can sometimes be the presenting symptom. The treatment of RTA depends on its severity. If the potassium level is very low, then the patient is given potassium supplements. Alkaline (basic; that is, the opposite of acidic) agents (sodium bicarbonate) are given to correct the acidity of the blood to prevent the formation of renal stones.

Another rare abnormality of the renal tubules in Sjögren's is nephrogenic diabetes insipidus. In this condition the renal tubules become insensitive to the effects of antidiuretic hormone (made in the pituitary gland at the base of the brain) and as a result cannot concentrate the urine. Patients with nephrogenic diabetes insipidus complain of thirst and of passing large amounts of urine frequently. The diagnosis is suspected if the urine remains dilute when the patient is deprived of water (when a normal person becomes dehydrated, the kidneys try to save water by concentrating the urine). Nephrogenic diabetes insipidus can be treated by a number of means, including diuretics, nonsteroidal anti-inflammatory drugs, and a low-salt, low-protein diet.

The glomeruli, which also form part of the kidney filtering mechanism, are rarely affected in Sjögren's. However, antibodies produced by the immune system can become deposited on the glomeruli and cause inflammation (glomerulonephritis). As a result, the function of the kidneys deteriorates. This can be detected on routine testing of a urine sample and by looking at the blood tests and observing a deterioration of kidney function. Symptoms include high blood pressure and leg swelling due to fluid retention (edema). Glomerulonephritis is rare in patients with Sjögren's and occurs mainly in patients who also have other overlapping conditions such as SLE, cryoglobulinemia (a condition whereby protein complexes circulating in the blood become deposited during cold weather), or vasculitis (inflammation of blood vessels). If left untreated, glomerulonephritis may lead to severe kidney failure. Therefore, in a patient with suspected glomerulonephritis, a kidney biopsy should be performed to confirm the diagnosis and assess the severity of the kidney disease. Treatment is then given in the form of corticosteroids as well as other immunosuppressive drugs such as cyclophosphamide (Cytoxan) or rituximab (Rituxan).

Inflammation of the bladder, known as interstitial cystitis, can occur in patients with Sjögren's. The symptoms are increased frequency and painful urination and pain in the lower abdomen over the bladder area.

Gastrointestinal Tract

In Sjögren's, the exocrine glands of the gastrointestinal tract can also be affected. The cells lining the esophagus (the muscular tube connecting the mouth and the stomach) produce less mucus, and the esophagus becomes dry, just like the mouth. This can lead to difficulty in swallowing. Difficulty in swallowing can also be caused by abnormal muscle contractions of the esophagus or by a lack of the normal contractions that move the food down the esophagus to the stomach. This condition, which can affect up to one-third of patients with Sjögren's, is known as esophageal dysmotility.

The diagnosis of dysmotility is made by measuring the pressure inside the wall of the esophagus during swallowing (manometry). When the wall of the esophagus contracts abnormally, treatment is aimed at relaxing the smooth muscle of the esophagus. Nitroglycerine and calcium channel blockers may be helpful.

On the other hand, when the muscle tone in the wall of the esophagus is reduced, gastric juice moves up the esophagus, producing a burning sensation behind the breastbone (heartburn) and chest pain. This is known as gastroesophageal reflux. Prolonged reflux can be treated by the use of antacids. Antacids form a "raft" that floats on the surface of the stomach contents to reduce reflux and protect the lining of the esophagus. Severe gastroesophageal reflux and esophagitis are best treated by the use of drugs that reduce acid production by the stomach. These include H_2-receptor antagonists (ranitidine [Zantac]) and proton pump inhibitors (omeprazole [Prilosec], among others).

A proportion of patients with Sjögren's have reduced acid secretion by the stomach. This is a result of longstanding inflammation that destroys the cells that produce acid (known as chronic, atrophic, gastritis), an immune process similar to the one that destroys the salivary glands. Atrophic gastritis can cause indigestion (dyspepsia) and pain over the upper part of the abdomen. Diagnosis is made by endoscopy. This is performed by a gastroenterologist with the patient awake but slightly sedated (conscious sedation). The stomach is visualized by inserting an elastic tube with a camera at its end (fiberoptic endoscope) through the mouth into the stomach. A biopsy often is taken to confirm the diagnosis. Unfortunately, once the acid-producing cells of the stomach are damaged, it is often too late to give any treatment.

However, other conditions associated with atrophic gastritis can be prevented. Destruction of the cells that produce acid in the stomach can prevent absorption of vitamin B_{12}, which is important in the production of red blood cells and the function of nerve cells. This vitamin deficiency can result in a form of anemia known as pernicious anemia. Pernicious anemia can be diagnosed by a simple blood test and can be successfully treated by monthly B_{12} injections.

In Sjögren's, involvement of other exocrine glands such as the pancreas can sometimes occur. Most of the time, this does not cause any symptoms. However, in some cases, the pancreas cannot secrete its digestive enzymes, and then diarrhea and steatorrhea (floating, fatty stools) occur. Pancreatic enzyme insufficiency can be treated by the regular administration of oral pancreatic enzymes with meals.

Acute inflammation of the pancreas, known as pancreatitis, rarely has been described in Sjögren's patients. This condition presents with abdominal pain, nausea, and vomiting. Laboratory tests show elevation of amylase, an enzyme produced in the pancreas that can be measured in the blood serum. Amylase is produced by the salivary glands as well as the pancreas. A quarter of patients with Sjögren's may have a raised serum amylase level due to salivary gland inflammation rather than due to acute pancreatitis.

Liver

In studies of Sjögren's patients, approximately 6% have been found to have autoimmune liver disease. The main two conditions associated with Sjögren's are chronic active hepatitis and primary biliary cirrhosis.

Primary biliary cholangitis (PBC, formally known as primary biliary cirrhosis) is a chronic disease that affects mainly middle-aged women. It is caused by inflammation around the channels that transport bile from the liver into the intestine, the bile ducts. As a result, these ducts become blocked and bile builds up in the liver and spills into the blood. In the late stages of the disease, the liver becomes scarred. This is known as cirrhosis. In the early stages, the main symptoms of PBC are due to the accumulation of bile acids and salts in the blood. Patients complain of generalized itching and tiredness. Later on in the disease they develop jaundice (yellow tinge of the skin and the eyes), pale stools, and dark urine. In the late stages, cirrhosis can cause accumulation of fluid in the abdomen (ascites) and internal bleeding from buildup of pressure in the veins of the esophagus (esophageal varices).

The diagnosis is suspected when a patient with Sjögren's has these symptoms and abnormal liver function test results. There is also a specific blood test for the diagnosis of PBC, the presence of anti-mitochondrial antibodies. However, a liver biopsy is usually necessary to confirm the diagnosis and to evaluate if the disease is in its early or late stages. This involves removing a small piece of liver, using a needle, under a local anesthetic.

The lack of bile salts in the intestine results in reduced absorption of fat and the fat-soluble vitamins A, D, E, and K. Vitamin D deficiency can result in weakening of the bones (osteoporosis) and fractures. Vitamin K deficiency can result in problems with blood clotting. Therefore, patients with PBC benefit from taking calcium plus vitamin D supplements to strengthen their bones, as well as vitamins A, E, and K.

Because the cause of PBC is not known, there is no curative treatment for the disease; the only definite treatment is liver transplantation. However, the prognosis of PBC varies greatly from one patient to another. Many patients lead active lives with few symptoms for 10 to 20 years. In some patients, however, the condition progresses more rapidly, and liver failure may occur in just a few years.

Ursodeoxycholic acid has been shown to improve liver function as well as reduce progression of the disease in patients with PBC. Treatment of pruritus is often a challenge in PBC. The mainstay is cholestyramine (Questran), a resin that forms a complex with bile acids in the intestine, promoting their excretion in stools.

In chronic autoimmune hepatitis (CAH), the immune system continuously attacks the liver cells, and as a result scarring of the liver (cirrhosis) can occur. In general, CAH can be caused by hepatitis viruses, by drugs, or by an unknown mechanism that dysregulates the immune system. The last of these is the case in Sjögren's patients. CAH is suspected in a patient with Sjögren's when liver function test results become abnormal without the patient taking any new drugs. Evidence pointing toward an autoimmune active hepatitis is the finding of antibodies in the blood against smooth muscle or liver/kidney microsomes. Typical symptoms are fatigue, malaise, fever, and loss of appetite. The diagnosis is confirmed by liver biopsy. CAH can be treated with corticosteroids and other immunosuppressive drugs such as azathioprine (Imuran, Azasan).

Heart

Involvement of the heart is rare in Sjögren's. Some Sjögren's patients have been found to have a small amount of fluid around the heart, known as pericardial effusion. This is caused by inflammation of the lining around the heart (pericarditis). It is usually detected by chance on routine ultrasound scanning of the heart (echocardiogram), as most patients are asymptomatic. Patients with Sjögren's who have lupus are more likely to develop pericarditis that gives rise to symptoms. This usually occurs during a lupus flare. The symptoms are typically of left-sided chest pain that changes with posture. When the patient is examined using a stethoscope, a characteristic sound, known as a "rub," can be heard at the left edge of the sternum. An electrocardiogram may show typical changes of pericarditis, and examination of the heart using echocardiography reveals fluid around the heart. Lupus patients mostly develop small to medium-sized collections of fluid around the heart that have no bearing on the heart function. However, very rarely, if there is a large amount of fluid around the heart, the pumping action of the heart can be impaired, and the patient can develop heart failure. Patients with RA and Sjögren's can also develop pericardial effusions during a flare of the RA. However, it has been estimated that during the course of their disease, fewer than 10% of RA patients have a clinical episode of pericarditis.

Corticosteroids are given to treat small to medium-sized pericardial effusions; for large effusions, draining of the fluid using a needle may be necessary.

Congenital Heart Block

When the fetus is inside the womb, its heart beats regularly as a result of its natural pacemaker. However, a condition known as congenital heart block can occur in which this pacemaker fails and the heart rate drops dangerously low. There are two types of congenital heart block: incomplete and complete. With complete heart block, insertion of an artificial pacemaker is necessary after delivery.

Almost all babies born with congenital heart block have mothers who carry anti-Ro (SSA) antibodies, whereas 75% have mothers with anti-LA (SSB) antibodies. Most of these mothers have these antibodies without having any symptoms of an autoimmune disease. These antibodies, which are common among Sjögren's patients (see later in the chapter), are thought to cross the placenta and bind onto the fetal heart, preventing the normal development of the pacemaker.

Up to 75% of Sjögren's patients have anti-Ro (SSA) antibodies and up to 40% have anti-La (SSB) antibodies. However, if a woman who has Sjögren's and anti-Ro antibodies becomes pregnant, the risk of having a fetus with congenital heart block is only 1% to 2%. If she has anti-La (SSB) antibodies in addition to anti-Ro (SSA) antibodies, the risk of having a fetus with congenital heart block is 3%. The risk is much higher if she has previously given birth to a baby with congenital heart block. For this reason, the fetuses of anti-Ro- and anti-La-positive mothers need to be closely monitored after the 16th week of gestation for signs of heart block, the most severe of which is slowing of the heart rate. If heart block is detected and is of the reversible form, treatment can be given with corticosteroids that cross the placenta (dexamethasone).

Nervous System

Patients with Sjögren's can have disease of the nervous system. The peripheral nerves that control sensation can be damaged by the immune system. This is known as sensory neuropathy. Patients with sensory neuropathy initially complain of numbness or tingling at the tips of their toes. Also, they may notice alterations in the appreciation of pain and temperature and a burning sensation. The problem is usually symmetrical. It can progress very slowly to involve the fingers of both hands. In most patients, the symptoms are mild and not disabling. Approximately 40% of patients improve spontaneously. Rarely, a Sjögren's patient has a severe sensory neuropathy that interferes with the ability to walk.

The diagnosis is usually made by examination of the peripheral nerves. Patients may have reduced sensation in the hands and feet in a "glove and stocking" pattern as well as reduced sensation of vibration and toe position (proprioception). The reflexes may also be absent. However, the physical examination can be normal. The results of neurologic testing by electrical stimulation of the nerves, called electromyography (EMG) and nerve conduction studies, are typically normal. Biopsy of the skin with counting of the nerve endings is diagnostic but unavailable in most medical centers. As most patients have mild symptoms, no specific treatment is usually given for peripheral sensory neuropathy in Sjögren's. For patients with severe symptoms, treatment may prove difficult. There are some therapies that can be tried, such as intravenous immunoglobulin or plasmapheresis.

Sometimes an individual nerve that controls the movement of one muscle can be affected, and this can result in weakness of the muscle. One such example is if a patient suddenly develops foot drop on one side (mononeuritis). The cause of this problem is inflammation in the blood vessel supplying the individual nerve, known as vasculitis. Vasculitis can be treated with corticosteroids or other drugs that suppress the immune system. If the treatment is given early, the nerve can recover from the damage and the muscle weakness can resolve.

The cranial nerves (the nerves supplying the face) can also be affected in Sjögren's. Most commonly the sensory branch of the trigeminal nerve is affected. This supplies the sensation around the eyes, nose, cheeks, and mouth. In Sjögren's, the symptoms of trigeminal neuropathy are numbness or tingling around the mouth and the cheeks. The area around the eye is less commonly involved. Pain may be present but usually is not severe.

In carpal tunnel syndrome, a common complication in Sjögren's, inflamed tissue in the forearm presses against the median nerve, causing pain, numbness, tingling, and sometimes muscle weakness in the thumb and index and middle fingers. The symptoms are often worse at night. The diagnosis is confirmed by nerve conduction studies. Night splints can help alleviate the symptoms. Also, corticosteroid injections into the carpal tunnel can give temporary relief for up to a few months. Such injections can be repeated once or twice, but if the symptoms persist, surgery may be necessary. The surgical procedure, known as carpal tunnel decompression, involves making a small cut on the inside of the wrist to free the tissues that press the median nerve. This can be done under local anesthesia on an outpatient basis and is usually very successful.

Sjögren's has been reported to affect the brain. However, this point will remain controversial until further studies are done. In studies of Sjögren's patients all over the world, a variety of neurologic symptoms originating from the brain have been recorded. For example, some patients have been noted to have symptoms of epilepsy, stroke, multiple sclerosis, or Parkinson's disease. However, no consensus has been reached as to the proportion of Sjögren's patients affected by diseases of the brain, or even whether these problems are more common among Sjögren's patients than those without Sjögren's. That is, although these neurologic diseases are noted to occur in Sjögren's patients, they may not necessarily be caused by Sjögren's.

There is an association of Sjögren's and neuromyelitis optica (NMO, or Devic's syndrome). NMO was once thought to be a rare variant of multiple sclerosis but is now considered a distinct disease. NMO patients have inflammation of the optic nerve and the spinal cord, which can lead to blindness and paralysis, respectively. Both these manifestations have been reported in Sjögren's. A significant percentage of NMO patients have anti-Ro present in their serum, and some Sjögren's patients with neurologic disease have autoantibodies binding a protein called aquaporin-4. These antibodies are common among those with NMO.

Some Sjögren's patients have been noted to have memory or concentration problems or symptoms of anxiety and depression. Again, the percentages quoted in studies vary (7–80%). Part of the problem is that the symptoms can be quite subtle and not easily recognized—sometimes reported by patients as "brain fog." Memory or concentration problems can also sometimes be a manifestation of anxiety or depression, so patients have to be carefully evaluated by a psychologist or psychiatrist. If anxiety or depression is confirmed, therapy in the form of psychological counseling or drugs (antidepressants) may be of benefit. Also, patients with isolated memory or concentration problems may improve with the help of mental exercises prescribed by specially trained psychologists.

Blood Vessels

As mentioned earlier, inflammation of the blood vessels known as vasculitis can occur in Sjögren's patients and cause mononeuritis. Vasculitis of blood vessels supplying blood to the skin (cutaneous vasculitis) is fairly common in Sjögren's and results in a raised red rash called palpable purpura. When a biopsy specimen is examined under the microscope, inflammatory cells surround small blood vessels in a condition known as leukocytoclastic vasculitis. Most patients only have single episode of this rash, which is usually treated with a short course of corticosteroids. Vasculitis of larger blood vessels is rare but can occur among those with Sjögren's. This involvement of larger vessels, called systemic vasculitis, can resemble a disease called polyarteritis nodosum and can involve the intestines, pancreas, heart, and/or lungs. Organ disease such as this generally requires immunosuppressive therapy with corticosteroids initially and then other agents such as cyclophosphamide.

Summing Up

Major body organs can be affected in one-third of Sjögren's patients. Involvement of the lungs usually produces mild symptoms requiring no more than symptomatic treatment. Interstitial lung disease occurs rarely and requires treatment with corticosteroids and immunosuppressive drugs. Involvement of the kidneys can manifest as interstitial nephritis, which is usually benign and requires no treatment. Very rarely it may cause kidney damage, which can be reversed if treated early with corticosteroids. More severe disease such as glomerulonephritis sometimes occurs, requiring treatment with corticosteroids and immunosuppressive drugs. Esophageal dysmotility can cause difficulty in swallowing as well as acid reflux. The latter can be treated with drugs that reduce acid production by the stomach. More rarely, indigestion can be due to atrophic gastritis. This can result in pernicious anemia, which is treated with regular vitamin B_{12} injections.

Primary biliary cholangitis rarely occurs in association with Sjögren's and has a variable prognosis. Ursodeoxycholic acid administration can delay the progression of the disease. Hepatitis also rarely occurs, and it can be treated with corticosteroids and immunosuppressive drugs. Pericarditis usually occurs in patients with Sjögren's and SLE and can be successfully treated with corticosteroids.

The most common disease of the peripheral nerves in Sjögren's is carpal tunnel syndrome. It can be treated with corticosteroid injections or surgery. Peripheral sensory neuropathy can occur in Sjögren's, and it is usually mild and not disabling. Very rarely vasculitis can result in mononeuritis or a condition resembling polyarteritis nodosum. Either usually can be reversed by treatment with corticosteroids and immunosuppressive drugs. Involvement

Table 14.2 Tools for Diagnosis of Internal Organ Involvement

Organs Involved in Sjögren's	How to Diagnose If an Organ Is Involved
Lung	Lung function test Computed tomography (CT) scan
Kidney	Urinalysis Blood tests Kidney biopsy
Esophagus	Manometry
Stomach	Gastroscopy
Pancreas	Blood tests
Liver	Blood tests Liver biopsy
Heart	Electrocardiogram (ECG) Blood tests Echocardiogram
Nerves	Nerve conduction studies
Brain	Magnetic resonance imaging (MRI) scan

of the brain is controversial. A variety of symptoms, such as memory problems, anxiety, and depression, are more common in Sjögren's patients. Other more severe symptoms of epilepsy, stroke, and multiple sclerosis have been reported and may possibly be caused by Sjögren's (Table 14.2). NMO and Sjögren's may be related.

For Further Reading

Aiyegbusi O, McGregor L, McGeoch L, et al. Renal disease in primary Sjogren's syndrome. *Rheumatol Ther.* 2021;8(1):63–80. doi:10.1007/s40744-020-00264-x.

Birnbaum J. Peripheral nervous system manifestations of Sjogren syndrome: Clinical patterns, diagnostic paradigms, etiopathogenesis, and therapeutic strategies. *Neurologist.* 2010;16(5):287–297. doi:10.1097/NRL.0b013e3181ebe59f.

Hatzis GS, Fragoulis GE, Karatzaferis A, et al. Prevalence and long-term course of primary biliary cirrhosis in primary Sjögren's syndrome. *J Rheumatol.* 2008;35(10):2012–2016.

Kassan SS, Moutsopoulos HM. Clinical manifestations and early diagnosis of Sjögren's syndrome. *Arch Intern Med.* 2004;164(12):1275–1284.

Nannini C, Jebakumar AJ, Crowson CS, et al. Primary Sjögren's syndrome 1976–2005 and associated interstitial lung disease: A population-based study of incidence and mortality. *BMJ Open.* 2013;3(11):e003569.

Ramos-Casals M, Brito Zeron P, Seror R, et al. Characterization of systemic disease in primary Sjögren's syndrome: EULAR-SS Task Force recommendations for articular, cutaneous, pulmonary and renal involvements. *Rheumatology.* 2015;54(12):2230–2238.

Retamozo S, Acar-Denizli N, Rasmussen A, et al. Systemic manifestations of primary Sjogren's syndrome out of the ESSDAI classification: Prevalence and clinical relevance in a large international, multi-ethnic cohort of patients. *Clin Exp Rheumatol.* 2019;37 Suppl 118(3):97–106.

Scofield RH. Vasculitis in Sjögren's syndrome. *Curr Rheumatol Rep.* 2011;13(6):482–488.

Vivino FB. Sjögren's syndrome: Clinical aspects. *Clin Immunol.* 2017;182:48–54.

15

Dry Mouth

Ava J. Wu and Troy E. Daniels

Dry mouth is a common complaint, with an estimated 25 million Americans or 15% of adults afflicted. The range of experience varies from a temporary, minor annoyance to a serious, likely irreversible complication of a disease process. The symptom of dry mouth is often referred to as xerostomia. It is usually caused by a gradual decrease in the amount and quality of saliva produced by the salivary glands but paradoxically may be associated with normal salivary gland function. Because it is a subjective perception, the symptom of dry mouth may not be experienced by all patients who have abnormal salivary function. As a result, it is important for patients with Sjögren's to be professionally examined for clinical signs of decreased salivary function, whether they have dry mouth symptoms or not. Strategies may then be initiated to increase oral comfort and, most importantly, prevent irreversible damage to the teeth. Most Sjögren's patients experience some degree of continuous or long-term dry mouth.

What Is Dry Mouth?

The sensation of dry mouth in any group of individuals is represented by a spectrum of severity. Typically, a complaint of dry mouth will be associated with one or more of the following: a feeling of cotton in the mouth; tongue and cheeks stick to the top of the mouth or the teeth; sores inside the mouth or at the corners of the lip; difficulty with swallowing, eating dry food, or talking; abnormal taste; burning of the tongue or inside of the mouth; and dental cavities occurring at the gum line of the teeth despite diligent oral hygiene. At the other end of the spectrum are individuals who did not realize that they had dry mouth until they developed dental problems. It is important to realize that dry mouth is a symptom that usually indicates that the salivary glands are malfunctioning by producing less saliva that

Ava J. Wu and Troy E. Daniels, *Dry Mouth* In: *The Sjögren's Book*. Edited by: Daniel J. Wallace, Oxford University Press.
© Sjögren's Foundation 2022. DOI: 10.1093/oso/9780197502112.003.0015

is also qualitatively deficient (i.e., missing or altered amounts of proteins or enzymes). As noted later in the chapter, there are various causes of dry mouth, making it important for individuals experiencing it to determine its cause with their physician.

The Salivary Glands and Saliva

Saliva is produced by three major pairs of salivary glands (parotid, submandibular, and sublingual) and hundreds of minor salivary glands located throughout the mouth. All of these glands may be affected in Sjögren's. The right and left parotid glands are located in the cheek area in front of the ears and are responsible for making a serous or watery saliva. The saliva from the parotid glands enters the mouth at the parotid papillae located on the inner cheek opposite the upper molar teeth. The submandibular and sublingual glands are located underneath the floor of the mouth and tongue. The submandibular and sublingual glands produce a thicker saliva that exits into the mouth underneath the tongue. Saliva is mainly water but contains a complex array of proteins in very small amounts that have important functions, described later in the chapter.

Protecting, Lubricating, and Cleansing the Oral Mucosa

Saliva coats the tissue of the mouth and ingested food, allowing the mucosa and food to move smoothly over the teeth. This moist coating facilitates chewing and swallowing and acts as a barrier to irritating and harmful substances contained in food. The saliva coating all the oral surfaces greatly facilitates speech.

Protecting Against Dental Caries (Decay)

Dental caries results from the exposure of teeth to acids produced by bacteria attached to the tooth surface. As discussed later, normal saliva has the ability to help wash away the bacteria, counter the effects of the acid produced by the bacteria, and repair the damage produced by the acid.

Maintaining a Neutral pH

Normal saliva contains several chemical systems called buffers that can neutralize the potentially damaging acidity from bacteria, foods, beverages, and gastric reflux on the teeth.

Dental Remineralization

Normal saliva is a reservoir of calcium and phosphate ions that replenish these elements as they are lost from the tooth surface. This is essentially a tooth surface "repair" at a microscopic level.

Protection Against Infection by Bacteria, Yeasts, and Viruses

There are several protein components in normal saliva (e.g., lactoferrin, peroxidase, histatins, and secretory leukocyte protease) that have antibacterial, antifungal, or antiviral properties. Secretory IgA is a unique antibody found in saliva that can coat many oral bacteria, interfering with their ability to adhere to teeth.

Aiding Digestion and Taste

The initial stages of digestion occur in the mouth by way of the enzymes contained in saliva. Taste buds, which are located in the mouth, can respond only to dissolved substances. Saliva enhances the sense of taste by both dissolving and beginning the digestion of solid foods. The solvent and digestive roles of saliva allow the taste buds to convey food flavors and enhance enjoyment of a meal.

Thus, quantitative and qualitative changes in saliva resulting from diminished salivary gland function in Sjögren's lead to a loss of oral protection and oral comfort.

Causes of Dry Mouth

While there are many causes of dry mouth (Box 15.1), the most common one is chronic use of prescription medication. Hundreds of medications have been associated with varying degrees of dry mouth (Box 15.2). Clinical experience also suggests that dry mouth may occur as a result of interactions between medications not usually associated with dry mouth alone. In most cases, the drugs causing dry mouth do so through their effect on nerves that regulate salivary function. The use of prescription drugs often exacerbates dry mouth in patients with Sjögren's. Accordingly, patients should review with their physicians any prescription drugs they are taking to determine if those medications are contributing to their dry mouth. Often there are alternative or equivalent drugs available. Temporary symptoms of dry mouth, such as when taking over-the-counter medication for cold symptoms, should not be a problem. However, if chronic drug-induced dry mouth persists for many

---

Box 15.1 Causes of Dry Mouth

Temporary dry mouth
- Effect of short-term medication use (e.g., antihistamine)
- Viral infection (e.g., mumps)
- Dehydration
- Psychogenic condition (e.g., anxiety)

Chronic dry mouth
- Effect of chronically administered drugs (see Box 15.2)
- Chronic diseases
  - Sjögren's
  - Sarcoidosis
  - HIV or hepatitis C infection
  - Depression
  - Diabetes mellitus, uncontrolled
  - Amyloidosis (primary or secondary)
  - Central nervous system diseases
  - Rarely, an absent or malformed salivary gland
- Other effects of treatment
  - Therapeutic radiation to the head and neck
  - Graft-versus-host disease (following bone marrow transplant)

Box 15.2 Medications with Anticholinergic Effects

Antidepressants: amitriptyline (++++), clomipramine (++++), doxepin (+++), imipramine (+++), desipramine (++), nortriptyline (++), selegiline (0), tranylcypromine (+), mirtazapine (+), nefazodone (0), trazadone (0), bupropion (+), duloxetine (+), venlafaxine (+)

Antipsychotics: thioridazine (++++), clozapine (++++), chlorpromazine (+++), olanzapine (++), perphenazine (++), aripiprazole (+), fluphenazine (+), haloperidol (+), quetiapine (+), risperidone (+), thiothixene (+), ziprasidone (+).

Antihistamines/antiemetics: brompheniramine(+++), chlorpheniramine(+++), dexchlorpheniramine (+++), carbinoxamine (++++), clemastine (++++), diphenhydramine (++++), pyrilamine (+/0), tripelennamine (+/0), promethazine (++++), cyproheptadine (+++), phenindamine (+++), azelastine (nasal only, +/0), cetirizine (+/0), levocetirizine (+/0), desloratadine (+/0), fexofenadine (+/0), loratadine (+/0)

Antiacne: isotretinoin

Antianxiety: alprazolam, hydroxyzine

Bronchodilator: ipratropium, tiotropium, albuterol

Drugs for bladder overactivity: oxybutynin, tolterodine, trospium, solifenacin, darifenacin

Decongestant: pseudoephedrine

Anti-Parkinson's: benztropine, trihexyphenidyl, selegiline

Opioids: meperidine

Muscle relaxant: cyclobenzaprine

Rating of anticholinergic (drying) effects: ++++, high; +++, moderate; ++, low; +, very low; 0, absent

For consistency and clarity, all drugs are listed by their generic names. There are hundreds of drugs associated with dry mouth, but with most of them the symptom is generally mild and occurs in a small minority of patients taking the drug, or the drug is not prescribed for chronic use. This list includes the categories of drugs that most commonly cause significant dry mouth but is not all-inclusive. When questions arise, patients should consult with their physician or a reliable drug information source.

Source: Wells BG, Dipiro JT, Schwinghammer TL, Dipro CV. Pharmacotherapy Handbook, 7th ed. Mcgraw Hill, 2009. Used with permission.

---

weeks or months, detrimental changes will begin to occur to the teeth and oral function.

Sjögren's is a systemic autoimmune disease that prominently attacks the salivary glands and lacrimal glands, compromising their function. A type of white blood cell (lymphocyte) enters these glands, replaces normal salivary gland cells that produce saliva (acinar cells), and affects the function of the duct cells that deliver the secretion to the mouth. Sjögren's patients may have an antibody in their bloodstream that can affect the nerves controlling salivary function. The onset and progression of dry mouth in patients with Sjögren's is usually gradual, and most patients cannot determine exactly when it began. It may progress until little or no saliva is produced, but more commonly patients' symptoms and salivary dysfunction progress to some intermediate point and do not progress further.

Radiation to the head and neck for cancer treatment causes direct damage to the salivary glands, greatly reducing their function.

Dry mouth can also be caused by other chronic systemic diseases such as sarcoidosis, HIV, or hepatitis C infection, uncontrolled diabetes, or depression. Previous medical treatment such as radiation therapy to the head and neck, bone marrow transplantation (graft-versus-host disease), or chemotherapy for treating malignancies can directly damage the salivary glands and result in decreased salivation (see Box 15.1). The effects of such treatment can be either temporary or permanent, depending on the type and intensity of the treatment.

Oral Problems Associated with Dry Mouth

The importance of saliva to our quality of life is not appreciated until it is reduced or missing. Progressive loss of saliva production and quality correspondingly decreases the protection and comfort afforded by normal saliva, as listed earlier. The most severely affected patients do not produce measurable amounts of saliva, even with stimulation, but the majority of patients retain some residual salivary gland function, ranging from a small amount to almost normal. The most common oral problems associated with chronic dry mouth are oral discomfort, dental caries, oral fungal infections, halitosis (bad breath), and, in about one-quarter of patients, enlargement of major salivary glands.

Oral Discomfort

The sensation of dry mouth does not occur until saliva production drops to about half of that person's normal value. The feeling of oral dryness in Sjögren's often develops over a period of months or years; sudden-onset oral dryness is rare. Occasionally, an individual with Sjögren's is not aware of being dry until asked if she can eat a cracker without supplemental water to aid swallowing. The severity of oral dryness in Sjögren's may fluctuate, but it usually does not include periods of time during the day where the mouth feels normal.

Normally, little saliva is produced during sleep, so it is common for everyone to feel some oral dryness in the morning or on awakening during the night. However, this symptom may be more severe in patients with Sjögren's and should be managed at night with small amounts of a commercial saliva substitute, instead of water, to avoid sleep disruption caused by the urge to urinate following water intake.

Dental Caries

The process of tooth decay is caused by interactions between several types of bacteria commonly found in the mouth and sugar present in the diet of most individuals. These bacteria form colonies or plaques that coat the teeth so rapidly that they can be seen by the unaided eye after a day or two without tooth-brushing. Sucrose (common table sugar) and other carbohydrates can be digested by these bacteria, allowing the organisms to proliferate and release acid as a byproduct. The acid progressively erodes the mineral content of the tooth surface, the first stage of dental caries.

For individuals with deficient saliva, dental caries can progress rapidly, even in those with good oral hygiene. The pattern of dry mouth caries is distinctive, occurring in areas typically thought to be accessible to cleaning. These caries are mostly located on the necks of the teeth near the gum line and are called root caries (Figure 15.1), and also on the cusp tips of back teeth

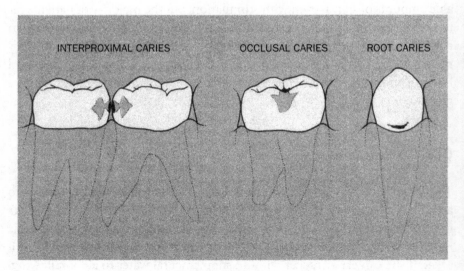

Figure 15.1 Locations of dental caries: interproximal occlusal, cusp tip, and root caries.

or biting edges of front teeth. Importantly, these caries also occur along the margins between existing crowns or fillings and the tooth, ultimately causing those restorations to fail and need replacement. The location of dry mouth caries differs from dental caries in individuals with normal saliva but inadequate oral hygiene. These caries usually occur between teeth and in the pits and fissures on the chewing surfaces of the back teeth, called interproximal or occlusal caries (see Figure 15.1). Insufficient saliva contributes to caries in several ways: a decreased ability to buffer acid that is produced by bacteria next to the tooth surface; an insufficient reservoir of calcium and phosphate ions to replenish that naturally lost from the tooth surface; a reduction of antimicrobial proteins; and reduced oral cleansing from the lack of saliva flowing across the oral surfaces.

A dental caries typically causes no symptoms until it penetrates through the outer enamel surface of the tooth into the inner dentin layer. Dental enamel is dense and composed almost entirely of nonorganic material, like ivory. The inner dentin is like bone with many organic components, including nerves, which can transmit the sensation of pain, heat, and cold. Thus, when decay enters the dentin layer, the tooth may become sensitive to heat, cold, and sweets. If untreated, the caries can progress to the tooth interior, the pulp composed of soft tissue, nerves, and blood vessels. Involvement of the pulp is usually associated with spontaneous pain. From the pulp, invading bacteria can expand into bone surrounding the root tip, causing a painful abscess.

An early dental caries appears as a flat, whitish spot (decalcification) on the tooth's surface. As the process continues, there is a progressive loss of tooth structure, and the cavity can appear tan to black in color. It is now believed that the early caries process (white spot) can be significantly slowed or reversed with the preventive strategies of remineralization (e.g., topical fluoride application).

Fungal Infections

About one-third of patients with long-term salivary deficiency will develop symptoms of burning on their tongue or elsewhere in their mouth and/or intolerance to acidic or spicy foods. These symptoms are usually caused by localized infection of the lining of the mouth by different species of the fungus *Candida*. This organism is often found normally in the mouth, but susceptible individuals with decreased saliva production may experience an overgrowth of these organisms. When this occurs in dry mouth patients, the affected tissue of the mouth will be red. The tongue may appear red, lose its normal carpet-like texture, and develop grooves. Other affected areas develop well-defined or diffuse red areas caused by thinning of the mucosa (atrophy). These intra-oral changes are often associated with redness or crusting at the corners of the lips, called angular cheilitis. This combination of clinical features is called erythematous candidiasis. Effective treatment with antifungal medication will lead to complete restoration of the mucosal color and elimination of the burning despite an ongoing salivary deficiency. However, in a few individuals, this condition will recur or persist; treatment can be repeated as often as necessary.

Oral Functional Problems

It is common for patients with Sjögren's to have difficulty swallowing dry foods, when there is insufficient saliva to adequately moisten the food bolus. They may have difficulty speaking because the tongue and lips get stuck to the teeth and palate. This can be overcome temporarily with frequent small sips of water, the use of a secretagogue, or sugar-free hard candy or gum to stimulate saliva production. Sjögren's patients wearing complete dentures often experience problems from the lack of oral lubrication that causes the tongue to continually move the lower denture from its normal position, decreasing its stability. Where it is possible, surgical implants can be considered for the lower jaw as a means to increase denture stability.

Periodontal Disease

Because chronic inflammatory periodontal disease is a very common disease worldwide, it is sometimes assumed that patients with Sjögren's will be at increased risk to develop this disease. However, most of the research that has examined this question has not shown that frequency or severity of periodontal disease is greater in the Sjögren's population than in the general population. Perhaps there is greater awareness of the beneficial effects of good oral hygiene in patients with Sjögren's.

Halitosis (Bad Breath)

Halitosis can occur when there is an overgrowth of certain types of odor-causing bacteria in the teeth or oral soft tissue. These bacteria can be the result of active dental caries, active periodontal or gum disease, inadequate oral hygiene, or deficient saliva. The problem is managed by appropriate dental or periodontal treatment to eradicate the underlying infection, along with regular and careful oral hygiene.

Salivary Gland Enlargement

Salivary gland enlargement or swelling occurs in about one-quarter of patients with Sjögren's, while the majority of the general population never experiences this change. The enlargement is usually gradual in onset and without symptoms or with only slight discomfort. It can slowly regress and recur over a period of several months or become chronic. In rare cases, the swelling can rapidly grow if it transforms into a malignant condition, usually lymphoma. In patients experiencing prolonged salivary gland enlargement, it may be appropriate to consider other causes of the enlargement by way of magnetic resonance imaging (MRI), fine-needle aspiration cytology, and/or salivary gland biopsy.

Diagnostic Testing of Dry Mouth

Dry mouth resulting from Sjögren's and other causes can be evaluated by both dentists or physicians using a combination of methods.

Symptoms and Follow-Up Questions

In evaluating oral symptoms experienced by individuals with Sjögren's, it is helpful to ask if the mouth feels dry while eating dry or solid food such as a cracker. Typically, saliva is stimulated by the smell and taste of food as well as the physical act of chewing. A positive answer suggests that the salivary glands are not producing enough fluid to allow for adequate wetting of the ingested food to facilitate softening, initial digestion, and the movement of the mass from the mouth into the throat and then the esophagus.

Salivary and Oral Examination

In examining patients suspected of having Sjögren's, the major salivary glands may exhibit evidence of tenderness, changes in consistency, or enlargement.

Saliva expressed from the major gland ducts intraorally may exhibit changes in its clarity, viscosity, and wetting ability. The oral mucosa may exhibit changes in its lubricity (normal wet and slippery vs. dry and sticky) and its color. The tongue may exhibit changes described previously. The pattern and extent of dental caries must be noted, as described earlier.

Salivary Flow Rate Measurement

Salivary gland function is most easily assessed by collecting saliva over a specified amount of time. The collection can be made of whole saliva (from all major and minor salivary glands) by simply expectorating (spitting) into a pre-weighed cup. This can be done to assess the severity of salivary gland dysfunction and monitor the progression of disease severity over time, and the effects of treatment. There is no universally accepted measure that defines normal salivary function, but an unstimulated whole salivary flow rate less than 0.1 mL/min is widely accepted as a threshold of abnormal function. A reduction in salivary flow rate may be caused by many different conditions and is not diagnostically specific for Sjögren's.

Scintigraphy

This test measure the rate at which a small amount of injected radioactive material is taken up from the blood into the salivary glands and secreted into the mouth. It is another method to measure salivary gland function and is usually done in a hospital setting. All four of the major salivary glands are evaluated at the same time during this test.

Sialography

This technique uses a liquid radiographic contrast medium injected into a salivary duct, followed by an X-ray image of the gland to show the ductal structures. This technique is useful to explore duct obstructions and distinguish between chronic inflammatory changes and neoplasms but is limited in its ability to provide diagnostically specific information regarding Sjögren's. Sialography in patients with significant salivary hypofunction must be done with a water-based contrast medium to avoid the risk of a chronic foreign body reaction coming from the use of an oil-based contrast medium leaking outside the ducts.

Ultrasound and MRI

These noninvasive imaging techniques can determine structural abnormalities in the salivary glands. Ultrasound examinations may be helpful in identifying vascular or cystic lesions. MRI is an excellent technique for imaging masses or tumors in the salivary glands, particularly as part of a presurgical evaluation. There have been only a few studies examining these techniques in the context of defining Sjögren's-specific features. Ultrasound for the diagnosis of the salivary component of Sjögren's has been more widely used than MRI and is more specific for Sjögren's diagnosis, while MRI is used less frequently, is more expensive, and only used to obtain very specific information.

Sialochemistry

Sialochemistry examines saliva for the presence and amount of particular substances. It has been used to compare saliva samples from normal individuals to those with Sjögren's with the hope of identifying differences that can be used as diagnostic criteria for Sjögren's. Differences between normal and Sjögren's saliva have been identified but have not yet been tested in large trials.

Minor Salivary Gland Biopsy

This test, also known as the lip biopsy, is currently considered the "gold standard" for diagnosing the salivary component of Sjögren's. Using local anesthesia, a small, superficial incision is made on the inner surface of the lower lip to directly visualize and remove at least five of these small glands. There are hundreds of these minor salivary glands located throughout the mouth; they are between 1/16 and 1/8 inches (1–3 mm) in diameter. This technique is preferable to the punch biopsy technique, which is a blind procedure and thus may not yield a sufficient sample of minor salivary glands; it may also endanger sensory nerves in the area. A pathologist will examine the glands for the presence of changes characteristic of the salivary component of Sjögren's (focal lymphocytic sialadenitis) or occasionally of other diseases.

Summing Up

Sjögren's affects the salivary glands, which are responsible for making and secreting a complex fluid that provides a multitude of protective and essential functions. The reduction or loss of saliva results in a decrease of these essential functions and significant oral discomfort and pathology. However, loss of saliva and a complaint of "dry mouth" can be the result of diverse causes (see Box 15.1). Because some of these causes will require different treatment, it is important to evaluate the cause of a complaint of dry mouth and the severity of salivary dysfunction. With this knowledge, individualized preventive measures may be promptly initiated to reduce symptoms and to minimize the impact of dry mouth on the oral cavity.

For Further Reading

Daniels TE. Evaluation, differential diagnosis, and treatment of xerostomia. *J Rheumatol.* 2000;61(Suppl):6–10.

Daniels TE, Wu AJ. Xerostomia—clinical evaluation and treatment in general practice. *J Calif Dent Assoc.* 2000;28(12):933–941.

Sreebny LM. A useful source for the drug–dry mouth relationship. *J Dent Educ.* 2004;68(1):6–7.

Wells BG, Dipiro JT, Schwinghammer TL, Dipro CV. *Pharmacotherapy Handbook* (7th ed.). McGraw-Hill; 2009.

16

Dry Eye

Cintia S. de Paiva, Reza Dana, and Gary N. Foulks

Dry eye, also called keratoconjunctivitis sicca (KCS), is a component of the dryness (sicca) that characterizes Sjögren's. There are greater than 20 million dry eye sufferers in the United States, and approximately 4 million of these people also have Sjögren's.

A recent survey of the members of the Sjögren's Foundation determined that dry eye is one of the most common symptoms in patients with Sjögren's (92%). Since the tears serve to protect the front of the eye and provide a smooth surface that maintains clear vision and comfort, the tear film is an essential feature of the healthy eye. However, disruption of the tear film (either quantity or quality) produces discomfort and disturbance of vision and possible damage to the ocular surface. The ocular surface consists of the conjunctiva (the mucous membrane covering the outside of the eyeball and the inner lining of the eyelids) and the cornea (the central transparent part of the eyeball that helps focus the entering light rays). Dry eye syndrome includes a variety of disorders that affect the ocular surface, both conjunctiva and cornea.

The definition of dry eye as proposed by the International Dry Eye Workshop (DEWS) in 2017 is:

Dry eye is a multifactorial disease of the ocular surface characterized by a loss of homeostasis of the tear film, and accompanied by ocular symptoms, in which tear film instability and hyperosmolarity, ocular surface inflammation and damage, and neurosensory abnormalities play etiological roles.

The dry eye associated with Sjögren's is generally more severe and requires more intensive therapy.

Cintia S. de Paiva, Reza Dana, and Gary N. Foulks, *Dry Eye* In: *The Sjögren's Book*. Edited by: Daniel J. Wallace, Oxford University Press. © Sjögren's Foundation 2022. DOI: 10.1093/oso/9780197502112.003.0016

What Causes Dry Eye?

The tear film that covers the surface of the eye usually is uniformly spread across the eye in a very stable layer. The tear film has been described as consisting of three layers: (1) a superficial lipid layer, (2) a middle aqueous layer, and (3) a deep mucin layer (Figure 16.1). However, recent studies suggest that there is significant interaction between the proteins and lipids in the aqueous layer. The aqueous layer forms the greatest bulk of the tear film and is secreted by the lacrimal (tear-producing) glands (Figure 16.2).

The aqueous layer contains water-soluble factors and electrolytes that wet the ocular surface and provide nutrition to the cornea and mechanical clearing of debris and microorganisms. The proteins contained in the aqueous layer inhibit the growth of organisms and contain growth factors for the ocular surface cells. Disruption of the tear film either because of inadequate secretion of tears (aqueous-deficient dry eye) or excessive evaporation of the tear fluid (evaporative dry eye) can result in dry spots and damage to the ocular surface. One of the most common causes of evaporative dry eye is obstruction of the lipid-producing glands in the eyelid (meibomian glands; see Figure 16.2). Both aqueous-deficient and evaporative dry eye frequently occur in patients with Sjögren's and can occur together.

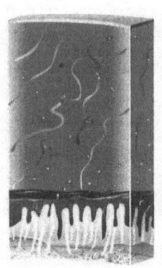

Superficial lipid layer
~0.1–0.2 microns thick

Aqueous layer
~7–8 microns thick

Adsorbed mucin layer
over 1 micron thick

Microvilli of epithelium
extend into and stabilize
mucin layer

Figure 16.1 Layers of the tear film: superficial lipid layer, middle aqueous layer, and deeper mucin layer. Interactions of lipids with proteins do occur within the aqueous layer.

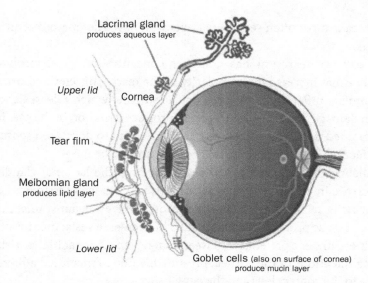

Lacrimal gland
produces aqueous layer

Upper lid

Cornea

Tear film

Meibomian gland
produces lipid layer

Lower lid

Goblet cells (also on surface of cornea)
produce mucin layer

Figure 16.2 Cross-section of the eye showing structures producing the tear film. Lacrimal glands produce aqueous tears. Meibomian glands produce lipids. Goblet cells in the conjunctiva produce mucin.

What Damage Can Occur to the Surface of the Eye from Dry Eye?

When the tear film is unstable or too concentrated, it can damage the surface of the eye, its cells, or its nerves. Loss of the lubricating ability of the tear film results in a greater blink-induced shear force of the eyelid against the ocular surface. This increased shear force can cause changes in the cells of the ocular surface. The normal tear film also contains growth factors that are required for surface cell healing; deficiency of these factors contributes to impaired healing of the damaged surface in dry eye patients. Therefore, a concentrated tear film can also impact the ocular surface cells.

The corneal epithelium (the most superficial cell layer) provides a protective barrier between the environment and the underlying structures of the eye. In moderate to severe dry eye, there is increasing loss of corneal epithelial cells, which are replaced by smaller epithelial cells, or there may be loss of cells to cause persistent epithelial defects since the normal healing process is impaired. In severe cases of dry eye, corneal defects may enlarge and deepen to produce corneal ulcers that lead to thinning of the cornea. Such ulcers, although usually sterile, may become secondarily infected. In the most severe cases, the cornea can thin considerably (melt) and even perforate. Melting of the cornea is most often seen in patients who have rheumatoid arthritis and Sjögren's.

The dry eye tear film has a higher concentration of electrolytes and molecules that increase the osmolarity of the tears. This elevated osmolarity can stimulate inflammation in the ocular surface, which releases chemicals that can damage the corneal surface and produce irritation in the eye. In time, the combined damaging effects on the cornea lead to decreased sensation of the surface of the eye, which further retards normal healing.

Paralleling the decrease in tear secretion from the lacrimal glands, there is a decrease in certain enzymes in tears (lysozyme, lactoferrin, and others) and normally secreted antibodies that protect the eye against infection. The absence of these protective agents results in decreased resistance to infection. In addition, dry eye patients who wear contact lenses are at higher risk of developing infections of the cornea, presumably due to increased adherence of bacteria to the contact lens and the ocular surface.

How Does One Recognize Dry Eye?

The patient's history is extremely important in diagnosing dry eye. Most symptoms in patients with KCS result from instability of the tear film producing discomfort and fluctuation of vision for prolonged reading or near tasks. Further symptoms occur because the lubrication of the surface is inadequate, resulting in a reduced ability of the ocular surface to respond normally to environmental challenges. Symptoms vary from one patient to another depending upon the severity of the dryness and the patient's tolerance for ocular discomfort. Patients often use the word "dryness" to describe their symptoms but may have difficulty defining exactly what it means. Burning, itching, a sensation of a foreign object in the eye, a sandy sensation, light sensitivity, and blurred vision may also be reported. Some patients describe their discomfort as fatigue of the eye.

The principal function of the tear film is to maintain a smooth, clear refractive corneal surface in a hostile external environment. Any adverse effect on the corneal regularity and clarity will interfere with vision; instability of the tear film is such an adverse event. Thus, blurred vision, particularly for near tasks or prolonged reading, may also be one of the initial complaints in a dry eye patient. It is somewhat like looking through a dirty windshield. If the dry eye is due to evaporation, then the vision may be improved by blinking frequently. Patients may also complain of excess secretion of mucus, heaviness of the eyelids, and inability to produce tears when crying.

In some cases, there is "wet dry eye," which is caused by a compensatory increase in tear secretion due to irritation. Associated inflammation of the surface of the eye may cause pain and redness. Pain may also be due to filaments that are strands of adherent mucus covered by epithelial cells on the corneal surface (Figure 16.3).

Dry eye patients are highly sensitive to winds and drafts and cold environments. They often volunteer that they are intolerant to air conditioning and riding in a car with the window down. Reading is often difficult for dry eye sufferers, as is prolonged work at a computer. Some patients complain that they have discomfort on awakening, which may be due to further decreased tear production during sleep. Still, most patients describe increasing discomfort as the day progresses, mainly if they have been doing prolonged computer work or reading. Smoke in the air is almost universally intolerable to tear-deficient patients.

Patients may not be able to produce tears in response to an irritant or emotional situation. For example, the inability to cry when peeling onions or when hurt suggests a severe compromise of lacrimal gland function. Some patients will report having used artificial tears or ointments for relief of symptoms. Although most patients with dry eye will improve with topical lubricant therapy, excessive use of artificial tears containing preservatives

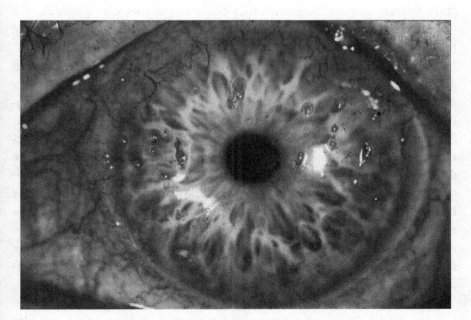

Figure 16.3 Filamentary keratopathy. Strands of mucus adherent to cornea. Filamentary keratopathy is often accompanied by conjunctival redness.

may worsen the symptoms. In addition, some systemic medications such as antihistamines and antidepressants may worsen symptoms by decreasing tear production.

A history of other associated systemic signs of dryness is essential in identifying the sicca condition. Dry mouth or vaginal dryness can be other signs of Sjögren's. Patients with severe dry mouth may have difficulty swallowing crackers, bread, or meat without additional fluids. Such patients are also at risk of dental and gum disease due to lack of saliva. Women may experience a decrease in vaginal secretions, which can lead to sexual dysfunction. It is helpful to know if there is a family history of any blood relatives with dry eye, Sjögren's, collagen vascular disease, or another eye disease.

Evaluation of Dry Eye

Clinical Examination

A complete clinical examination is advisable as part of the evaluation of dry eye. Facial skin must be inspected for evidence of rosacea, which is a skin condition commonly associated with meibomian gland dysfunction and evaporative dry eye. Rosacea causes redness in the skin around the eyes, nose, and chin. Salivary gland enlargement may occur in patients with Sjögren's. The thyroid gland also should be examined for signs of enlargement or presence of nodules as this may be seen in Sjögren's as well.

Examination of the eye includes the evaluation of the lacrimal glands to determine whether there is enlargement or signs of inflammation. Redness of the eyes due to dilated conjunctival blood vessels can be a sign of inflammation of the surface of the eye, which occurs in moderate to severe dry eye. A detailed examination of the ocular surface, including cornea and conjunctiva, is best done with magnification using the slit-lamp biomicroscope in the doctor's office. Distortion of the light reflexes on the cornea indicates disruption of the tear film or damage to the superficial cells of the cornea. There may be excess mucous fragments or debris in the tear film. Sometimes mucous strands stick to the cornea at sites of focal desiccation, and surface cells extend onto the strand, making it very adherent to the cornea. Filaments can cause discomfort or even pain when blinking pulls on the strand. This condition is called filamentary keratopathy.

The health of the meibomian glands in the eyelid must be examined to determine if thick, turbid secretions obstruct the glands. Foam in the tear film suggests meibomian gland dysfunction. The eyelid margins are examined for thickening of the lid margin, increased blood vessels, broken or missing eyelashes, or other signs of inflammation (blepharitis) in the eyelid.

Tear Function Testing

Schirmer Test

The Schirmer test is the most traditional test to determine the level of tear production. Small strips of filter paper 35 mm long are placed on the lateral lower eyelid margin of both eyes and left in place for 5 minutes (Figure 16.4). Then, the amount of wetting of the strip is measured; less than 7 millimeters of wetting suggests dry eye. There is significant variability in this test, however, and it can be affected by environmental conditions of temperature and humidity and the level of room illumination.

Tear Osmolarity Testing

Tear osmolarity testing measures the concentration of the tear film, which can be elevated in either aqueous-deficient or evaporative dry eye. In-office testing is now available and provides an easy, rapid, and reliable measure of tear function (Figure 16.5). Since increased tear osmolarity plays an essential

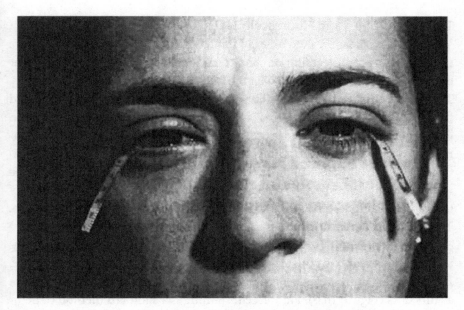

Figure 16.4 Schirmer test. Tear production is measured by the length of wetting of a filter strip positioned at the lower end of the eyelid.

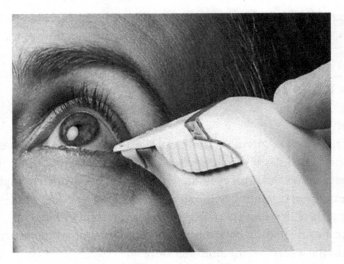

Figure 16.5 Osmolarity testing using the TearLab Osmometer, which collects a minute amount of tears

role in damage to the ocular surface, this test can be a valuable diagnostic test and a potential monitor of the effectiveness of therapy. However, there is considerable variability in this test.

Tear Breakup Test and Fluorescein Test

Measurement of tear breakup time is a standard part of the evaluation of dry eye since instability of the tear film is a characteristic of both forms of dry eye. The tear breakup time measures of how well the cornea remains moist between blinks. Typically, the test is done by instilling a small amount of fluorescent dye called fluorescein into the tear film. This is an orange dye that fluoresces green when illuminated by a blue light and is used in both the tear breakup test and the fluorescein test. To determine tear breakup time, after instillation of the dye, the patient is asked to blink several times. The observer at the slit-lamp biomicroscope will measure the time between when the patient blinks and the first evidence of tear film disruption, seen as a dark spot in the otherwise green-colored tear film. The normal tear breakup time is considered more than 10 seconds.

Fluorescein staining of the surface of the eye is an effective way to determine the stability of the tear film and the integrity of the ocular surface. Fluorescein staining reveals disruptions of the cells of the surface of the eye as tiny dots (Figure 16.6). Fluorescein staining is a standard method of demonstrating damage to the surface of the eye, and it is usually performed when also measuring the tear breakup time.

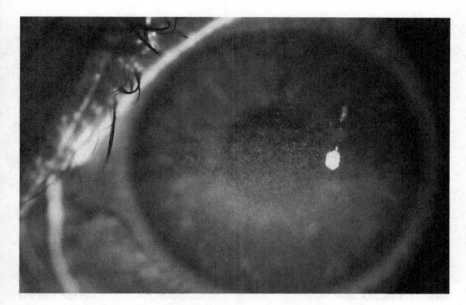

Figure 16.6 Fluorescein staining of cornea. Note tiny dots over the pupil.

Rose Bengal and Lissamine Green Test

Rose bengal and lissamine green dyes are used to determine if surface cells of the eye have lost their normal mucin coating. Both stains demonstrate similar abnormalities, but rose bengal provides a more intense pink stain while lissamine green provides a more subtle blue stain of damaged or mucin-deficient cells (Figure 16.7). Rose bengal has the disadvantage of stinging on application, whereas lissamine green is less irritating. Since the loss of the protective mucin covering of the cells is a feature of dry eye, these dyes help determine the severity of the dryness and the degree of damage to the conjunctiva.

Laboratory Tests

Tear Lysozyme and Lactoferrin

Tear lysozyme and lactoferrin levels can be measured by several methods. Normal tear lysozyme levels are between 2 and 4 mg/mL. Normal lactoferrin level is above 0.9 mg/mL. KCS results in decreased levels of these antibacterial enzymes.

(a)

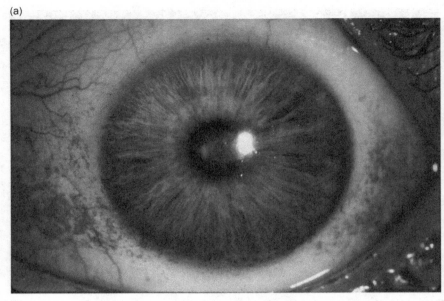

(b)

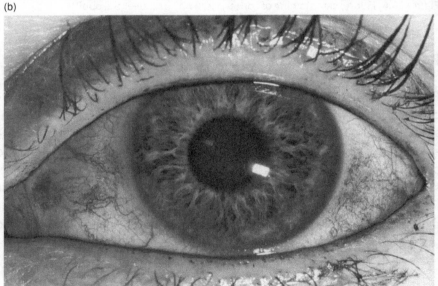

Figure 16.7 Rose bengal (**a**) and lissamine green (**b**) staining of the conjunctiva.

Tear Proteins

Tear protein analysis can be performed by several different tests. Electrophoresis is a method to separate various proteins in tears using electric gradients. Enzyme-linked immunosorbent assay (ELISA) testing identifies proteins by using antibodies directed against specific proteins in the tear film. Protein array analysis can measure large numbers of proteins and identify patterns associated with dry eye. Decreased levels of the goblet-cell specific mucin MUC5AC have been demonstrated in tears of patients with Sjögren's.

Conjunctival Impression Cytology

Conjunctival impression cytology is a method of sampling superficial cells of the surface of the eye using the application of a specific filter paper to the anesthetized surface of the eye. In addition to detecting characteristics of cells of the surface that can indicate the presence of dry eye, the test measures the number of active goblet cells in the conjunctiva that release mucin into the tear film. The number of goblet cells is reduced in dry eye and Sjögren's.

Conditions That Mimic Dry Eye

Certain eye conditions may produce a sensation of dryness. Blepharitis (inflammation of the eyelid) is a very common condition that can mimic dry eye due to the similarity of symptoms. Patients with blepharitis have symptoms of burning and scratchiness of the eye that are worse on awakening and are associated with crusting of the eyelashes. There is only a modest response to use of artificial lubricants, and treatment is more effective with eyelid hygiene done regularly. It is important to recognize that blepharitis and dry eye can coexist.

In allergic conjunctivitis, symptoms are primarily itching. A history of hay fever, asthma, or atopic dermatitis can be present. Typically, there are fine strands of mucus in the tear film with redness of the eyes. The Schirmer test is normal or high due to reflex tearing, and there is usually no fluorescein, rose bengal, or lissamine green staining of the surface. Allergy and dry eye often coexist. Also, systemic anti-allergy medications can exacerbate dryness by reducing tear production.

A variety of conditions that disturb the surface of the eye may be perceived as dryness, such as viral infections, contact lens irritation, and medication-induced irritation. The lack of aqueous tear secretion in KCS results in an inability to dilute or wash away substances that contact the eye either on purpose, such as medications or lubricants, or inadvertently, such as cosmetics to the face and eyelids. Some medications and preservatives in medications or lubricants can cause tear film and surface epithelial abnormalities. Discontinuing such exposure reduces or reverses the toxic effects to the surface and the symptoms they produce.

Social Aspects of Dry Eye

Dry eye can produce chronic symptoms of ocular dryness and discomfort that can be debilitating. When severe, the symptoms may affect the patient's psychological or emotional health and the ability to work. Because of the chronic nature of the problem, many patients experience periods of discouragement and depression. Physicians caring for Sjögren's patients must recognize this aspect of the illness and encourage their patients to pursue activities to the greatest degree possible while complying with recommended treatments. Patients need to remain hopeful since advances in understanding dry eye disease and Sjögren's are continually being made. New therapies are forthcoming, and the management of the disease is improving.

Summing Up

Dry eye (KCS) is one of the most bothersome complaints of Sjögren's patients. It represents the failure of tears to protect the eye and provide a smooth corneal surface. KCS is a consequence of aberrant interactions between proteins and lipids in the aqueous layer of the tear film. Diagnosed by clinical examination, tear function testing, and laboratory analysis of tears, KCS requires that other common conditions such as allergies or blepharitis are ruled out, along with the use of drying medication.

For Further Reading

American Academy of Ophthalmology. Preferred practice pattern: Dry eye, 2018. https://www.aao.org/preferred-practice-pattern/dry-eye-syndrome-ppp-2018

Craig JP, Nichols KK, Akpek EK, et al. TFOS DEWS II definition and classification report. *Ocul Surf.* 2017;15(3):276–283.

Pflugfelder SC, Beuerman RW, Stern ME, eds. *Dry Eye and Ocular Surface Disorders.* Marcel Dekker; 2004.

Sjögren's Foundation. Living with Sjögren's: Summary of Major Findings, 2016. https://www.sjogrens.org/sites/default/files/inline-files/LivingwithSjogrens-8.5x11Bifold-2020_1.pdf

PART IV
DIAGNOSIS

17

Diagnostic and Classification Criteria for Sjögren's

Matthew Makara

Diagnosing a patient with Sjögren's can be different depending on whether the diagnosis is for ongoing management in a physician's office or is for participation in a clinical trial. For the former, the diagnostic criteria are much looser and include the expert opinion of the diagnosing physician. For the latter, official, validated classification criteria are used, which are much more stringent. This chapter will discuss both diagnostic and classification criteria for Sjögren's, including key differences and why and how they are used in clinical and research settings.

Diagnostic Criteria

By definition, diagnostic criteria are a set of signs, symptoms, and tests developed for use in routine clinical care to guide the care of individual patients.

As those familiar with Sjögren's likely know, determining and receiving a Sjögren's diagnosis can often be a difficult and time-consuming process for a variety of reasons, one of which is that there is no single test to confirm the diagnosis. Though complicated, clinicians consider a variety of factors when evaluating a patient for Sjögren's, which may include both objective tests and subjective findings. Objective tests may include blood tests (e.g., anti-SSA/Ro or anti-SSB/La), eye tests (e.g., Schirmer test), and oral tests (e.g., salivary flow). Subjective tests may include questions related to ocular symptoms (e.g., how long have you been experiencing dry eye?) and oral symptoms (e.g., how long have you been experiencing dry mouth?).

These are just a few, but often key, examples of what a clinician may consider when ruling out or arriving at a Sjögren's diagnosis. The following chapters in this section will provide further, detailed information on the measures used for diagnosing Sjögren's, including lab tests, imaging, and biopsy.

Matthew Makara, *Diagnostic and Classification Criteria for Sjögren's* In: *The Sjögren's Book*. Edited by: Daniel J. Wallace, Oxford University Press. © Sjögren's Foundation 2022. DOI: 10.1093/oso/9780197502112.003.0017

Classification Criteria

Fundamentally different from diagnostic criteria are classification criteria, which are standardized definitions primarily intended to enable clinical studies to have uniform cohorts for research. Classification criteria are often stricter than diagnostic criteria as there has to be absolute certainty that a patient being included in a study meets all of the necessary criteria.

For patients, it is important to understand that classification criteria are not used to diagnose a disease. Even if you are diagnosed with a disease, you may still not meet the classification parameters necessary for inclusion in a study.

In Sjögren's, various sets of classification criteria have been in use over the past few decades, including the 2002 American-European Consensus Group (AECG) criteria, the 2012 American College of Rheumatology (ACR) criteria, and, most recently, the 2016 ACR-European League Against Rheumatism (EULAR) criteria (Shiboski, 2016). The latter represent the most current and widely used classification criteria in Sjögren's, so we will describe this set in more detail.

Using and building upon the previous methods used to develop classification criteria in Sjögren's, the 2016 ACR-EULAR Classification Criteria is a single set of validated data-driven consensus classification criteria developed by a group of international experts representing a variety of medical and research specialties. As seen in Table 17.1, the 2016 ACR-EULAR criteria use five objective items, each with a weighted score. Two items—(1) labial salivary gland with focal lymphocytic sialadenitis and focus score of at least 1 and (2) being positive for anti-SSA/Ro—are weighted with a higher score, 3, than the remaining three items, which are each scored as 1. Therefore, for a patient to be classified as having Sjögren's, one of these items must be included to achieve a total score of at least 4.

Summing Up

- Diagnostic criteria are used to diagnose a patient in a clinical setting. In Sjögren's, this requires that a clinician analyze and interpret a number of different variables, including both objective and subjective measures.
- Classification criteria are used to categorize patients in a research setting, which helps in the development of more useful research studies and clinical trials. Classification criteria are not used to diagnose a disease.
- Even if a person is diagnosed with a disease, they may not meet all classification criteria for inclusion in a research study of that disease.

Table 17.1 ACR-EULAR Classification Criteria for Sjögren's

The classification of Sjögren's applies to any individual who meets the inclusion criteria,[1] does not have any condition listed as exclusion criteria,[2] and who has a score ≥4 when summing the weights from the following items:

Item	Weight/Score
Labial salivary gland with focal lymphocytic sialadenitis and focus score ≥1[3]	3
Anti-SSA (Ro) +	3
Ocular staining score ≥5 (or van Bijsterfeld score ≥4) on at least one eye[4]	1
Schirmer ≤5 mm/5 min on at least one eye	1
Unstimulated whole saliva flow rate ≤0.1 mL/min[5]	1

[1]Inclusion criteria: These criteria are applicable to any patient with at least one symptom of ocular or oral dryness, defined as a positive response to at least one of the following questions: (1) Have you had daily, persistent, troublesome dry eyes for more than 3 months? (2) Do you have a recurrent sensation of sand or gravel in the eyes? (3) Do you use tear substitutes more than 3 times a day? (4) Have you had a daily feeling of dry mouth for more than 3 months? (5) Do you frequently drink liquids to aid in swallowing dry food?; or suspicion of Sjögren's from the ESSDAI questionnaire (at least one domain with positive item).

[2]Exclusion criteria: Prior diagnosis of any of the following conditions would exclude diagnosis of Sjögren's and participation in Sjögren's studies or therapeutic trials because of overlapping clinical features or interference with criteria tests: history of head and neck radiation treatment; active hepatitis C infection (with positive PCR); acquired immunodeficiency syndrome; sarcoidosis; amyloidosis; graft-versus-host disease; IgG4-related disease.

Note: Patients who are normally taking anticholinergic drugs should be evaluated for objective signs of salivary hypofunction and ocular dryness after a sufficient interval off these medications for these components to be a valid measure of oral and ocular dryness.

[3]The histopathologic examination should be performed by a pathologist with expertise in the diagnosis of focal lymphocytic sialadenitis, and focus score count (based on number of foci per 4 mm^2) following a protocol described in: Daniels TE, Cox D, Shiboski CH, et al. Associations between salivary gland histopathologic diagnoses and phenotypic features of Sjögren's syndrome among 1,726 registry participants. *Arthritis Rheumatol.* 2011;63(7):2021–2030. doi:10.1002/art.30381

[4]Ocular staining score described in Whitcher JP, Shiboski CH, Shiboski SC, et al. A simplified quantitative method for assessing keratoconjunctivitis sicca from the Sjögren's Syndrome International Registry. *Am J Ophthalmol.* 2009;149(3):405–415. van Bijsterfeld score described in van Bijsterveld OP. Diagnostic tests in the sicca syndrome. *Arch Ophthalmol.* 1969;82(1):10–14.

[5]Unstimulated whole saliva described in Navazesh & Kumar, 2008. Navazesh M. Methods for collecting saliva. *Ann N Y Acad Sci.* 1993;694:72–77.

Source: Shiboski CH, Shiboski SC, Seror R, et al. 2016 American College of Rheumatology/European League Against Rheumatism Classification Criteria for Primary Sjögren's Syndrome: A Consensus and Data-Driven Methodology Involving Three International Patient Cohorts. *Arthritis Rheumatol.* 2017 Jan;69(1):35–45. doi:10.1002/art.39859.

- The 2016 ACR-EULAR set of classification criteria represent the most current and widely used classification criteria for Sjögren's.

For Further Reading

Aggarwal R, Ringold S, Khanna D, et al. Distinctions between diagnostic and classification criteria? *Arthritis Care Res.* 2015;67(7):891–897. doi:10.1002/acr.22583

Baer AN. Diagnosis and classification of Sjögren's syndrome. UpToDate. https://www.upto-date.com/contents/diagnosis-and-classification-of-sjogrens-syndrome

Shiboski CH, Shiboski SC, Seror R, et al. 2016 American College of Rheumatology/European League Against Rheumatism classification criteria for primary Sjögren's syndrome: A consensus and data-driven methodology involving three international patient cohorts. *Arthritis Rheumatol.* 2017;69(1):35–45. doi:10.1002/art.39859

18

Laboratory Tests

Alan N. Baer

Laboratory testing helps the clinician establish the correct diagnosis of Sjögren's, determine involvement of internal organs, estimate the risk of lymphoma development, and monitor the disease and its treatments periodically. The testing is typically done as part of a broader evaluation to achieve these goals, including an interview with the physician, physical examination, imaging studies, biopsy, and occasionally more specialized testing (Box 18.1). Examinations of the eyes and mouth by eye care and oral medicine specialists may also be requested. This chapter reviews the more common laboratory tests used in Sjögren's patients, with an emphasis on how the clinician uses these tests. Subsequent chapters focus on other aspects of the diagnostic process.

Establishing the Diagnosis

The diagnosis of Sjögren's requires demonstration of an autoimmune basis for the presence of dry eyes and/or dry mouth. The current classification criteria for Sjögren's mandate that affected individuals have antibodies to a distinct small intracellular RNA–protein complex (termed SS-A), or that they have a lip biopsy that shows a characteristic pattern (termed focal lymphocytic sialoadenitis) and severity of inflammation, graded by a focus score of 1 or greater. Many Sjögren's patients have other immunologic abnormalities, evident on blood testing, that will lend support to the diagnosis. These include the presence of antinuclear antibodies, rheumatoid factor, an elevated level of serum immunoglobulins (antibody proteins), and occasionally a monoclonal protein.

SS-A and SS-B Antibodies

Antibodies are a large family of proteins in the blood that are capable of binding to molecular targets (termed antigens) on the surfaces of microorganisms, cells,

Alan N. Baer, *Laboratory Tests* In: *The Sjögren's Book*. Edited by: Daniel J. Wallace, Oxford University Press.
© Sjögren's Foundation 2022. DOI: 10.1093/oso/9780197502112.003.0018

Box 18.1 Diagnostic Testing in Sjögren's

Establishing the diagnosis of Sjögren's
- Mandatory tests
  - Positive test for anti-SS-A antibodies

OR

  - Lip biopsy showing focal lymphocytic sialoadenitis with focus score of 1 or greater
- Tests to exclude Sjögren's mimics
  - IV blood test
  - Hepatitis C blood test
  - Chest X-ray and/or angiotensin-converting enzyme (ACE) level
- Serum IgG4 level
- Diagnostic test results that support diagnosis of Sjögren's
- Abnormal salivary gland ultrasonography
- High titer of antinuclear antibodies
- Positive test for rheumatoid factor
- Elevated serum IgG levels
- Low complement C3 and/or C4 levels
- Low white blood cell count (leucopenia)

Defining internal organ involvement
- Careful history and physical examination
- Blood tests: complete blood counts, urinalysis, blood chemistries
- Additional tests will depend on findings from initial evaluation.

Monitoring disease progression and risk for lymphoma
- Routine blood tests: complete blood counts, urinalysis, blood chemistries
- Parotid ultrasonography and/or sialometrics
- Immunoglobulin quantitation
- Serum protein electrophoresis and/or immunofixation electrophoresis
- Serum cryoglobulins
- Serum C3 and C4 levels

and blood proteins. Each antibody protein has a binding site that can only attach to a very specific molecular target. However, the large array of such antibody proteins in our blood ensures that a diverse and large number of molecular targets can be recognized. Binding of such molecular targets is an essential step in our defense against infections and cancer. Cells that produce antibodies against molecular targets on our own tissues are actively eliminated from our bodies, particularly early in life. If this mechanism goes awry, then we may form antibodies to self-material and be susceptible to autoimmune disease.

SS-A and SS-B antibodies are examples of two antibodies that bind molecular targets within our own cells. The SS-A and SS-B targets (also known respectively as Ro and La) are proteins that are attached to a strand of ribonuclear material (RNA). These RNA–protein complexes can be located in either the nucleus or the cytoplasm of the cell. Since they can be found in the nucleus, they are one of the potential targets of antinuclear antibodies, present in patients with systemic autoimmune diseases, such as systemic lupus erythematosus, Sjögren's, and scleroderma. Since the SS-A and SS-B RNA–protein complexes are normally contained within the cell, they are not accessible to antibodies in the blood. However, these proteins are clustered in packets and brought to the surface of the cell during the process of cellular death. It is hypothesized that this process (termed apoptosis) may allow susceptible individuals to form antibodies to the SS-A and SS-B proteins.

SS-A antibodies are found in approximately 60% to 80% of Sjögren's patients (Table 18.1). SS-B antibodies are less common, being found in approximately

Table 18.1 Features of Sjögren's Patients, Defined by 2016 ACR-EULAR Classification Criteria (co-published by the American College of Rheumatology and the European League Against Rheumatism)

Feature	Hopkins Sjögren's Center[1] (N = 408)	SICCA Registry[2] (N = 1,578)
Age (years, mean ± standard deviation)	53 ± 10	
Women (%)	91	93
ANA (%)	85	
ANA ≥ 1:320 (%)	60	59
SS-A antibodies (%)	89	74
SS-B antibodies (%)	29	49
Centromere antibodies (%)	5	
Rheumatoid factor (%)	55	61
Hypergammaglobulinemia (%)	42	55
Monoclonal protein (%)	12	
Low C4 (%)	15	18
Leucopenia (%)	25	

[1] Patients of the Jerome L. Greene Sjögren's Syndrome Center at Johns Hopkins, December 2018.

[2] Shiboski CH, Baer AN, Shiboski SC, et al. Natural history and predictors of progression to Sjögren's syndrome among participants of the SICCA Registry. *Arthritis Care Res.* 2018;70:284–294.

30% to 50% of Sjögren's patients. SS-A antibodies thus occur commonly by themselves; however, it is very uncommon for SS-B antibodies to occur alone. Accordingly, 20% to 40% of Sjögren's patients may lack SS-A and/or SS-B antibodies. The finding of SS-A and/or SS-B antibodies is not specific to Sjögren's patients. These antibodies may also be found in patients with systemic lupus and occasionally in other autoimmune diseases, such as myositis. Additionally, they may be found in approximately 1 in 200 healthy women.

SS-A and SS-B antibodies are commonly detected using either an enzyme-linked immunosorbent assay (ELISA, Figure 18.1) or a multiplex flow immunoassay (MFIA, Figure 18.2). These testing methods measure the binding of serum antibodies to purified SS-A and SS-B proteins that are bound to the surface of plastic wells or tiny beads. Results are typically reported as positive or negative along with an index. These two assay methods are preferred by most large laboratories since they are automated and easily quantifiable. The advantage of MFIA is that it can test for multiple antibodies in a single specimen, using only a small amount of serum. It is also performed on a highly automated and high-throughput system. However, both assay systems can sometimes detect weak and nonspecific binding of other serum antibodies to the SS-A and SS-B targets, leading to a false-positive test result. It is thus prudent to have the test repeated at a different laboratory if a positive result does not correlate with the clinical findings.

Common Blood and Urine Test Abnormalities in Sjögren's Patients

Certain abnormalities in the blood and urine are commonly seen in patients with Sjögren's. Their presence can thus lend support to the diagnosis. The following tests are routinely performed in the evaluation of a patient with suspected Sjögren's.

1. The **complete blood count** (CBC) determines the number of red cells (RBCs), white cells (WBCs), and platelets as well as the level of hemoglobin (oxygen-carrying protein in red cells) in the blood. A low number of WBCs (leucopenia) can be found in approximately 15% to 20% of Sjögren's patients, but this is usually not associated with an increased risk of infection. Anemia, defined by a low hemoglobin level and low number of red blood cells, is less common.

2. The **complete metabolic panel** (i.e., blood chemistries) measures the electrolytes as well as chemicals or proteins in the blood that reflect

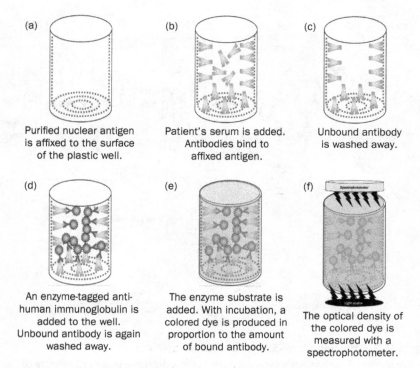

(a) Purified nuclear antigen is affixed to the surface of the plastic well.

(b) Patient's serum is added. Antibodies bind to affixed antigen.

(c) Unbound antibody is washed away.

(d) An enzyme-tagged anti-human immunoglobulin is added to the well. Unbound antibody is again washed away.

(e) The enzyme substrate is added. With incubation, a colored dye is produced in proportion to the amount of bound antibody.

(f) The optical density of the colored dye is measured with a spectrophotometer.

Figure 18.1 ANA detection using ELISA

The ELISA test is often performed using a plastic plate with 96 wells like the one shown. Purified nuclear antigen is affixed to the surface of the plastic well. In a multi-step process, a patient's serum sample can be tested for the presence of antibodies that bind specifically to the nuclear antigen. Detection of this binding requires the use of a commercially available antibody to human immunoglobulin that is generated in an animal (such as a rabbit or goat) and subsequently tagged with an enzyme. Akin to the formation of a sandwich, this commercially available antibody binds to those in the patient's serum that have attached to the nuclear antigen on the surface of the plastic wells. In the next step, the enzyme converts an added colorless substrate (chromogen) to a colored product, and the amount of chromogen produced indicates the amount of antibody–antigen binding in the well.

the function of the kidneys, liver, and immune system. In Sjögren's, the total protein level may be elevated, reflecting the increase in antibody (or immunoglobulin) levels in the blood. The serum bicarbonate or carbon dioxide level may be low, reflecting a disorder of the kidney that may occur in Sjögren's known as renal tubular acidosis. An elevation of the creatinine level indicates the presence of kidney dysfunction, a rare complication of Sjögren's. Elevation of the liver enzymes, alkaline

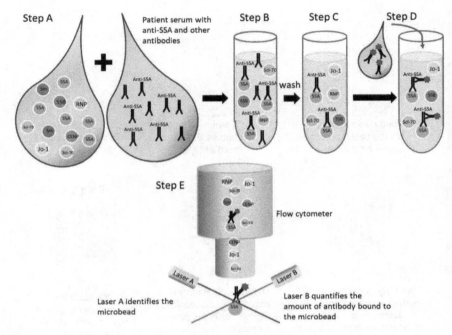

Figure 18.2 Detection of anti-SSA antibodies using MFIA

Step A: A drop of the patient's serum is mixed with a drop of a standard mixture of microbeads. Each microbead in this mixture is coated with a specific antigen protein (e.g., SSA, SSB, Sm, RNP, Scl-70, CENP, and Jo-1); up to 13 can be included in current assays used in clinical laboratory testing. Microbeads coated with each of the antigens are also impregnated with a unique fluorescent dye, allowing the machine to distinguish them in Step E, after they are illuminated by a laser beam. Step B: Antibodies to SSA in the patient's serum (if present) bind to microbeads coated with the SSA protein. After Step B, the microbeads are washed, removing all antibody proteins that have not been bound by a microbead. The result is the mixture seen in Step C. In Step D, a reagent is added to the microbead mixture; this reagent is composed of antibodies to the human immunoglobulin molecule, created in a rabbit or other animal. Each of these antibodies is coupled with a molecule (a fluorochrome, shown as a red star) that fluoresces when hit by laser light, allowing its detection in Step E. Since the antibodies to SSA are an immunoglobulin protein, they will be bound by this anti-human immunoglobulin antibody. In Step E, the microbead mixture is passed through a flow cytometer, a machine that can characterize each bead as it passes single file through a laser detector. Two lasers are used; one identifies the bead based on the color of its impregnated dye and the other quantifies the amount of the fluorochrome (red star molecule) on the bead surface (representing tagged anti-SSA antibodies).

phosphatase, aspartate aminotransferase (AST), and alanine aminotransferase (ALT) can be seen in liver diseases, including different forms of autoimmune hepatitis that can complicate Sjögren's (e.g., primary biliary cholangitis).

3. The **antinuclear antibody (ANA) test** is positive in the majority of Sjögren's patients. However, a positive ANA test is also common in healthy individuals. The ANA test is most commonly performed using a technique that involves immunofluorescent staining of human cells grown in tissue culture (Figure 18.3). With this test, a positive result is listed as the last dilution of serum that results in visible staining of the nucleus of the cultured human cell. Typical dilutions are 1:40, 1:80, 1:160, 1:320, and 1:640. Positive ANA test results of 1:80 and 1:160 may be seen in up to 15% and 5% of healthy individuals, respectively. A negative ANA test does not exclude the diagnosis of Sjögren's; some of these individuals may still have SS-A and/or SS-B antibodies. With the immunofluorescent staining test, the pattern of nuclear staining is reported. Most Sjögren's patients have either a speckled or homogeneous pattern. However, some patients may have a centromere pattern, denoting staining of centromere proteins in the mitotic spindle of dividing cells.

4. The **rheumatoid factor (RF) test** detects immunoglobulins in the blood that bind to other immunoglobulins, resulting in large protein complexes. RF is a characteristic feature of rheumatoid arthritis, being found in up to 80% of affected patients. However, it is also common in Sjögren's patients and in this setting does not indicate the presence of or predict the later development of rheumatoid arthritis.

5. The **erythrocyte sedimentation rate (ESR)** measures the degree to which whole blood, collected in tubes containing a chemical that prevents clotting (anticoagulant), separates into plasma (the upper layer) and packed red cells (the lower layer) over the course of 1 hour. The rate at which red cells settle to the bottom of the tube depends largely on the amount of fibrinogen protein in the blood. Fibrinogen binds to the surface of red cells and decreases their negative electrostatic charges, allowing the cells to aggregate and settle more quickly. The amount of fibrinogen produced by the liver increases with systemic inflammation. Thus, the ESR is a simple test for measuring the degree of inflammation. The ESR can also increase when there are higher levels of immunoglobulins in the blood, as is the case for some Sjögren's patients.

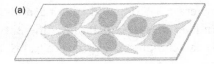

(a) Human tissue culture cells are grown on a glass slide.

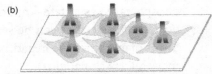

(b) The patient's serum, containing anti-nuclear antibodies, is layered over the cells. After a period of incubation, the serum is washed away. The antinuclear antibodies remain affixed to the nuclei of the cells.

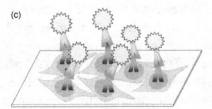

(c) An antibody labeled with a fluorescent chromophore and directed against human immunoglobulin, is layered over the cells. The antibody binds to the human anti-nuclear antibodies. The excess is washed away.

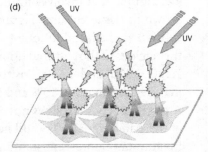

(d) When exposed to ultraviolet light, the chromophore emits yellow-green light, allowing visualization of the antibodies which have bound to the cellular nuclei.

Figure 18.3 Immunofluorescent staining technique for ANA detection
In this multi-step process akin to making a sandwich, the patient's diluted serum is layered over human tissue culture cells that have adhered to a glass slide. After a period of incubation, the patient's serum is washed away. ANA binding to the cellular nuclei is then detected with the use of a commercially available antibody to human immunoglobulin that is generated in an animal (such as a rabbit or goat) and subsequently tagged with fluorescein, a fluorescent dye. When viewed under a microscope equipped with special lighting, the fluorescent dye can be seen "staining" the cellular nuclei if ANAs were present in the patient's serum.

6. The **C-reactive protein (CRP) test** measures systemic inflammation. It is elevated most commonly in the setting of an infection or tissue injury, such as a myocardial infarction (heart attack). In the setting of autoimmune disease, the CRP may be elevated, but usually to a much lesser extent than during an infection.

7. **Urinalysis** detects a variety of abnormalities in the kidney or genitourinary system, including the bladder. Protein in the urine (proteinuria) is an indication of kidney disease, stemming from a disorder of either the glomerulus (the filtering structure) or the tubules (the structures within the kidney responsible for reabsorbing filtered salts, water, and acids from the initial blood filtrate). Blood in the urine may arise from

a glomerular disease or from a disorder in the urine collecting system or bladder (e.g., a kidney stone or tumor). WBCs in the urine denote the presence of inflammation or infection anywhere in the kidneys, urine collecting system, bladder, or urethra. The specific gravity is an indirect measure of the concentration of the urine. The pH indicates the extent of urine acidification. In Sjögren's, the most common abnormality is inflammation in the tissue surrounding the tubules (interstitial nephritis), and this may lead to poorly concentrated urine (with a low specific gravity), protein in the urine, and occasionally a high urine pH. Inflammation or damage in the glomerulus (glomerulonephritis) is a less common form of kidney disease in Sjögren's and is characterized by protein in the urine, occasionally with RBCs and/or WBCs.

8. The **immunoglobulin quantitation test** measures the levels of the most common types of immunoglobulins in the blood, known as IgG, IgM, and IgA. Some patients with Sjögren's have elevated levels of these immunoglobulins (termed hyperglobulinemia), reflecting overactivity of the immune system.

9. The **serum protein electrophoresis** and the **serum immunofixation electrophoresis** tests analyze the types of proteins present in the liquid phase of the blood (serum). These tests rely on an electric field to separate the proteins based on their electrical charge. In the diagnostic evaluation of a patient with Sjögren's, particular attention is paid to the immunoglobulins, proteins produced by plasma cells. Each of these cells creates a unique antibody, with a structure different from that produced by most other plasma cells. In approximately 10% of Sjögren's patients, a clone of plasma cells proliferates and produces increased amounts of one immunoglobulin, with identical structure and specificity. This is called a monoclonal protein. This monoclonal immunoglobulin protein can be detected and characterized with electrophoretic techniques that rely on its distinctive properties in an electrical field.

10. The **complement proteins, C3 and C4,** are part of a group of proteins that mediate tissue inflammation and damage in certain immunologic diseases, including Sjögren's. Low levels of these proteins generally reflect the ongoing utilization of these proteins in a process triggered by the binding of immunoglobulins to molecular targets in the serum (thereby forming immune complexes) or to targets on cellular surfaces. Very low levels of C4 can also reflect the genetic absence of this protein.

Some physicians may order a commercial panel of antibody and other tests in their evaluation of a patient with suspected Sjögren's or lupus. The

AVISE CTD™ (Exagen, Vista, CA) includes tests for antibodies seen in lupus, Sjögren's, antiphospholipid syndrome, and rheumatoid arthritis, in addition to measures of complement protein activation. The panel is specifically designed to provide a diagnostic likelihood of lupus but also includes tests relevant to the diagnosis of Sjögren's. The Sjö™ panel (IMMCO Diagnostics, Inc, Williamsville, NY) tests for antibodies to three mouse proteins—salivary protein-1 (SP-1), carbonic anhydrase-6 (CA6), and parotid salivary protein (PSP)—that appear before the development of anti-SSA/Ro antibodies in a mouse model of Sjögren's. The panel is marketed as having diagnostic utility as an early test for Sjögren's in humans, but this has not been proven. A high proportion of people with non-Sjögren's rheumatic conditions (such as osteoarthritis) have positive test results, thereby limiting the test's diagnostic specificity.

Exclusion of Sjögren's Mimics

Certain other diseases can mimic Sjögren's and should be excluded in the diagnostic evaluation of a patient with suspected Sjögren's. Hepatitis C and human immunodeficiency virus (HIV) infections can be excluded with blood tests. IgG4 plasmacytic infiltrative disease is characterized by elevated serum levels of IgG4 (a subclass of the IgG immunoglobulin family) and/or infiltration of the salivary or lacrimal glands with IgG4-producing plasma cells. Thus, a biopsy of the salivary or lacrimal glands may be required. Lymphoma requires biopsy of an enlarged salivary or lacrimal gland or lymph node for definitive diagnosis.

Defining the Extent of Disease Involvement

Sjögren's involves organs other than the salivary and lacrimal glands in up to 50% of patients. A search for this "extraglandular involvement" begins with the history and physical examination and is aided by basic laboratory tests, including a urinalysis and complete metabolic panel (see the list of tests earlier in the chapter). If there is concern about the presence of specific organ involvement, different test modalities may be employed. We will describe these briefly.

1. Skin involvement: Patients with Sjögren's may develop skin rashes, usually related to the presence of vasculitis or to the deposition of immune

complexes at the junction of the epidermis (outer layer of the skin) and the subjacent dermis (so-called interface dermatitis). A skin biopsy may be required for accurate diagnosis of these conditions. This is usually performed with a punch technique, in which a 3- to 4-mm cylindrical plug of anesthetized skin is removed and sent to the laboratory.

2. <u>Peripheral nervous system involvement</u>: Damage of the peripheral nerves ("peripheral neuropathies") can occur in Sjögren's as a result of diverse autoimmune mechanisms. Symptoms include burning pain or numbness of the hands and feet, weakness of the extremities, poor balance, and altered gait. The diagnosis of a peripheral neuropathy requires electrodiagnostic testing, including electromyography (EMG) and nerve conduction studies. These tests measure the electrical activity of muscles and nerves and are usually done at the same time. The nerve conduction study measures how quickly electrical impulses move along a nerve and can distinguish between neuropathies caused by damage to the nerve's axon and those caused by damage to the myelin sheath surrounding the nerve. The EMG measures the electrical activity of a muscle and provides information about the muscle itself and how well it receives stimulation from the nerve. Patients with Sjögren's may develop a peripheral neuropathy that only affects small nerve fibers. In such cases, the results of the EMG and nerve conduction studies may be normal, since these tests detect abnormalities in the large nerve fibers, responsible for vibratory and position sense. In such patients, injury to the small nerve fibers can be assessed with a series of skin biopsies taken from several sites in an arm or a leg. These skin biopsies are examined with special staining techniques to visualize the small nerve fibers that innervate the skin. An absence or decrease in the density of these nerve fibers in the epidermis (outer layer of the skin) is indicative of a small fiber neuropathy. Rarely, patients with a peripheral neuropathy may require a biopsy of the nerve to elucidate the cause of the neuropathy. The sural nerve (in the ankle) and the superficial radial nerve (wrist) are the sites most often used for biopsy.

3. <u>Central nervous system involvement</u>: Sjögren's may involve the central nervous system, such as the brain and the spinal cord. The types of involvement are diverse but usually involve focal areas of damage to the coatings of the nerve fibers (demyelination) or strokes. Magnetic resonance imaging (MRI) of the brain and a lumbar puncture ("spinal tap") are generally required to diagnose such involvement. In neuromyelitis optica, a distinctive form of central nervous system involvement in Sjögren's, there is demyelination of the optic nerves and spinal cord.

Patients with this disorder have antibodies to aquaporin-4, a water channel protein.

4. Lung involvement: Inflammation within the lung tissue (interstitial pneumonitis) may occur in Sjögren's, manifested by shortness of breath and cough. The diagnostic evaluation usually involves a chest X-ray, computed tomography (CT) scan of the lung, and pulmonary function testing. A biopsy of lung tissue may be required to differentiate the various types of lung inflammation that can occur in Sjögren's.

5. Kidney involvement: Inflammation of either the glomerulus (glomerulonephritis) or the supporting tissue of the kidney (interstitial nephritis) occurs in a small minority of patients with Sjögren's. An excess of protein in the urine or impairment of kidney function (i.e., elevated serum creatinine or decrease in glomerular filtration rate) may indicate either form of kidney disease. Interstitial nephritis may lead to a condition called renal tubular acidosis in which the kidney fails to reabsorb bicarbonate from the urine or to secrete hydrogen ions into the urine. Manifestations include a low serum bicarbonate level, a relatively high urine pH level, dilute urine, and excess urine concentrations of glucose, uric acid, phosphate, and amino acids. These types of kidney involvement can be detected initially with an analysis of the urine and the serum chemistries and creatinine. A kidney biopsy may be required for definitive diagnosis.

6. Liver involvement: Autoimmune hepatitis occurs in approximately 5% of Sjögren's patients. Symptoms, if present, usually include fatigue, itching, nausea, poor appetite, and abdominal pain. The diagnosis is first suggested by the finding of elevated liver function tests on blood chemistries (particularly the aminotransferases, ALT and AST). The finding of characteristic antibodies, such as anti-mitochondrial and anti-smooth muscle (actin) antibodies, supports the diagnosis. Confirmation requires a liver biopsy.

7. Gastrointestinal involvement: Sjögren's can affect the ability to chew, swallow, and digest food through a variety of mechanisms. Difficulty swallowing may relate to lack of saliva, dryness of the esophagus, or poor esophageal contractions. Poor digestion may result from impaired secretion of acid by the stomach or digestive enzymes by the pancreas. Absorption of nutrients can be impaired by the presence of a second autoimmune disease, celiac disease, which may occur in patients with Sjögren's. Testing for gastrointestinal involvement usually requires X-ray studies, endoscopy, and blood tests.

8. <u>Hematologic involvement</u>: Abnormalities of the blood counts, including low numbers of RBCs (anemia), WBCs (leucopenia), and platelets (thrombocytopenia), occur in a minority of Sjögren's patients. They may arise from a variety of mechanisms, not all of which are autoimmune. Thus, it is important that these abnormalities be evaluated carefully, since some may reflect nutritional deficiencies (e.g., low levels of iron, folic acid, vitamin B_{12}) or primary bone marrow disorders. The evaluation usually requires blood tests and occasionally a bone marrow aspiration.

Estimating the Risk of Lymphoma

Certain immunologic tests may help define whether there is a high risk for the development of lymphoma. These include the presence of low levels of the C4 complement protein, a monoclonal immunoglobulin, and serum cryoglobulins (serum proteins, often a mixture of monoclonal and non-monoclonal immunoglobulins, which precipitate in the cold). In addition, changes in some blood test results, such as a precipitous drop in immunoglobulin levels or blood counts, may suggest that a lymphoma is developing.

Monitoring Disease Progression

Sjögren's is a chronic disease that shows minimal progression over years of follow-up for most patients. Thus, measures of saliva and tear production often do not decline significantly over periods of greater than 5 years. However, it is important that patients with Sjögren's are evaluated on at least an annual basis in order to assess their oral and ocular health and monitor for the development of internal organ involvement and lymphoma. Additionally, patients taking hydroxychloroquine need to be examined by an eye care professional annually to make sure that there is no evidence of retinal damage, a rare complication of this treatment. This evaluation includes assessments of the visual fields using perimetry and an examination of the retina with optical coherence tomography. Laboratory monitoring every 2 to 3 months may also be required for patients taking immunosuppressive treatments for Sjögren's (e.g., methotrexate, leflunomide, azathioprine, and mycophenolate).

The periodic evaluation of a patient with Sjögren's generally involves a careful history and physical examination, including specialized examinations of the eyes (by an eye care professional) and the mouth (by a dentist).

Laboratory testing, such as a CBC, complete metabolic panel, and urinalysis, may serve to screen for internal organ involvement.

In some rheumatic diseases, there are blood tests that may be used to assess the overall activity of the disease and the patient's response to treatment. Examples include the ESR and CRP in rheumatoid arthritis and giant cell arteritis and complement levels and DNA antibody levels in systemic lupus. In Sjögren's, such a test does not exist.

Summing Up

The diagnosis and the management of Sjögren's require a variety of testing modalities, including blood and urine assays, tissue biopsies, and medical imaging. These tests are essential to establish the correct diagnosis, to define the extent of disease involvement, and to monitor for potential disease complications. Since Sjögren's is a heterogeneous disorder, the clinician must choose diagnostic testing based on the unique features of each patient. Ongoing research holds promise in defining molecular diagnostic tests that may refine the diagnosis of Sjögren's and better define the potential for certain disease complications.

For Further Reading

Daniels TE, Whitcher JP. Association of patterns of labial salivary gland inflammation with keratoconjunctivitis sicca. Analysis of 618 patients with suspected Sjögren's. *Arthritis Rheumatol.* 1994;37(6):869–877.

Emamian ES, Leon JM, Lessard CJ, et al. Peripheral blood gene expression profiling in Sjögren's. *Genes Immunol.* 2009;10(4):285–296.

Fritzler MJ, Pauls JD, Kinsella TD, Bowen TJ. Antinuclear, anticytoplasmic, and anti-Sjögren's antigen A (SS-A/Ro) antibodies in female blood donors. *Clin Immunol Immunopathol.* 1985;36:120–128.

Garcia-Carrasco M, Ramos-Casals M, Rosas J, et al. Primary Sjogren syndrome: Clinical and immunologic disease patterns in a cohort of 400 patients. *Medicine.* 2002;81(4):270–280.

Goeb V, Salle V, Duhaut P, et al. Clinical significance of autoantibodies recognizing Sjögren's A (SSA), SSB, calpastatin and alpha-fodrin in primary Sjögren's. *Clin Exp Immunol.* 2007;148(2):281–287.

Gottenberg JE, Cagnard N, Lucchesi C, et al. Activation of IFN pathways and plasmacytoid dendritic cell recruitment in target organs of primary Sjögren's. *Proc Natl Acad Sci USA.* 2006;103(8):2770–2775.

Ramos-Casals M, Brito-Zerón P, Perez-De-Lis M, et al. Sjögren syndrome or Sjögren disease? The histological and immunological bias caused by the 2002 criteria. *Clin Rev Allergy Immunol.* 2010;38(2–3):178–185.

Ramos-Casals M, Font J, Garcia-Carrasco M, et al. Primary Sjogren syndrome: Hematologic patterns of disease expression. *Medicine.* 2002;81(4):281–292.

Routsias JG, Tzioufas AG. Sjögren's: Study of autoantigens and autoantibodies. *Clin Rev Allergy Immunol.* 2007;32(3):238–251.

Solomon DH, Kavanaugh AJ, Schur PH. American College of Rheumatology Ad Hoc Committee on Immunologic Testing Guidelines. Evidence-based guidelines for the use of immunologic tests: antinuclear antibody testing. *Arthritis Rheumatol.* 2002;47(4):434–444. doi:10.1002/art.10561

Tzioufas AG, Voulgarelis M. Update on Sjögren's autoimmune epithelitis: From classification to increased neoplasias. *Best Pract Res Clin Rheumatol.* 2007;21(6):989–1010.

Voulgarelis M, Skopouli FN. Clinical, immunologic, and molecular factors predicting lymphoma development in Sjögren's patients. *Clin Rev Allergy Immunol.* 2007;32(3):265–274.

19
Assessing the Salivary Gland Component in Sjögren's

Biopsy and Imaging

Malin V. Jonsson, Kathrine Skarstein, and Chiara Baldini

Introduction

A common feature of Sjögren's is the symptom of oral dryness, or xerostomia. The assessment of salivary gland involvement in Sjögren's is commonly based on subjective symptoms of xerostomia and objective measures of reduced salivary secretion. Xerostomia is the subjective sensation of oral dryness and should not be confused with hyposalivation, the objective measurement of reduced salivary secretion.

Salivary gland tissue in Sjögren's is characterized by focal chronic inflammatory cell infiltrates, loss of saliva-producing acinar epithelial cells, and scar tissue (fibrosis). The minor labial salivary gland (LSG) biopsy has long been considered the "gold standard" for objective evaluation of the autoimmune salivary gland component of Sjögren's, but other methods are needed if a biopsy is inconclusive or cannot be performed.

The diagnostic evaluation and management of the oral component in a patient with Sjögren's is in many ways closely related to both the amount of saliva and the function of the major and minor salivary glands. The least invasive tool for determining dryness is interviewing the patient about relevant medical history, including the nature and duration of dryness symptoms. To obtain a quantitative measure of salivary gland function, unstimulated and stimulated sialometry (measure of saliva flow) is performed to determine possible hyposalivation. Before going on to the minor, or major, salivary gland biopsy, some centers now perform ultrasonography to evaluate the salivary gland organ involvement. Salivary gland involvement can also be evaluated by other imaging methods, such as sialography, magnetic resonance imaging (MRI), and computed tomography (CT).

Malin V. Jonsson, Kathrine Skarstein, and Chiara Baldini, *Assessing the Salivary Gland Component in Sjögren's*
In: *The Sjögren's Book*. Edited by: Daniel J. Wallace, Oxford University Press. © Sjögren's Foundation 2022.
DOI: 10.1093/oso/9780197502112.003.0019

By using these various tests the clinician in many cases can establish a correct diagnosis of Sjögren's, define the extent of disease involvement in the salivary glands, advise the patient on treatment or prevention of oral dryness symptoms and complications, and monitor overall disease progression. Doing analyses of saliva and salivary glands may also help to uncover disease mechanisms as well as markers for classifying individuals into stratified subpopulations that will benefit from specific intervention.

Minor LSG Biopsy

Biopsy of the minor salivary gland of the lower lip is widely used in the diagnosis of Sjögren's and has played an important role in classification of Sjögren's since it was first described over 40 years ago (Shiboski et al., 2017; Theander et al., 2011). A shallow 1.5- to 2.0-cm linear incision is made on the inner aspect of the lower lip, allowing the harvest of at least five minor salivary glands, each a sphere approximately 2.2 mm in diameter. The biopsy evaluation remains the best method for diagnosing the salivary gland component of Sjögren's, mainly because of its high disease sensitivity and specificity. The significant role of salivary gland biopsy is widely accepted in both the established 2002 American-European Consensus Group (AECG) classification criteria and in the newly proposed American College of Rheumatology-European League Against Rheumatism (ACR-EULAR) classification criteria. Also of importance is that LSG biopsies may have the potential to stratify and provide prognostic insights of Sjögren's patients.

A minor LSG biopsy is usually performed, although some centers prefer a parotid biopsy performed by an experienced clinician, which in their hands is associated with a lower complication rate. The most characteristic histopathologic feature in the minor salivary glands is the presence of dense, well-defined foci of mostly lymphocytes located around the striated ducts (Figure 19.1). A positive LSG biopsy has been defined as containing at least one focal mononuclear cell infiltrate per 4 mm^2 glandular tissue area (focus score $\geq$ 1). The focal infiltrate should contain 50 or more mononuclear cells in a periductal location, typically adjacent to normal-appearing acini.

As the focal infiltrates increase in size, lymphoid organization in the form of germinal center (GC)-like structures (Figure 19.2) may develop in approximately 20% to 25% of patients. These structures represent organized nests of cells involved in antibody production. The GC-like structures have been implicated in the development of Sjögren's-associated mucosa-associated lymphoid (MALT) lymphomas.

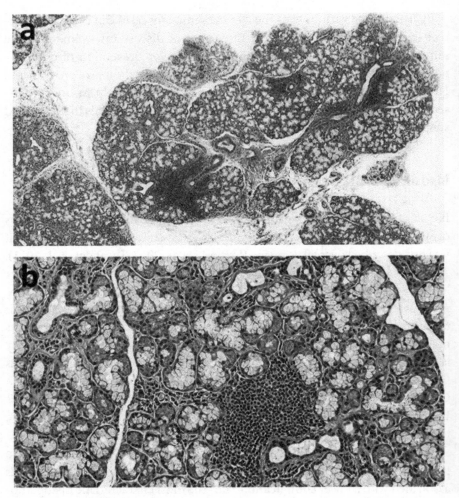

Figure 19.1 Sjögren's, minor salivary gland expression The histologic picture is typical. Dense, well-defined foci of mononuclear cells, dominated by lymphocytes, surround the ducts (**a**). Normal-appearing acinar structures appear in the periphery of the focal infiltrate (**b**).

Major Salivary Gland Biopsy

Studies have proposed that histopathologic evaluation of the parotid gland should be included in the classification criteria for Sjögren's as an alternative to labial glands. Given the fact that the parotid biopsy requires specific surgical skills and that a labial biopsy is more easily performed, labial gland biopsy is still preferred by most groups. However, recent studies

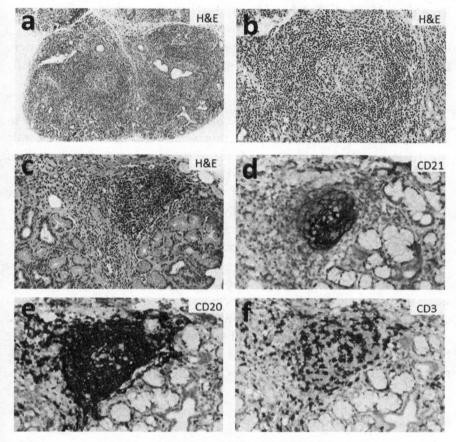

Figure 19.2 Sjögren's, minor salivary gland In late stage of disease only remnants of acini remain and the gland is replaced by a confluent infiltrate of lymphocytes (**a**). GC-like structures can be detected in some of the glands with extensive inflammation (**b**). In some cases the GC-like morphologic appearance is not so evident (**c**). Immunohistochemical staining with follicular dendritic cell maker CD21 (**d**), B-cell marker CD20 (**e**), and T-cell marker CD3 (**f**) may improve reliability and offer more consistent identification of GC-like structures.

underline the diagnostic potential of parotid gland tissue, including the possibility of detecting parotid MALT lymphoma at an earlier stage. Of particular interest is the possibility of repeated biopsies in the same parotid gland, which can facilitate evaluation of treatment efficacy in clinical trials and may also serve as a guide to disease stratification and personalized treatment. Nevertheless, the concordance between the parotid and the labial gland biopsy is debated, and there is a need for larger and comparative studies.

Imaging Modalities for Major Salivary Glands

In the diagnostic work-up in patients with xerostomia and/or hyposalivation, assessment of the major salivary glands can be performed by the currently available imaging techniques, based on the clinical diagnostic question:

- To quantify the function of the major salivary glands and determine if an impairment of salivary gland function is causing the patient's xerostomia
- To assess whether there is evidence of structural changes indicative of chronic inflammatory changes in the salivary glands
- To determine the presence of anatomic defects, such as a blocked salivary duct, as the basis for recurrent salivary gland swelling
- To evaluate whether swelling of one or more salivary glands is due to retention of saliva, infection, inflammation, or a tumor

To decide on the best imaging method, it is important that the treating physician makes a good description of the clinical findings and formulates a good clinical diagnostic question that the images can answer. Based on the clinical question, the radiologist or treating physician/rheumatologist can determine the most suitable imaging modality in line with radiation-protection principles, keeping the radiation dose "as low as reasonably achievable" (ALARA).

Sialoscintigraphy

Scintigraphy, or sialoscintigraphy in the case of salivary glands, is a nuclear medicine imaging modality that evaluates the function of the parotid and submandibular glands by the uptake and secretion of a radioactive tracer. Briefly, the patient receives an injection of a low-level radioactive tracer, commonly ^{99m}Tc-sodium pertechnetate, and is then monitored by a gamma camera that detects the radiation and produces an image. Imaging typically begins directly following the injection to observe the progressive accumulation of radioactive tracer in the glands. After 45 minutes, the patient is given a sour substance such as lemon juice or a hard lemon candy to stimulate salivary secretion and emptying of the salivary glands. Another set of images is then acquired for comparison. The entire process takes about 60 minutes. With the aid of a computer, the uptake and secretion of the radioactive tracer can be quantified for each of the major salivary glands. The level of radioactivity used to obtain the images is low, but for children and pregnant women, alternative tests should be considered (ALARA).

Conventional Sialography

Sialography involves infusion of a radiopaque contrast medium into the ductal system of one or several of the major salivary glands, providing a good illustration of the ductal structures. The test, which has long been considered the "gold standard" for showing ductal inflammatory changes, requires cannulation, the insertion of a small tube into the salivary duct. The contrast solution may be either water- or oil-based; the water-based one is preferred due to a higher risk of adverse reactions with the oil-based one. Immediately following retrograde injection of 0.2 to 1.5 mL of contrast medium into the main excretory duct of the parotid or submandibular gland (Stensen's or Wharton's duct, respectively), one or a series of images with different projections are taken. A couple of minutes after the intraglandular contrast is given, a new radiograph is taken with the same projection(s) to monitor the gradual washout of contrast. In cases of reduced function, contrast may be retained for several minutes, even up to an hour, and in this regard sialography can also be considered a functional test.

The images may show strictures of the ducts, dilatation of the terminal portions of the ducts, or blockages of the duct, such as stones or mucous plugs. If found, such anatomic alterations are not specific for Sjögren's. The typical imaging finding for Sjögren's is the "cherry blossom," "snowstorm," or "Christmas tree" pattern; the radiologic term is sialectasia—filling of contrast in the acini. A healthy gland more resembles a tree with a major stem branching off to finer and finer branches.

Sialography can be indicated in the evaluation of chronic inflammatory diseases and ductal pathology. However, in cases of acute infection, known sensitivity to iodine, or pending thyroid function tests, sialography is contraindicated. Sialography is also contraindicated in patients with severe glandular dysfunction, where instead MR-sialography may be an alternative imaging method.

Magnetic Resonance Imaging

The human body is composed primarily of water and thus hydrogen atoms. Using strong magnetic fields, electric field gradients, and radio waves, the properties of hydrogen atoms in different tissues within the body can be assessed by generating images of organs or segments of the body. Since the properties of atoms vary in the main tissues of the body (muscle, tendons, fat, brain, cerebrospinal fluid, blood) MRI is an excellent technique for imaging soft tissues, including the major salivary glands. MRI provides better tissue/contrast resolution than CT but poorer spatial/geometric resolution. The anatomic overview is similar, though MRI images are better for soft tissue such as muscle and fat and CT images are better for hard tissue such as bone and teeth.

Strengths of MRI include no ionizing radiation, and hence no radiation dose to the patient. Because its soft tissue contrast is superior to that of CT, the MRI technique may be particularly useful when the clinical findings and a history of a swollen salivary gland suggest the possibility of a tumor. For visualizing salivary glands, T1-weighted and T2-weighted images with fat suppression are used. In T1-weighted images, fat appears bright and water dark, and in T2-weighted images fat appears gray and water bright.

A further development of the MRI technique, MR-sialography, facilitates visualization of the larger salivary gland ducts and may be an alternative to conventional plain-film contrast sialography, especially if ductal catheterization is problematic or contraindicated. Before imaging, the patient is given lemon juice to stimulate secretion of saliva. Saliva within the ducts then functions as inherent contrast, enabling visualization of the ductal structures.

MR-sialography can be a suitable method for investigating the major salivary glands in the diagnosis of Sjögren's and has largely replaced conventional plain-film sialography. In healthy individuals the main duct and the primary branching ducts of the parotid glands are clearly visible, whereas in patients with Sjögren's, a punctate, globular, cavitary, or destructive appearance can be seen within the parotid glands, correlating well with findings in the minor salivary gland biopsy. However, MRI may not be readily available, it is expensive, and some patient may perceive it as claustrophobic.

Computed Tomography

Using a thin, fan-shaped beam of X-rays, the X-ray tube with its rays of detectors rotates multiple times around the object. Images are then reconstructed to obtain cross-sectional images of the body. X-rays, thus ionizing radiation, are used in both plain-film radiography and CT, but the radiation dose to the patient is significantly higher for a CT exam. CT can be used to visualize structures in and adjacent to the salivary glands. Depending on the imaging protocol, CT can display hard tissue such as calcified tissues, teeth, and bone, as well as minute differences in soft tissue densities. With CT, it is possible to visualize the parenchyma and the main duct of the major salivary glands, but visualization of the fine branching of the ducts requires infusion of a contrast medium (see the earlier section on sialography).

CT of the salivary glands is indicated in assessing acute inflammatory processes and abscesses, cysts, mucoceles, and tumors. For salivary tumors, however, other methods such as MRI and ultrasonography are more sensitive. CT can also be used to detect salivary duct stones.

Major Salivary Gland Ultrasonography

Ultrasonography is a non-invasive, non-irradiating imaging technique based on sound waves. Piezo-electric crystals emit and receive sound waves; the higher the frequency, the better the spatial resolution. The development of transducers has provided both high spatial (geometric) and tissue (contrast) resolution. The parotid and submandibular salivary glands are anatomically situated superficially and thus are well suited for high-frequency transducers. The technique is also readily available and "comfortable" for the patient.

The salivary ducts can be seen, but only if dilated due to retention of saliva. Doppler or color Doppler may be used to facilitate identification of vessels. With power Doppler, the power in the Doppler signal is encoded in color, depending on the amount of blood present. Combining gray-scale salivary gland ultrasound (SGUS) and the color/power Doppler technique has been suggested to provide more details with regard to the blood perfusion of soft tissues and may be of value for narrowing the differential diagnosis.

In the field of Sjögren's, major SGUS has received increasing attention over the last 10 years. The imaging technique shows promise both as part of the diagnostic work-up and in follow-up of natural history or treatment outcome. Parenchymal inhomogeneity and the occurrence of hypoechogenic areas in the glands (Figure 19.3) have been proposed as the best SGUS parameters related to Sjögren's diagnosis. However, several other aspects sometimes have been taken into consideration, such as gland size, hyperechogenic bands, visibility of the borders, and intraglandular calcification (De Vita et al., 1992). As a result, several different SGUS scores have been used over time (summarized in Table 19.1).

Compared to other available techniques (Table 19.2), major salivary gland function may be better evaluated by sialoscintigraphy, but the identification of Sjögren's-associated pathologic changes seems better with SGUS,

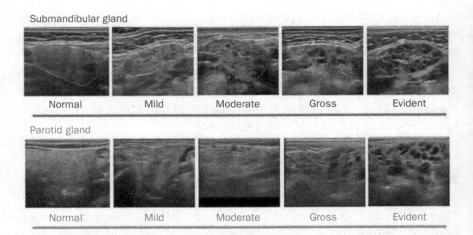

Figure 19.3 Representative images of major SGUS images from patients with Sjögren's. Parenchymal inhomogeneity mostly reflects salivary gland involvement in Sjögren's. The top row shows submandibular glands and the bottom row shows parotid glands, with normal-appearing morphology, mild changes, moderate changes, gross changes, and evident changes.

followed by sialography and sialoscintigraphy (Hocevar et al., 2005). Imaging of the parotid and submandibular glands using SGUS is also less invasive than sialoscintigraphy and salivary gland biopsy. Comparing SGUS and sialoscintigraphy, one study found that SGUS was better while another found SGUS equivalent to MRI. Use of ocular symptoms, oral symptoms, Schirmer's I-test and anti-Ro/SSA compared with use of SGUS, sialoscintigraphy, or minor salivary gland biopsy found that similar numbers of patients fulfilled criteria with positive SGUS and positive sialoscintigraphy, and slightly fewer with a positive minor salivary gland biopsy. The usefulness of SGUS in evaluating therapeutic response to new therapies in clinical trials is under active investigation, as is using SGUS not only for Sjögren's diagnosis but also for follow-up.

Childhood Sjögren's

In parallel, SGUS has also been proposed for the assessment of salivary gland involvement in childhood Sjögren's, a poorly defined and possibly underdiagnosed condition. The disease affects children and adolescents. A variety of organ systems may be affected, resulting in neurologic, dermatologic,

Table 19.1 SGUS Scoring Systems

Lead Author (year)	Scoring System	Calculation
De Vita (1992)	0: Normal 1: Mild: diffuse or localized small hypoechogenic areas 2: Evident: Evident multiple scattered hypoechogenic areas, usually of variable size and not uniformly distributed, and/or multiple or linear non-shadowing densities 3: Gross: Large circumscribed or confluent hypoechogenic areas, and/or gross linear densities, and/or multiple cysts or multiple calcifications, resulting in severe damage to the glandular architecture	Range: 0–6 Sum of the single scores (0–3) for each pair of parotid or submandibular glands. If homonymous glands are discordant for the degree of inhomogeneity, the higher degree should be considered in assessing the (0–3) single score.
Hocevar (2005)	*Parenchymal echogenicity* 0: Comparable to the thyroid gland 1: Decreased compared to the thyroid gland *Homogeneity* 0: Homogenous gland 1: Mild inhomogeneity 2: Evident homogeneity 3: Gross inhomogeneity *Presence of hypoechogenic areas* 0: Absent 1: A few, scattered 2: Several 3: Numerous *Hyperechogenic reflections* *Parotid glands* 0: Absent 1: A few, scattered 2: Several 3: Numerous *Submandibular glands* 0: Absent 1: Present *Clearness of salivary gland borders* 0: Clear, regular defined borders 1: Partly defined borders 2: Ill-defined borders 3: Borders not visible	Range: 0–48 Summation of grades for the five parameters for all four glands. Cut-off ≥ 17
Cornec (De Vita modified) (2013)	0: Normal 1: Small hypoechogenic areas without echogenic bands 2: Multiple hypoechogenic areas measuring <2 mm with echogenic bands 3: Multiple hypoechogenic areas measuring 2–6 mm with hyperechogenic bands 4: Multiple hypoechogenic areas measuring >6 mm or multiple calcifications with echogenic bands	Range: 0–16 In each patient, four grades are obtained (one grade per gland). The highest grade as well as the sum of the grades of the four glands are determined. Cut-off ≥ 2 in each gland (or 8 in the total score)

Continued

Table 19.1 *Continued*

Lead Author (year)	Scoring System	Calculation
Theander (2014)	0: If parenchyma is completely homogeneous 1: If mildly inhomogeneous 2: If several rounded hypoechoic lesions were present 3: If the rounded hypoechoic lesions were either numerous or confluent	Range: 0–3 Consider the highest score among four glands. A score of 0 or 1 is normal or unspecific. A score of 2 or 3 is abnormal and typical for Sjögren's.
Hammenfors (2015)	0: Normal 1: Few minor focal hypo-/anechoic areas 2: Aat least one of the glands was more severely affected with multiple focal hypo-/anechoic areas but some homogenous and normal-appearing salivary gland tissue remained 3: Gevidence of at least two of the glands with minimal normal-appearing glandular tissue remaining, as well as at least a grade 2 affection of the remaining gland(s)	Range: 0–3 Consider the highest score among four glands. A score of 0 or 1 is normal or unspecific. A score of 2 or 3 is abnormal and typical for Sjögren's.

musculoskeletal, vascular, gastrointestinal, respiratory, renal, and hematologic manifestations.

Diagnosis of Sjögren's is based on clinical symptoms and the presence of autoantibodies, after excluding infectious or lymphoproliferative diseases. Diagnosis, treatment, and follow-up of childhood Sjögren's are generally based on clinical experience from Sjögren's in adults, but compared to Sjögren's in adults, childhood patients with Sjögren's often display swelling of the major salivary glands as an initial symptom. Recurrent parotitis in childhood is most commonly of infectious origin or due to retention of saliva. In Sjögren's, parotid swelling usually precedes classic oral and ocular symptoms, while typical serologic findings may be absent. SGUS shows typical features of Sjögren's that can add useful information, and SGUS has been suggested as a routine imaging tool in patients with recurrent parotitis and autoantibodies.

For Further Reading

Astreinidou E, Roesink JM, Raaijmakers CP, et al. 3D MR sialography as a tool to investigate radiation-induced xerostomia: Feasibility study. *Int J Radiat Oncol Biol Phys.* 2007;68(5):1310–1319.

Carotti M, Ciapetti A, Jousse-Joulin S, Salaffi F. Ultrasonography of the salivary glands: The role of grey-scale and colour/power Doppler. *Clin Exp Rheumatol.* 2014;32(1 Suppl 80):S61–S70.

Table 19.2 Current Imaging Methods

Topic	Sialography	Sialoscintigraphy	MRI	US	Clinical Comparisons
Functional information	+(+) Detection of ductal structures	+++ Detection of isotopes	+(+) Examination of perfusion and diffusion	+ Perfusion	Sialoscintigraphy superior
Morphologic information	Filling of contrast in ductal structures	+ Low resolution	+++ Excellent both tissue and spatial resolution	++ Excellent tissue resolution, but problems with anatomic overview	MRI superior in resolution and in making anatomic "maps"
Existing experience	++	+++	+	++	Sialoscintigraphy is a well-established method. US is also widely used. MRI is expensive and time-consuming and is more commonly used for tumors.
Seeing the ducts	+++ Contrast sialography	-	+++ MRI sialography	(+) only if ducts are dilated	Contrast sialography and MR sialography both show the ductal structures.

Source: Geitung JT, Jonsson MV. Imaging technology in Sjögren's syndrome – Non-invasive evaluation of the salivary glands. In: Fox RI and Fox C, editors. Sjögren's syndrome: Pathogenesis and therapy. New York, Dordrecht, Heidelberg, London: Springer; 2011. ISBN: 978-1-60327-956-7, pp 83–9.

Carvajal Alegria G, Costa S, Jousse-Joulin S, et al. What is the agreement between pathological features of parotid gland and labial salivary gland biopsies? *Ann Rheum Dis*. 2018;77(7):e37.

Cornec D, Costa S, Devauchelle-Pensec V, et al. Do high numbers of salivary gland-infiltrating B cells predict better or worse outcomes after rituximab in patients with primary Sjögren's syndrome? *Ann Rheum Dis*. 2016;75(6):e33.

Cornec D, Jousse-Joulin S, Pers JO, et al. Contribution of salivary gland ultrasonography to the diagnosis of Sjögren's syndrome: Toward new diagnostic criteria? *Arthritis Rheum*. 2013;65(1):216–225.

De Vita S, Lorenzon G, Rossi G, et al. Salivary gland echography in primary and secondary Sjögren's syndrome. *Clin Exp Rheumatol*. 1992;10(4):351–356.

El Miedany YM, Ahmed I, Mourad HG, et al. Quantitative ultrasonography and magnetic resonance imaging of the parotid gland: Can they replace the histopathologic studies in patients with Sjögren's syndrome? *Joint Bone Spine*. 2004;71(1):29–38.

Haacke EA, van der Vegt B, Meiners PM, et al. Abatacept treatment of patients with primary Sjögren's syndrome results in a decrease of germinal centres in salivary gland tissue. *Clin Exp Rheumatol*. 2017;35(2):317–320.

Hammenfors DS, Brun JG, Jonsson R, Jonsson MV. Diagnostic utility of major salivary gland ultrasonography in primary Sjögren's syndrome. *Clin Exp Rheumatol*. 2015;33(1):56–62.

Hocevar A, Ambrozic A, Rozman B, et al. Ultrasonographic changes of major salivary glands in primary Sjögren's syndrome: Diagnostic value of a novel scoring system. *Rheumatology*. 2005;44(6):768–772.

Jonsson MV, Baldini C. Major salivary gland ultrasonography in the diagnosis of Sjögren's syndrome: A place in the diagnostic criteria? *Rheum Dis Clin North Am*. 2016;42(3):501–517.

Jousse-Joulin S, Nowak E, Cornec D, et al. Salivary gland ultrasound abnormalities in primary Sjögren's syndrome: Consensual US-SG core items definition and reliability. *RMD Open*. 2017;3(1):e000364.

Lieberman SM. Childhood Sjögren syndrome: Insights from adults and animal models. *Curr Opin Rheumatol*. 2013;25(5):651–657.

Milic VD, Petrovic RR, Boricic IV, et al. Diagnostic value of salivary gland ultrasonographic scoring system in primary Sjögren's syndrome: A comparison with scintigraphy and biopsy. *J Rheumatol*. 2009;36(7):1495–1500.

Milic V, Petrovic R, Boricic I, et al. Ultrasonography of major salivary glands could be an alternative tool to sialoscintigraphy in the American-European classification criteria for primary Sjögren's syndrome. *Rheumatology*. 2012;51(6):1081–1085.

Nieto-Gonzalez JC, Monteagudo I, Bello N, et al. Salivary gland ultrasound in children: A useful tool in the diagnosis of juvenile Sjögren's syndrome. *Clin Exp Rheumatol*. 2014;32(4):578–580.

Pijpe J, Kalk WW, van der Wal JE, et al. Parotid gland biopsy compared with labial biopsy in the diagnosis of patients with primary Sjögren's syndrome. *Rheumatology*. 2007;46(2):335–341.

Risselada AP, Kruize AA, Goldschmeding R, et al. The prognostic value of routinely performed minor salivary gland assessments in primary Sjögren's syndrome. *Ann Rheum Dis*. 2014;73(8):1537–1540.

Rubin P, Holt JF. Secretory sialography in diseases of the major salivary glands. *Am J Roentgenol Radium Ther Nucl Med*. 1957;77(4):575–598.

Shiboski CH, Shiboski SC, Seror R, et al. 2016 American College of Rheumatology/European League Against Rheumatism classification criteria for primary Sjögren's syndrome: A consensus and data-driven methodology involving three international patient cohorts. *Ann Rheum Dis*. 2017;76(1):9–16.

Theander E, Mandl T. Primary Sjögren's syndrome: The diagnostic and prognostic value of salivary gland ultrasonography using a simplified scoring system. *Arthritis Care Res*. 2014;66(7):1102–1107.

Theander E, Vasaitis L, Baecklund E, et al. Lymphoid organisation in labial salivary gland biopsies is a possible predictor for the development of malignant lymphoma in primary Sjögren's syndrome. *Ann Rheum Dis*. 2011;70(8):1363–1368.

Tonami H, Ogawa Y, Matoba M, et al. MR sialography in patients with Sjögren syndrome. *AJNR Am J Neuroradiol*. 1998;19(7):1199–1203.

20

The Difficult-to-Diagnose Sjögren's Patient

Astrid Rasmussen

Sjögren's is a complex disease that can manifest in a great variety of ways. Some patients may have dryness as the most prominent feature, while others can have life-threatening disease or considerable disability and involvement of multiple organs. The chameleonic nature of the disorder and the lack of a single diagnostic test often result in significant difficulty and delay in achieving a correct diagnosis. Reports from the past two decades suggested that a clinical diagnosis of Sjögren's is delayed for 6 to 10 years after the onset of symptoms. Those early years of disease are likely crucial for implementing effective treatment and preventive strategies to delay or avoid the accrual of damage to the affected organs. Major joint efforts by the research community and Sjögren's patient organizations, in particular the Sjögren's Foundation, have led to a significant reduction in the diagnostic delay. The Foundation's "2012 Breakthrough Goal" intended to shorten the time to diagnosis by 50%; at the 5-year mark of the initiative, the reported average time to diagnosis was down to 2.8 years. The strategies used to achieve this notable improvement have been centered around two main themes: (1) increased awareness and education of the public and healthcare professionals and (2) the development of novel guidelines to identify Sjögren's.

To address the question of diagnostic difficulties, it is first important to identify the factors that generate confusion. Top among them is the fact that Sjögren's shares many clinical and laboratory features with other autoimmune diseases, and several diseases may coexist in the same person. These closely related autoimmune diseases are rheumatoid arthritis (RA), systemic lupus erythematosus (SLE), and systemic sclerosis or scleroderma (SSc). Patients with Sjögren's, RA, SLE, and SSc have in common joint pain, arthritis, fatigue, abnormal antibodies in blood (mainly antinuclear antibody [ANA], rheumatoid factor [RF], anti-Ro/SSA, and anti-La/SSB), increased sensitivity to the sun, skin rashes, low cell counts in the blood, and other markers of autoimmunity. In some cases, the patient truly has only one of the diseases, but

Astrid Rasmussen, *The Difficult-to-Diagnose Sjögren's Patient* In: *The Sjögren's Book*. Edited by: Daniel J. Wallace, Oxford University Press. © Sjögren's Foundation 2022. DOI: 10.1093/oso/9780197502112.003.0020 it may be hard to determine which one. In other cases, up to one-third of patients in the case of RA for example, there is overlap with Sjögren's, and the diagnosis may end up being one of an overlap syndrome or Sjögren's in addition to RA. Unfortunately, at this point we still do not possess a single, "gold standard" diagnostic test for Sjögren's. But awareness and education about these confounding factors should be helpful, and hopefully in the near future, the unmet need for accurate and easily accessible diagnostic tests for Sjögren's will be resolved.

Differential Diagnosis: Is it Sjögren's or Something Else?

To understand which patients are most likely to be misdiagnosed with other autoimmune diseases, we undertook a study in 1,175 patients being evaluated for Sjögren's in a research clinic. We compared the signs and symptoms of patients who had previously received a diagnosis or suspected diagnosis of RA, SLE, or SSc with those who did not have such prior diagnoses. Of all the patients who had sicca symptoms, 524 (~45%) had been given an initial diagnosis different from Sjögren's, most commonly RA or SLE. Exhaustive investigation into their clinical problems revealed that only 130 (24.5%) actually had SLE or RA; close to half of all of the patients with dry eyes and dry mouth and a prior diagnosis of another autoimmune disease in reality had Sjögren's and the diagnosis had been missed or delayed. The factors that influenced the non-Sjögren's diagnoses were related to sociodemographic characteristics that have classically been associated with each of the other diseases: Being younger and female increased the likelihood of a suspicion of SLE, while being older and non-White increased the suspicion of RA. This was particularly evident in patients who had been tested for multiple antibodies and were negative for the classical Sjögren's anti-Ro/SSA and anti-La/SSB autoantibodies at their initial evaluation, probably biasing the diagnostic suspicion toward other diseases. Additionally, patients who tested positive for ANA were more likely to be told initially that they had SLE. While ANAs are present in more than 95% of SLE patients, they are also present in the majority of patients with Sjögren's; therefore, in patients with dry eyes or dry mouth, ANA positivity should not be considered sufficient to diagnose SLE. Similarly, the patients who tested positive for RF tended to be initially suspected of having RA. RF is identified in the blood of 70% to 90% of RA cases but is also quite common in Sjögren's (36–74%). Thus, neither ANA nor RF is sufficient to rule out Sjögren's.

Then there is the case of multiple overlapping autoimmune diseases. The coexistence of Sjögren's and SLE has ranged between 9% and 19% in several studies, and up to 34% of SLE patients report symptoms of dryness. When analyzed in the reverse direction, the most common autoimmune disease that Sjögren's patients develop is SLE. Sicca symptoms are present in 30% to 50% of patients afflicted by RA, and eventually 4% to 31% of those will have full-blown Sjögren's as well. When a patient suffers from overlapping conditions, two important factors must be kept in mind: They will need follow-up and management of both their conditions, and overlapping syndromes often have clinical peculiarities that are different from patients with a single disease. All these findings highlight that, in clinical practice, there are diagnostic challenges that require experience and a high level of suspicion on the part of the clinician.

Clinical Diagnosis Versus Research Classification

For research purposes, consistent identification of well-characterized and homogeneous patients is paramount to ensure valid results and to protect study participants from exposure to unjustifiable risks in clinical trials. With these goals in mind, several research classification methods for Sjögren's have been described. However, the rigor required for research is not equivalent to what is desirable in clinical practice. The clinician and the patient suffering from symptoms related to Sjögren's should find a balance between obtaining support and treatment for milder or less well-defined cases (which would not meet the research classification definitions) and over-diagnosing any person with dry eyes or dry mouth as having an autoimmune condition. While it may be tempting to use research definitions to solidly diagnose Sjögren's in the clinic, an additional drawback is that the classification criteria require a multidisciplinary team and invasive procedures that are often inaccessible in clinical practice. Nevertheless, the criteria can be used as a frame of reference for the clinician, and judicious, stepwise approaches using some of the criteria items can be of great help when the diagnosis is not obvious.

More than a dozen research classification systems have been developed, but until quite recently, the most widely used were the 2002 revised American European Consensus Group (AECG) classification criteria. A modified version was sponsored and approved by both the American College of Rheumatology and the European League Against Rheumatism in 2016 (ACR-EULAR criteria).

The 2002 AECG and 2016 ACR-EULAR criteria are designed to evaluate patients presenting with symptoms of dry eyes or dry mouth or clinical suspicion of Sjögren's. To determine whether complaints of dry eyes or dry mouth rise to the level of true sicca, six standardized questions are used as a screening tool. The tests used in the criteria are measurement of the volume of tears produced in 5 minutes (Schirmer's I-test); evaluation of damage to the surface of the eye through staining of the ocular surface and visualization with a slit-lamp exam (van Bijsterveld or Ocular Staining Score); and measurement of the volume of saliva produced in 15 minutes (whole unstimulated salivary flow). Formal evaluation of autoimmunity requires the identification of auto-antibodies in blood, specifically anti-Ro/SSA and in some cases anti-La/SSB, and determining whether there are abnormal numbers and conglomerates of lymphocytes (a type of white blood cell) in the salivary glands (focus score). This is done by performing a biopsy of the lower lip to obtain a few minor salivary glands and observing them under the microscope. A person is classified as having Sjögren's when they meet a minimum of four criteria (AECG) or points (ACR-EULAR); either an abnormal result on the minor salivary gland biopsy or positive anti-Ro/SSA in blood is required. A description of classification criteria can be found in the chapter on classification (see Chapter 17).

From Research to the Doctor's Office

As mentioned earlier, the question then becomes how to translate this research tool into clinical practice for better and more timely diagnoses. Given that these criteria were developed by expert clinicians and that the criteria have very good agreement with clinical judgment, modified versions should be applicable for the practicing clinician. Several ideas come to mind, including a stepwise process for patient assessment in which the least invasive and most accessible tests are used as screening measures. The obvious place to start would be to use the six standardized questions of the AECG criteria to determine if the suspicion of Sjögren's warrants additional investigation.

Next, measurements of saliva and tear production are non-invasive tests that can easily be performed in a regular clinical practice without specialized training or equipment. The saliva is collected in a pre-weighed container; the patient is asked to let saliva pool in the mouth and then drool into the container periodically for 15 minutes. The container with the collected saliva is weighed again and the result is subtracted from the initial weight of the empty container. The result in grams is a good estimate of the volume of saliva produced in mL; any value of 1.5 mL or less is suggestive of Sjögren's. The

Schirmer's test, which should be performed without local anesthesia, is used to quantify the tear production by letting filter-paper strips marked with a scale from 0 to 35 mm become impregnated with tears for 5 minutes. This is done for both eyes; if the strip from either eye is impregnated to 5 mm or less in 5 minutes, the tear production is considered abnormal.

Corroboration of autoimmunity by testing for autoantibodies against ANA, RF, Ro/SSA, and La/SSB in blood is the next step. This is a minimally invasive procedure that only requires a blood draw and is also accessible for most clinicians. A patient describing ocular and oral symptoms of dryness, and who has an abnormal Schirmer's I-test or salivary flow and presence of anti-Ro/SSA or anti-La/SSB in serum, can be diagnosed with Sjögren's without the need for additional invasive or specialized procedures.

If additional tests are needed, and the clinical suspicion is not sufficient for the clinician to be comfortable with a diagnosis of Sjögren's, referral for more specialized studies that are not painful should be the next step. The two main avenues to pursue are the ocular exam by an eye specialist and ultrasound of the salivary glands. Both the ocular surface staining and tear break-up time, performed by a professional with adequate training, and the ultrasound evaluation of the parotid and submandibular salivary glands in search of Sjögren's-specific findings are significantly less invasive than the biopsy and have the built-in benefit of screening for disease-related ocular damage and the potential detection of tumors that may occur in the salivary glands of Sjögren's patients.

In a non-research setting, the salivary gland biopsy becomes the definitive or necessary test only for patients who do not have Sjögren's autoantibodies or when the clinician is concerned about the risk of lymphoma (a cancer of the lymphatic system). The biopsy can be done for the minor salivary glands of the lip or the parotid glands. The lip glands are often the glands of choice because they are easily accessible and there is no visible scar resulting from their removal because they are obtained from the inside of the mouth. In trained hands, the procedure is very safe and bleeding or infections are rare, although there is a small risk of damage to local nerves. The alternative is to biopsy the parotid glands, which are located over the jaw and in front of the earlobe. They are biopsied by making a small incision below and slightly behind the earlobe, and a few stiches are necessary. The resulting scar is small but not completely invisible; the risk of facial nerve damage is also present, but complications are rare. Advocates of parotid gland biopsies note that lymphomas associated with Sjögren's are most often localized in these glands, and therefore the parotid should be the tissue to biopsy. Also, each lip gland is removed in its entirety, so the exact same gland cannot be biopsied more than once for purposes of follow-up. The opposite is the case with the parotid glands; they are large, superficial, and easily accessible, and can therefore be biopsied more than once if necessary.

Atypical and Extreme Cases of Sjögren's

Among the patients who are difficult to diagnose are those whose symptoms and clinical findings are at the extremes of the Sjögren's spectrum and those who have diseases that may mimic classical sicca or extraglandular Sjögren's features and that may not be autoimmune in nature. The differential diagnosis for these patients requires a higher level of suspicion and diligence on part of the medical team to ensure that an accurate diagnosis is reached.

When the disease manifests mildly or the complaints are mostly restricted to dryness, patients are often dismissed as having "just a nuisance disease" or no Sjögren's at all. It is common to learn that middle-aged females with vaginal and skin dryness accompanying ocular and oral dryness and possibly fatigue have been told that their dryness is related to menopause and that no further diagnostic work-up is warranted. Similarly, in areas with a high prevalence of seasonal allergies that are treated with antihistamine drugs, the cause of dryness can be difficult to distinguish: Sicca may be a secondary effect of the medications, but a patient with allergies and dryness can also suffer from Sjögren's. In these instances, an attentive professional should rule out Sjögren's when the patient does not improve after temporarily suspending the allergy medications, or if additional features such as joint pain and fatigue are present. Another often-overlooked cause of sicca localized to the eye and mouth is radiation therapy of the head and neck, which can cause permanent damage to the salivary glands and reduced saliva production.

On the opposite side of the clinical spectrum, severe Sjögren's that affects organs other than the eyes and mouth can also be hard to pinpoint. Some patients with Sjögren's first present with aggressive disease that affects the lungs, kidneys, brain, or nerves or even manifests as lymphoma; in such cases, little attention may be given to a history of dry eyes and dry mouth, resulting in delayed suspicion of Sjögren's.

Among non-autoimmune diseases that should be suspected when there are unusual symptoms or in patients with known risk factors are infectious diseases. The most relevant ones to screen for are hepatitis C virus (HCV), human immunodeficiency virus (HIV), and human T-lymphotropic virus type 1 (HTLV-1).

Chronic infection with hepatitis C may present with Sjögren's-like symptoms in up to 10% to 12% of infected patients; these include sicca symptoms, fatigue, joint pain, and abnormalities in the salivary glands. Additionally, about half of all HCV-positive subjects have abnormal auto-antibodies in blood that can also be found in Sjögren's, such as RF and anti-thyroid antibodies. Given that there are now effective treatments for HCV infection and that untreated chronic HCV can result in irreversible liver damage, cirrhosis, and liver cancer, screening for HCV is advisable in patients with suspected Sjögren's.

Acute or early infection with HIV can also mimic autoimmune diseases, manifesting with ulcers in the mouth, fatigue, joint pain, enlarged lymph nodes, and fever; the symptoms of sicca are less prominent, but there may be swelling of the parotid gland. Screening for HIV is warranted if there is any suspicion of associated risk factors so that transmission prevention and treatment can immediately be implemented.

HTLV-1 is a virus that causes symptoms in only about 5% of those infected but can result in a wide range of clinical manifestations, the most severe of which are leukemia and a type of progressive paralysis. Some HTLV-1-infected patients have Sjögren's features including dry eyes and mouth, scarring of the surface of the eye, joint pain, Raynaud's, and abnormalities in the salivary gland biopsy. These Sjögren's-like patients with HTLV-1 sometimes go on to develop paralysis as well. Unfortunately, no therapy has proven effective for such a complication, but symptomatic treatment that includes steroids can reduce disability and improve quality of life.

Two noninfectious disorders in which immune cells infiltrate the salivary and lacrimal glands must also be considered in the differential diagnosis: IgG4-related disease (IgG4-RD) and sarcoidosis.

IgG4-RD should be suspected in patients who have swelling of the lacrimal or salivary glands, in particular when the salivary glands that are located below the chin and jawline (submandibular salivary glands) are bilaterally swollen, or when the tear glands are so enlarged that they are easily visible. A peculiarity of IgG4-RD is that there is only mild eye and mouth dryness despite very enlarged glands, and, in general terms, those affected do not have Sjögren's autoantibodies in their blood. An additional clue to IgG4-RD is when the patient with glandular enlargement also has a history of pancreatitis. The disease is diagnosed by biopsy of the affected gland and measurement in blood of the IgG4 subtype of immunoglobulin.

Sarcoidosis is a disease that causes "clumps" or clusters of abnormal tissue in the body called granulomas. These granulomas, depending on their number, size, and location, can prevent organs from functioning properly and cause swelling. The most commonly affected organ is the lung, but between 5% and 10% of patients with sarcoidosis have granulomas in salivary or lacrimal glands. The result can be enlargement of the glands and Sjögren's symptoms, including sicca and arthritis. Rarely, sarcoidosis can present with acute bilateral swelling of the parotid, submandibular, and lacrimal glands accompanied by fever, which is very uncommon in Sjögren's. In most cases, a plain chest X-ray will show enough findings to guide the diagnosis of sarcoidosis, but sometimes a gland biopsy is necessary to make the distinction with Sjögren's.

Finally, enlargement of the glands may be due to lymphoma, a cancer that can appear in the absence of Sjögren's but for which Sjögren's patients have an elevated risk. Therefore, persistently enlarged glands justify doing a biopsy to ensure that a tumor is not being missed.

While this is by no means an exhaustive list of the situations in which Sjögren's is not readily suspected or could be hard to diagnose, the most important lesson to derive is that knowledge and awareness about Sjögren's by not only healthcare providers but also patients and their advocates is crucial for opportune diagnosis, treatment, and prevention of complications.

Summing Up

- Sjögren's is a complex disease with numerous manifestations and features, many of which are shared with other autoimmune diseases. There is no single diagnostic test. These are major contributors to the difficulty and the delay in diagnosis that are often seen.
- Relying on research classification criteria for a diagnosis has drawbacks, including the need for a multidisciplinary team and invasive procedures, both of which depend on accessibility.
- Implementing a stepwise approach to patient assessment can help overcome barriers to a timely and accurate diagnosis. For example, begin with the least invasive and most accessible tests and proceed to incorporate additional tests as needed to help confirm or rule out a diagnosis of Sjögren's.
- Extreme symptoms and clinical findings as well as differential diagnoses further contribute to the difficulty in accurately diagnosing Sjögren's. These situations require a higher level of diligence by the medical team.
- Increased education and awareness by all stakeholders is important to further improve our abilities to diagnose, treat, and prevent Sjögren's-related complications.

For Further Reading

Brito-Zeron P, Baldini C, Bootsma H, et al. Sjogren syndrome. *Nat Rev Dis Primers.* 2016;2:16047.

Mariette X, Criswell LA. Primary Sjögren's syndrome. *N Engl J Med.* 2018;378:931–939.

Rasmussen A, Radfar L, Lewis D, et al. Previous diagnosis of Sjögren's syndrome as rheumatoid arthritis or systemic lupus erythematosus. *Rheumatology.* 2016;55:1195–1201.

Shiboski CH, Shiboski SC, Seror R, et al. 2016 American College of Rheumatology/European League Against Rheumatism classification criteria for primary Sjögren's syndrome: A consensus and data-driven methodology involving three international patient cohorts. *Arthritis Rheumatol.* 2017;69:35–45 and *Ann Rheum Dis.* 2017;76:9–16.

Vitali C, Bombardieri S, Jonsson R, et al. Classification criteria for Sjögren's syndrome: A revised version of the European criteria proposed by the American-European Consensus Group. *Ann Rheum Dis.* 2002;61:554–558.

21

Diseases Associated with Sjögren's

Janet Lewis and Frederick B. Vivino

Sjögren's may occur in isolation or it may be found in association with another autoimmune disease. About half of those with Sjögren's have Sjögren's alone and about half have another major rheumatic, autoimmune disease with their Sjögren's. Examples of autoimmune disorders associated with Sjögren's include rheumatoid arthritis (RA) and systemic lupus erythematosus (SLE). Symptoms and signs caused by these associated autoimmune disorders can have an impact on treatment and potential complications in people with more than one related disease. Early and accurate diagnosis of associated autoimmune conditions is key to the successful management and long-term outcomes of Sjögren's. The signs, symptoms, and relationship of these disorders to Sjögren's are discussed in this chapter.

Definitions and Terms

An autoimmune disease is the result of the immune system attacking the cells, tissues, and organs of the body. Often these diseases are associated with autoantibodies in the blood (i.e., antibodies directed against one's own cells or tissues). The term "autoimmune connective tissue disorder" or "collagen vascular disease" refers to a group of chronic, autoimmune, inflammatory diseases that affect the connective tissues of the body. The autoimmune response results in inflammation, which can affect various organs in the body. Common symptoms of connective tissue disorders include arthritis (swelling of the joints), joint pain, muscle pain/inflammation, Raynaud's phenomenon (see later in the chapter), skin rashes, fatigue, interstitial lung disease (scarring of the lungs), esophageal dysmotility (disordered contraction of the esophagus), acid reflux, and kidney disease. Other internal organs may also be affected.

Janet Lewis and Frederick B. Vivino, *Diseases Associated with Sjögren's* In: *The Sjögren's Book*. Edited by: Daniel J. Wallace, Oxford University Press. © Sjögren's Foundation 2022. DOI: 10.1093/oso/9780197502112.003.0021

Connective Tissue Disorders

The connective tissue disorders that are most commonly associated with Sjögren's include RA, SLE, scleroderma, polymyositis, dermatomyositis, mixed connective tissue disease, undifferentiated connective tissue disease, and vasculitis.

Rheumatoid Arthritis

RA is the most common autoimmune rheumatic disease and may affect up to 1% to 1.5% of the North American population. It occurs most often in people 40 to 60 years old but may develop at any age, even in children. It is more common in women than men, with a female-to-male ratio of 2.5 to 1. As the name implies, the target organ for inflammation in RA is the joint, particularly the joint lining (the synovium). RA patients typically develop painful swelling of small and large joints over a period of weeks to months. It typically is a symmetrical polyarthritis, meaning that it affects multiple joints on both sides of the body. The onset of joint symptoms is usually gradual, occurring over weeks to months, but in rare cases this process occurs more acutely. The proximal interphalangeal and metacarpophalangeal joints (the two sets of knuckle joints closest to the wrist) of the hands as well as the wrists, elbows, shoulders, hips, knees, ankles, and feet are often affected. People with RA often have associated fatigue and generalized morning stiffness that can limit mobility and lasts 45 to 60 minutes or longer before maximal improvement. In some cases, subcutaneous nodules (firm lumps underneath the skin) called rheumatoid nodules develop. Often these are located on the hands or near the elbows, but they also can be found on areas that are pressure points.

Box 21.1 describes the clinical and laboratory features used in the diagnosis of RA. The diagnosis of RA is based on clinical findings, laboratory studies, X-rays, and joint fluid analysis. The latter test is performed by taking a small sample of synovial fluid from a swollen joint to look for inflammation and to rule out infection and other causes of arthritis. The diagnosis of RA requires the presence of arthritis symptoms for at least 6 weeks. A blood test for rheumatoid factor (RF) is positive in up to 85% of patients with RA. Although helpful in the diagnosis of RA, serum RF is not specific for this disease and may occur in Sjögren's as well as other connective tissue diseases. A second blood test for RA is the anti-cyclic citrullinated peptide (CCP) antibody. CCP antibodies occur with a similar frequency as RF in people with RA but are felt to be more specific for this disease. This means that CCP antibodies are

---

Box 21.1 2010 American College of Rheumatology (ACR)-European League Against Rheumatism (EULAR) Classification Criteria for Rheumatoid Arthritis

A. Joint involvement

1 large joint: 0 points

2–10 large joints: 1 point

1–3 small joints (with or without involvement of large joints): 2 points

4–10 small joints (with or without involvement of large joints): 3 points

>10 joints (at least 1 small joint): 5 points

B. Serology (at least 1 test result is needed for classification)

Negative RF *and* negative ACPA: 0 points

Low-positive RF *or* low-positive ACPA: 2 points

High-positive RF *or* high-positive ACPA: 3 points

C. Acute-phase reactants (at least 1 test result is needed for classification)

Normal CRP *and* normal ESR: 0 points

Abnormal CRP *or* abnormal ESR: 1 point

D. Duration of symptoms

<6 weeks: 0 points

>6 weeks 1 point

Add score of categories A–D; if greater than or equal to 6 points, the patient can be considered to have definite RA unless there is another explanation for their arthritis.

Source: Jonathan Kay, Katherine S. Upchurch, ACR/EULAR 2010 rheumatoid arthritis classification criteria, *Rheumatology*, Volume 51, Issue suppl_6, December 2012, Pages vi5–vi9.

---

uncommonly found in conditions other than RA. Up to 20% of people with RA may test negative for both RF and CCP antibodies. X-rays in chronic cases of RA often show symmetrical narrowing of joint spaces due to cartilage loss, thinning of bone around inflamed joints (periarticular osteopenia), and erosions. Erosions (little holes at the edges of the bone ends) are a sign of joint damage from RA. In a subset of patients with RA the inflammation can affect other organs such as the lungs and eyes. About 35% of people with RA have Sjögren's. An inflammatory polyarthritis that resembles RA can develop in people with Sjögren's, but it is typically not as severe as RA and generally bone erosions are not observed.

Most cases of RA require aggressive treatment, including multiple mediations and physical therapy to prevent disability, deformity, and other complications. Nonsteroidal anti-inflammatory drugs (NSAIDs) (e.g., ibuprofen), oral and intra-articular steroids, hydroxychloroquine (Plaquenil), methotrexate, leflunomide (Arava), and the TNF-α inhibitors (etanercept [Enbrel], infliximab [Remicade], adalimumab [Humira], golimumab [Simponi], certolizumab pegol [Cimzia]) are the most commonly used treatments. Rituximab (Rituxan), abatacept (Orencia), and tofacitinib (Xeljanz) are also used. Patients who fail to respond to medical therapy eventually may require joint replacement surgery.

Systemic Lupus Erythematosus

SLE is a chronic autoimmune rheumatic disorder characterized by immune complex (antigen–antibody complexes) deposition in various tissues. These deposits result in inflammation that can affect multiple organs and lead to damage or even organ failure. SLE is associated with antinuclear antibody (ANA) production in the blood. In North America, lupus affects approximately 0.05% of the general population and preferentially strikes young women (female-to-male ratio is 8:1) in the 15- to 40-year old age group, especially African Americans. Less commonly, SLE occurs among men, children, older adults, and other ethnic/racial groups. Lupus can run in families.

Because lupus patients may manifest a myriad of findings, diagnosis can be challenging. Several different classifications are used as guidelines in the diagnosis of SLE. The Systemic Lupus International Collaborating Clinics (SLICC) criteria are one of the more commonly used sets of criteria for research classification and also provide a useful framework for diagnosis (Box 21.2).

The most characteristic skin and mucous membrane abnormalities include the malar rash, discoid rash, skin photosensitivity, oral ulcers, or nasal ulcers. The malar or butterfly rash looks like a red patch over the nasal bridge, nose, and cheeks in the shape of a butterfly and heals without scarring. In contrast, discoid lupus causes raised, pink to red plaques on the head and extremities. These plaques are often associated with scaling and follicular plugging (skin pores/hair follicles develop dark spots), which can result in loss of pigmentation, scarring, and/or loss of hair. In some instances, patients with lupus develop severe skin rashes in sun-exposed areas (photosensitive rashes) following brief exposure to the sun or ultraviolet light. Some of the less common lupus rashes can present as hives or blisters or resemble the lesions of psoriasis, which can add to the challenge of making a diagnosis of lupus. Painless or painful oral and nasal ulcers can also occur.

The diagnostic hallmark of SLE is the presence of ANAs, found in 95% or more of patients. Cases of ANA-negative lupus (i.e., patients with clinical

Box 21.2 2012 SLICC Criteria for the Classification of SLE

Clinical criteria

1. —Acute cutaneous lupus
2. —Chronic cutaneous lupus
3. —Nonscarring alopecia
4. —Oral or nasal ulcers
5. —Arthritis
6. —Serositis
7. —Renal disorder
8. —Neurologic disorder
9. —Hemolytic anemia
10. —Leukopenia of lymphopenia
11. —Thrombocytopenia

Immunologic criteria

1. —Positive ANA
2. —Positive anti-dsDNA
3. —Positive anti-Sm
4. —Positive antiphospholipid antibodies
5. —Low complement levels
6. —Positive direct Coombs test

Note: A patient is classified as having SLE if he or she satisfies four of the clinical and immunologic criteria used in the SLICC classification criteria, including at least one clinical criterion and one immunologic criterion. Alternatively, according to the SLICC criteria, a patient is classified as having SLE if he or she has biopsy-proven nephritis compatible with SLE in the presence of ANAs or anti-dsDNA antibodies.

Source: Petri M, Orbai AM, Alarcón GS, et al. Derivation and validation of the Systemic Lupus International Collaborating Clinics classification criteria for systemic lupus erythematosus. *Arthritis Rheum.* 2012;64(8):2677–2686. doi:10.1002/art.34473

lupus but a negative ANA blood test) are uncommon but have been described. The common marker autoantibodies for Sjögren's, anti-SSA and anti-SSB, are also found in 15% to 45% of SLE patients. Anti-Sm antibodies, another type of autoantibody, are very specific for SLE but are found in less than 30% of patients with SLE. Anti–double-stranded-DNA antibodies occur in less than 60% of patients with SLE. In some lupus patients, the level of anti–double-stranded DNA antibodies may rise with disease flares and fall during periods of remission. Like anti-Sm antibodies, anti–double-stranded DNA antibodies are fairly specific for SLE and, thus, are not commonly found in other autoimmune diseases, although they have been reported in a few patients with Sjögren's.

Constitutional symptoms in lupus include fevers, weight loss, malaise, and fatigue. Internal organ involvement in SLE also can cause serious and sometimes life-threatening complications. Interstitial lung disease (scarring of the lungs), pleurisy (inflammation of the lining around the lung), pleural effusions, pneumonitis (lung inflammation), and pulmonary hemorrhage all cause shortness of breath and, in the most severe cases, can lead to respiratory failure. Pericarditis (inflammation of the heart lining) and pericardial effusions (fluid surrounding the heart) can cause chest pain and shortness of breath. Heart failure, valvular heart disease, and accelerated coronary atherosclerosis also can occur. Acute or chronic kidney inflammation (lupus nephritis) can lead to loss of kidney function. Signs of kidney involvement include abnormal amounts of protein, cells, and/or casts (clumps of white or red blood cells) in the urine as well as a rise in the serum creatinine level, which is a measure of kidney function. In the most severe cases, lupus nephritis may rapidly progress, and prompt recognition and treatment are needed to prevent permanent kidney damage that can lead to kidney failure requiring dialysis.

Serious complications can also develop as a result of central nervous system involvement. Lupus can cause seizures, psychosis, coma, stroke, mini-stroke, mood disorders, confusion, cognitive dysfunction, severe headaches, chorea (movement disorders), transverse myelitis (spinal cord damage due to inflammation), and abnormalities of the cranial nerves. Peripheral neuropathies also occur.

Musculoskeletal manifestations of lupus are common and include joint and muscle pain. The arthritis of SLE often affects the same joints that are affected by RA. It can cause deformities similar to those seen in RA but rarely causes erosions noted by X-ray.

Blood abnormalities in lupus include autoimmune hemolytic anemia (low red blood cell count due to destruction of the red blood cells) and thrombocytopenia (low platelets). In these conditions the body forms antibodies against its own red blood cells or platelets. The anemia can cause fatigue and shortness of breath, while the low platelet count can cause bleeding.

The 10-year survival rate in lupus is approximately 90%. While SLE can be a serious disease, many patients with SLE have mild cases (e.g., skin rashes, joint pain) that do not require treatment with potent immunosuppressive drugs. Skin rashes, hair loss, and oral ulcers often can be effectively managed with hydroxychloroquine, other antimalarial drugs, and/or topical steroids. Hydroxychloroquine and NSAIDs alleviate arthritis and joint or muscle pain. Use of oral steroids (e.g., prednisone), intravenous steroids, and/or more toxic immunosuppressives (e.g., azathioprine [Imuran], cyclophosphamide [Cytoxan], mycophenolate [Cellcept]) is indicated in patients who fail to respond to more conservative measures or develop life-threatening problems such as hemolytic anemia, severe thrombocytopenia, or disease of the heart, lungs, kidneys, or central nervous system. Belimumab (Benlysta) is a newer biologic medication that can be effective in controlling manifestations of SLE.

Scleroderma

Scleroderma (also known as systemic sclerosis) is an autoimmune rheumatic disease characterized by progressive thickening of the skin. Scleroderma can also cause fibrosis (scarring) of the internal organs and thickening of small blood vessels. It is an uncommon disorder that affects only a small percentage of the general population (0.02–0.075%), with peak occurrence at ages 35 to 65 years and a female preponderance. In the early stages it causes puffiness of the hands, later followed by skin thickening of the fingers and toes. The skin on the digits becomes tight and shiny, like leather (sclerodactyly), and this process gradually spreads up the arms and legs to involve the face and, occasionally, the trunk as well. Diagnosis can be made by skin biopsy or documentation of skin involvement and typical features by an experienced clinician. Diagnosis of scleroderma requires the presence of one major and two minor criteria (Box 21.3).

Patients are classified into disease subsets and prognostic categories according to the degree of skin involvement and autoantibody profile. Limited scleroderma and diffuse scleroderma are the two main subsets of scleroderma. People with limited scleroderma have skin thickening limited to the distal limbs (below the elbows and knees) without truncal involvement. About 40% to 50% of people with limited scleroderma test positive for the anti-centromere antibody. Skin involvement of the face may occur. CREST syndrome is a type of limited scleroderma. The letters in CREST stand for calcinosis cutis (calcium deposits in the skin), Raynaud's phenomenon, esophageal dysmotility (disordered contractions of the esophagus), sclerodactyly, and telangiectasia (small dilated blood vessels in the skin and mucous membranes). People with diffuse scleroderma have more widespread skin thickening that affects the hands and feet and often extends above the elbows and knees. Additionally it may affect the skin on the trunk. Roughly 20% to 30% of people with diffuse scleroderma test positive for an antibody called anti-Scl-70. In general, diffuse scleroderma tends to result in more complications due to greater internal organ disease.

Box 21.3 2013 American College of Rheumatology (ACR)-European League Against Rheumatism (EULAR) Criteria for the Classification of Systemic Sclerosis

---

A. Skin thickening

Skin thickening of the fingers of both hands extending proximal to the metacarpophalangeal (MCP) joints: 9 points

Skin thickening of the fingers that does not extend proximal to the MCP joints: 4 points

Puffy fingers: 2 points

B. Fingertip lesion

Digital tip ulcers: 2 points

Digital pitting scars: 3 points

C. Telangiectasias: 2 points

D. Abnormal nailfold capillaries: 2 points

E. Pulmonary arterial hypertension and/or interstitial lung disease: 2 points

F. Raynaud's phenomenon: 3 points

G. +Scleroderma-related antibodies (anti-centromere, Scl70, or RNP polymerase III): 3 points

Add up the points in each category. For categories A and B, count only 1 item within each category using the item with the highest number of points.

If the score adds up to 9 or more points, this is considered to be definite systemic sclerosis.

These criteria should not be used for people who have a systemic sclerosis-like disorder. Alternatively, according to the SLICC criteria, a patient is classified as having SLE if he or she has biopsy-proven nephritis compatible with SLE in the presence of ANAs or anti-dsDNA antibodies.

Source: van den Hoogen F, Khanna D, Fransen J, et al. 2013 classification criteria for systemic sclerosis: an American college of rheumatology/European league against rheumatism collaborative initiative. *Annals of the Rheumatic Diseases* 2013;72:1747–1755.

Raynaud's phenomenon (cold-induced color changes in the fingers) is discussed later in the chapter and may predate the onset of scleroderma by months to years. In addition to skin thickening, patients can also develop itching, malaise, fatigue, arthritis, and musculoskeletal pain. Involvement of the gastrointestinal tract can cause difficulty swallowing due to esophageal dysmotility (disordered contractions of the esophagus) and severe gastroesophageal reflux disease (GERD). Involvement of the lungs can lead to shortness of breath. Diffuse scleroderma is associated with interstitial fibrosis (scarring of the lung tissue), and limited scleroderma is associated with pulmonary hypertension (high blood pressure in the blood vessels in the lungs) in a relatively small number of patients. Pericarditis, pericardial effusions (fluid around the heart), heart rhythm abnormalities, and heart failure can result from inflammation and scarring of cardiac tissue. Severe hypertension can be associated with sudden and rapidly progressive renal failure (scleroderma renal crisis); this is a medical emergency that requires aggressive management of blood pressure and may necessitate dialysis if not quickly brought under control. Muscle weakness due to myositis (muscle inflammation) can also occur.

Symptomatic treatments for scleroderma are available and used according to organ involvement. Some patients will note spontaneous improvement of skin thickening. Medications such as methotrexate or mycophenolate mofetil can be of benefit for some of the manifestations of scleroderma. Acid reflux is treated by dietary modification and use of proton pump inhibitors (e.g., omeprazole [Prilosec]). Angiotensin-converting enzyme (ACE) inhibitors (e.g., captopril) can control blood pressure and preserve kidney function if initiated early in scleroderma renal crisis.

Raynaud's Phenomenon

Raynaud's phenomenon is defined as cold-induced color changes of the fingers, toes, nose, or earlobes that result from spasm and/or thickening of small arteries at involved sites. It can exist as an isolated problem (primary Raynaud's disease) or in association with any of the connective tissue disorders, including Sjögren's (secondary Raynaud's). Individuals with scleroderma tend to have particularly severe Raynaud's symptoms. People with Raynaud's typically develop blanching (white coloration) of part of the fingers or involved areas after exposure to cold, followed by cyanosis (bluing) and later erythema (redness) upon rewarming. Sometimes episodes can be induced by nicotine from cigarettes or emotional stress. Primary Raynaud's disease usually affects young women and may be annoying to the patient but seldom causes significant discomfort or permanent damage. In contrast, secondary Raynaud's may cause a significant disruption of blood flow to the tissue to the extent that it results in complications such as digital ulcers, infections, loss of fingertip pads or bone, and even digital gangrene (blackening of the fingers due to death of the tissue). People with Raynaud's should avoid the cold and other precipitating factors. Medications such as calcium channel blockers (e.g., nifedipine [Procardia]), which relax the blood vessels, and antiplatelet agents such as aspirin, which help prevent clots, can be of benefit for Raynaud's symptoms. Phosphodiesterase inhibitors, which are used to treat erectile dysfunction (e.g., sildenafil [Viagra]), may also provide relief. Very severe cases may require use of intravenous medications, nerve blocks, or surgical amputation.

Polymyositis and Dermatomyositis

Polymyositis and dermatomyositis represent a group of autoimmune rheumatic diseases that cause skeletal muscle weakness. These diseases are due to inflammation of the muscles (myositis). Dermatomyositis also causes a characteristic rash. These disorders affect 0.05% to 0.08% of the population, with peak age at onset of 10 to 15 years in children and 45 to 60 years in adults. The female-to-male ratio is 2:1. Polymyositis is more common than dermatomyositis in adults, but the reverse is true for children.

Symptoms of muscle weakness typically develop slowly over weeks to months. Usually the muscle weakness is symmetrical (affects both sides of the body) and affects the proximal muscles (large muscles around the hips and shoulders) rather than the distal muscles of the limbs. Muscle involvement may cause difficulty getting up from a chair, climbing stairs, walking, or raising an arm to comb the hair or lift an object overhead. The myositis may spread to muscles that control breathing or swallowing, resulting in shortness of breath or dysphagia (difficulty swallowing). Other problems can include fatigue, arthritis, joint and muscle pain, Raynaud's, interstitial lung disease, acid reflux, esophageal dysmotility, and heart failure. Sjögren's can complicate polymyositis and dermatomyositis, and myositis can occasionally be a manifestation of Sjögren's.

People with dermatomyositis exhibit one or more of several characteristic rashes. These include a heliotrope rash (lilac discoloration of the eyelids), Gottron's sign/papules (a scaly, red rash over the knuckles that may be raised), shawl sign (redness of the upper back, posterior shoulders, and back of the neck), and the V sign (redness of the anterior neck and upper chest). Children with dermatomyositis often develop ectopic calcifications (painful calcium deposits of the skeletal muscle and subcutaneous tissues). The diagnosis of polymyositis and dermatomyositis is suspected when the skeletal muscle enzymes (creatine phosphokinase [CPK] and aldolase) are elevated in the blood of a person with proximal muscle weakness. An electromyographic (EMG) study will demonstrate abnormal electrical activity of the muscles and will help eliminate other causes of the weakness. Magnetic resonance imaging (MRI) of the muscles shows inflammation and can be useful to help determine the best site for muscle biopsy. The diagnosis is confirmed by biopsy of an involved muscle that shows damage and infiltration of muscle fibers by lymphocytes and other inflammatory cells.

Most patients with polymyositis and dermatomyositis respond to treatment with high-dose oral and/or intravenous steroids followed by physical therapy for gait training and muscle strengthening. Patients who fail to respond to steroids or develop unacceptable side effects may be treated with other immunosuppressive agents, including methotrexate, azathioprine, cyclosporine, and intravenous gamma globulin.

Mixed Connective Tissue Disease

Mixed connective tissue disease, as originally described, denotes a subset of connective tissue disease patients whose blood contains high titers (large amounts) of anti-ribonucleoprotein (anti-RNP) antibodies. Patients typically manifest features of several different connective tissue diseases, including RA, SLE, scleroderma, and polymyositis/dermatomyositis. Sjögren's may also occur. The most common signs and symptoms include puffy hands, sclerodactyly, Raynaud's, skin rashes, pleurisy, polyarthritis, dysphagia, acid reflux, myalgias, and myositis. In some patients the disease evolves over time into classic lupus or scleroderma, and the results of autoantibody testing may change. When patients meet diagnostic criteria for only two different collagen vascular diseases at the time of diagnosis, the term "overlap syndrome" is preferred.

Sjögren's with Other Major Rheumatic Disease: Clinical Manifestations, Diagnosis and Prevalence

The onset of Sjögren's among connective tissue disease patients is highly variable. Sjögren's has been reported to occur anywhere from 1 to 40 years after diagnosis of another major rheumatic disorder but occurs in the majority of people about 5 to 10 years after diagnosis of another connective tissue disease. Sicca symptoms, when Sjögren's is diagnosed in patients with another related disorder, are generally milder than those who have Sjögren's alone. Additionally, salivary gland swelling, lymphadenopathy (enlargement of the lymph nodes), and lymphomas appear more frequently in patients who have Sjögren's that does not occur in the setting of another major rheumatic disease.

Some studies suggest that dry eye occurs more commonly than dry mouth in lupus and RA patients with Sjögren's, while in patients with scleroderma and Sjögren's, the reverse seems true. Interestingly, in scleroderma, Sjögren's occurs more commonly among the limited variant than the diffuse form of the disease. Treatments for these patient groups are typically directed toward the underlying disease. However, all rheumatic disease patients with dryness may benefit from therapy with secretagogues and other measures for dryness.

The prevalence of Sjögren's in autoimmune collagen vascular disorders is variable and depends on how this diagnosis is made. When older diagnostic criteria were applied to large patient populations, prevalence figures for Sjögren's of 31%, 20%, and 20% were reported in patients with RA, SLE, and scleroderma, respectively. According to one survey, anti-SSA and anti-SSB are normally present in Sjögren's and SLE, as described earlier, but become more prevalent in all patient groups with the development of Sjögren's: RA (24% in primary/6% in secondary), SLE (73%/46%), and scleroderma (33%/18%). Studies of positive lip biopsies in the same patient groups suggest prevalence figures that are even higher: RA 35%, SLE 18% to 90%, and scleroderma 17% to 51%. Interestingly, the proportion of patients with positive lip biopsies in these studies was always substantially higher than the number of patients with symptoms. Future studies of prevalence using the new classification criteria will provide more precise information on prevalence.

How Sjögren's May Influence the Expression of Other Connective Tissue Diseases

Little information is available regarding the influence of secondary Sjögren's on the course of other connective tissue diseases. In RA patients the coexistence of secondary Sjögren's reportedly has little effect on the course of arthritis or other clinical manifestations. However, dryness of the gastrointestinal tract from Sjögren's could potentially exacerbate a variety of problems common to these disorders, including reflux, dysphagia, dyspepsia (indigestion), and constipation. Respiratory dryness from Sjögren's could not only aggravate chronic cough due to interstitial lung disease but also predispose to recurrent respiratory infections. In lupus, some studies have suggested that secondary Sjögren's is associated with an increased incidence of erosive polyarthritis, an uncommon complication of SLE. In scleroderma it has been reported that the subset of patients with scleroderma and secondary Sjögren's (particularly the CREST variant) were at increased risk of developing vasculitis (inflammation of the blood vessels). It has also been reported that autoimmune liver disease, particularly primary biliary cirrhosis, was more common in scleroderma patients with secondary Sjögren's compared to scleroderma patients alone.

Antiphospholipid Antibody Syndrome

Antiphospholipid antibody syndrome (APS) is an autoimmune disorder characterized by recurrent arterial and venous thromboses (blood clots) and/or recurrent spontaneous abortions (miscarriages) associated with the presence of antibodies to phospholipids in the blood. It can occur by itself as a primary disorder (primary APS) or in association with connective tissue diseases (secondary APS), most notably SLE. APS can occur in Sjögren's, although it does so less frequently than in SLE. Manifestations of APS include deep venous thromboses (blood clots) in the arms and legs, pulmonary emboli (blood clots in the lungs), strokes, mini-strokes, or recurrent miscarriages (usually in the later stages of pregnancy). To make a diagnosis of APS, blood clots must be documented by objective medical testing, and antibody presence is demonstrated when one or more of the following tests is positive: anticardiolipin antibodies, anti-B_2 glycoprotein I antibodies, or lupus anticoagulant. Platelet counts may be low in APS. It is not uncommon for people with Sjögren's to have positive anticardiolipin and/or anti-B_2 glycoprotein I antibodies, but they may never develop blood clots or experience a miscarriage. The presence of anticardiolipin and/or anti-B_2 glycoprotein I antibodies without a history of a thrombotic event or miscarriage is not sufficient to make a diagnosis of APS.

The primary treatment for APS is lifelong anticoagulation with blood thinners such as heparin or warfarin. Other causes of blood clots and pregnancy loss must always be excluded in the diagnostic evaluation.

Vasculitis

Vasculitis is a broad term that describes a heterogeneous group of about 30 collagen vascular disorders that cause blood vessel inflammation with subsequent damage to the vessel wall, tissue necrosis from ischemia (poor blood supply due to the damaged blood vessels), and in some cases organ injury that can lead to organ failure. Clinical manifestations vary according to the site of involvement. It can be localized to a single organ or cause systemic disease. Vasculitis can exist as a primary disorder (e.g., polyarteritis nodosa) or occur as a complication of another connective tissue disease, including Sjögren's. It can sometimes be precipitated by infections or medications. Vasculitic disorders are grouped according to (1) the size and type of vessel involved, (2) the type of cells that cause the vessel inflammation, (3) etiology, and (4) affected organs.

The subset of Sjögren's patients with extraglandular manifestations (i.e., serious internal organ disease) seem to be at greatest risk to develop vasculitis. Laboratory clues may include the appearance of cryoglobulins in the blood (proteins that precipitate out in the cold); high levels of anti-SSA antibodies; elevation of serum IgG, elevation of the erythrocyte sedimentation rate, decreased levels of complement C_3 or C_4; or positive anti-neutrophil cytoplasmic (ANCA) antibodies. However, like other patient groups, the definitive diagnosis of vasculitis in Sjögren's can only be made by biopsy of an involved organ or by doing an arteriogram. The biopsy should show invasion and/or damage of blood vessel walls by inflammatory cells. An arteriogram (an imaging study performed by injecting radiopaque contrast dye into an artery) may show abnormalities of vessel shape, including aneurysms, segmental narrowing, or dilatation.

The skin is the most common site of vasculitis in Sjögren's. Cutaneous vasculitis affects small vessels (arterioles, capillaries, venules) and typically causes raised reddish-purple spots on the legs, called palpable purpura. These lesions may be painful or pruritic. Other vasculitic rashes in Sjögren's can include urticaria (hives), skin ulcers, or erythema multiforme (red spots of variable size and shape). Vasculitic involvement of small to medium-sized arteries in Sjögren's will occasionally affect the nervous system and cause strokes, mini-strokes, or peripheral neuropathies. A particular type of peripheral neuropathy, mononeuritis multiplex, is highly suggestive of vasculitis and is suspected when the patient develops foot drop associated with patchy loss of sensation in the lower extremities. The diagnosis is confirmed by performing an EMG/nerve conduction study of the legs followed by biopsy of the sural nerve in the calf. Vasculitis of the medium-sized arteries of abdominal organs is rare in Sjögren's but can cause life-threatening complications. The diagnosis is proven by arteriography or examination of tissue specimens obtained during emergency surgery.

Treatments for vasculitis vary with the organs involved but in some cases requires long-term treatment with potent immunosuppressive medications. Therefore, every effort should be made to obtain a proper diagnosis at the time of initial presentation and exclude other disorders that cause similar symptoms but require different treatments.

Undifferentiated Connective Tissue Disease

This term describes a group of individuals who exhibit signs and symptoms of connective tissue disease as described earlier and are ANA-positive. These patients fail to meet the diagnostic criteria for any one specific disorder. They may complain of sicca symptoms, but lip biopsies are typically negative. In some cases, a change over time in clinical features or autoantibody profile may yield a specific diagnosis. Treatments vary according to major symptoms.

Evolution of Sjögren's into Other Disorders

Patients with various connective tissue disorders, including Sjögren's, can share overlapping clinical and laboratory features, and sometimes it is difficult to establish a definitive diagnosis. RA, for example, may be complicated by Sjögren's, and initial manifestations of Sjögren's when occurring alone can include a rheumatoid-like polyarthritis with RF in the blood. The presence of anti-SSA and anti-SSB antibodies in both Sjögren's and SLE suggests a common pathogenic mechanism. Manifestations of autoimmune diseases can change over time. It has been observed that a patient can present with one autoimmune disease and then their symptoms may evolve into a classic presentation of a different autoimmune disease and the initial autoimmune disease appears to fade away. All of this can make the diagnosis of autoimmune disease quite challenging as well as reinforce the need to continue to reassess the autoimmune disease over time, particularly if new symptoms develop that are atypical for the initial disease.

Other Autoimmune Disorders Associated with Sjögren's

Other autoimmune disorders that primarily affect a single organ system may coexist with Sjögren's but are not strictly classed among the connective tissue diseases (Box 21.4).

Any patient with a known autoimmune disease is at increased risk for developing a second autoimmune disorder. Autoimmune disorders (but not always the same disease) typically run in families. This phenomenon occurs due to common inheritance of immune response genes that predispose to one or more of these disorders. A second autoimmune disease can be difficult to diagnose in Sjögren's because symptoms often begin insidiously and overlap with those of Sjögren's. Some of these disorders are discussed next.

Hashimoto's Thyroiditis

This autoimmune disease can be associated with Sjögren's and cause thyroid enlargement (goiter), thyroid nodules, and most commonly hypothyroidism (underactive thyroid). Hypothyroidism can also result from other etiologies and causes fatigue, dry skin, coarse hair, constipation, headaches, arthralgias, myalgias, facial swelling, cognitive dysfunction, and hoarseness. Hypothyroidism is diagnosed by blood tests (high thyroid stimulating hormone [TSH], low or normal free T_4). Hashimoto's is confirmed by the presence of one or more thyroid autoantibodies in the blood, including anti-microsomal and anti-thyroid peroxidase antibodies. It is treated with thyroid hormone replacement. Frequent monitoring of thyroid function tests is required.

Celiac Disease

Celiac disease (a.k.a. celiac sprue, non-tropical sprue, or gluten-sensitive enteropathy) is a common autoimmune disease that targets the small intestine and may cause multiple organ problems. It can present in children and adults and is now thought to affect as many as 1% of people in the United States. It often runs in families as certain genes predispose to this disorder. Celiac

---

Box 21.4 Autoimmune Diseases Associated with Sjögren's

- Hashimoto's thyroiditis
- Graves' disease
- Primary biliary cirrhosis
- Chronic active autoimmune hepatitis
- Addison's disease
- Celiac sprue
- Multiple sclerosis
- Myasthenia gravis
- Pernicious anemia

disease can be an isolated problem or coexist with other diseases, including Sjögren's. Celiac disease is caused by an abnormal immune response to gluten, a protein found in wheat, barley, and rye. Repeated exposure to dietary gluten stimulates an inflammatory reaction in the small intestine that leads to malabsorption, nutrient deficiencies, and other health problems.

Symptoms may include weight loss, abdominal pain, diarrhea, bloating, anemia (especially iron-deficiency anemia), vitamin D deficiency, osteoporosis, fatigue, headaches, neurologic problems, and dermatitis herpetiformis (itchy bumps or blisters on the skin). Celiac disease is most often diagnosed by blood tests or a biopsy of the small intestine. Serum IgA anti-tissue transglutaminase and IgA anti-endomysial antibodies have the highest sensitivity and specificity. For patients who are IgA-deficient (up to 1:500 individuals), an IgG anti-tissue transglutaminase and IgG anti-endomysial antibody test should be done. An intestinal biopsy will show lymphocyte infiltration of epithelial cells or the lamina propria (inflammation of the intestinal lining cells or layer below) and shrinkage/flattening of internal villi (finger-like projections of intestinal surface that absorb nutrients). Genetic testing is also available.

Currently the major treatment is to follow a life-long gluten-free diet. Consultation with a registered dietitian can be extremely helpful. Other resources are available. In most cases, strict adherence to the diet will lead to complete resolution of symptoms over weeks to months. Some diagnostic test results may also improve or normalize. Therefore, all diagnostic testing should ideally be completed before initiation of the diet.

Fibromyalgia

Fibromyalgia is not considered an autoimmune disease but nevertheless represents an important comorbidity in Sjögren's that can exacerbate pain, fatigue, and cognitive dysfunction. Fibromyalgia appears to be due to an abnormality of pain processing in the central nervous system. Besides disturbed sleep, patients also note whole-body pain, morning stiffness, fatigue, and modulation of symptoms by the weather (symptoms are usually worse on cold, damp days). Patients frequently have trouble falling asleep or staying asleep or experience nonrestorative sleep (i.e., waking up tired). Other symptoms can include numbness and tingling of the extremities, dry eyes, dry mouth, and "brain fog" (memory loss, difficulty with concentration).

Fibromyalgia can be easily misdiagnosed as Sjögren's or vice versa or can coexist with Sjögren's. It can be found in 47% to 55% of patients with Sjögren's, depending on the study. Fibromyalgia may be associated with a variety of other disorders, including irritable bowel syndrome (spastic colon), bladder pain syndrome, temporomandibular joint syndrome (TMJ), migraines, depression, and costochondritis.

The diagnosis of fibromyalgia is based on clinical findings. On physical examination, numerous "tender points" (localized areas of muscular tenderness) are found. Despite patient complaints of joint swelling and tingling of the extremities, no objective abnormalities of the joints or nervous system are typically observed on physical examination.

Blood tests are usually done to rule out other causes of muscle pain (e.g., hypothyroidism, vitamin D deficiency). In certain individuals, sleep studies are performed to look for potentially treatable causes of disturbed sleep such as sleep apnea, upper airway resistance syndrome, restless leg syndrome, or periodic limb movement disorder of sleep. In fibromyalgia, the most commonly observed sleep study pattern is termed "alpha wave intrusion in delta non-REM sleep." A similar pattern may also be observed in other patients with chronic pain syndromes. Specific treatments are generally directed at finding ways to promote restful sleep, palliate pain, and improve patient function.

Summing Up

A variety of connective tissue diseases and other disorders (both autoimmune and non-autoimmune) can coexist with Sjögren's and add to the patient's burden of illness. Each of these conditions presents unique challenges that affect the diagnosis and management of Sjögren's. The American College of Rheumatology's website contains information on a number of autoimmune disorders for patients/caregivers.

For Further Reading

Anaya J-M, Rojas-Villarraga A, Mantilla RD, et al. Polyautoimmunity in Sjogren syndrome. *Rheum Dis Clin North Am.* 2016;42:457–472.

Klippel J, Stone J, Crofford L, White P, eds. *Primer on the Rheumatic Diseases* (13th ed.). Arthritis Foundation; 2008.

Theander E, Jacobsson LTH. Relationship of Sjögren's syndrome to other connective tissue and autoimmune disorders. *Rheum Dis Clin North Am.* 2008;34:935–947.

22

Childhood Sjögren's

Scott M. Lieberman, Sara M. Stern, and Jay Mehta

While often considered a disease of adulthood, Sjögren's can and does occur in children. One of the first reported cases of Sjögren's in a child was published in the mid-1960s and described a 10-year-old girl with parotid gland swelling and arthritis (inflammation of the lining of the joint causing swelling, pain, and stiffness). Since then, while hundreds of cases of Sjögren's in children have been published, this disease is still largely under-diagnosed in children. Part of the challenge of diagnosing these children is the frequent lack of classic Sjögren's symptoms of profound eye and mouth dryness. Because Sjögren's often presents differently in children than in adults, the criteria developed and often used to diagnose Sjögren's in adults are not adequate to diagnose Sjögren's in children. This may be due to the difficulty in performing some of the testing procedures in young or anxious children. Also, children likely represent an earlier stage of disease and lack the degree of damage that develops after decades of dryness and inflammation, so even when tests are performed, the results may not be abnormal to the same degree as in adults. We are currently working to develop new child-specific criteria for diagnosis of Sjögren's, but at present no such criteria have been widely accepted.

When Do Kids Get Sjögren's?

Sjögren's in children may occur any time during childhood but is not present at birth and is exceedingly rare in the first year of life. The mean age at diagnosis reported for Sjögren's in children has ranged from 10 to 12 years, but children may be diagnosed at nearly any age in childhood from less than 1 year old to 18 years old. Similar to Sjögren's in adults, Sjögren's in children is more commonly diagnosed in females, with a male:female ratio of 1:5 to 1:12.

Scott M. Lieberman, Sara Stern, and Jay Mehta, *Childhood Sjögren's* In: *The Sjögren's Book*. Edited by: Daniel J. Wallace, Oxford University Press. © Sjögren's Foundation 2022. DOI: 10.1093/oso/9780197502112.003.0022

Symptoms and Other Features

Dry Eyes and Dry Mouth

Unlike Sjögren's in adults, the disease in children often does not present with symptoms of profound dryness. By this, we mean that children are rarely brought to the doctor specifically because they complain of very dry eyes or very dry mouth. However, if asked the right questions, it turns out that many children with Sjögren's actually do have some manifestations suggesting some degree of decreased tears or decreased saliva, the features that cause the symptoms of dryness in adults. Specifically, approximately 50% of children with Sjögren's may have features reflecting "dryness" when they are diagnosed, but these may not be evident unless asked specifically about having recurrent dental cavities, having to wake in the middle of the night to take drinks, having to take drinks to aid in swallowing of particularly dry foods (breads or crackers, for example), having to regularly use rewetting drops to help their irritated eyes, or having the feeling of "sand" or "grittiness" in their eyes. Notably, many children who answer yes to these questions may answer no when asked if they experience any symptoms of dry eyes or dry mouth. Still others may attribute eye symptoms to seasonal allergies or other irritants and not appreciate that their tear-producing glands are not functioning properly. Even though dryness may occur in children with Sjögren's, it is rare that children have severe eye damage when they are first diagnosed with Sjögren's.

Salivary Gland Swelling

The main glands that produce saliva are the parotid glands, located at the angle of the jaw just underneath the skin and soft tissue layers in the cheeks. One of the most common features of Sjögren's in children is inflammation of these parotid glands, often presenting as painful swelling of the cheeks that may affect one side or both sides at the same time. Some children have significant pain with mouth opening or eating when this occurs. Some have fevers when this occurs as well. The painful swelling may last a few days to a few weeks before improving. Because viral and bacterial infections can cause similar painful swelling, children are often treated with a course of antibiotics when this first occurs. Because these swelling episodes tend to resolve after 1 to 2 weeks, it is often assumed that the antibiotics made the swelling go away. Only after repeated episodes do the patients, the parents, or the doctors begin to question whether these are truly infections. Or, in some cases, the child is not given antibiotics and the swelling resolves in the same amount of time, suggesting that the symptoms are not due to a bacterial infection. The recurrent nature of these episodes makes infection less likely, but when this occurs for the first time it is common and necessary for the doctor to consider the possibility of infection to prevent missing treating something that requires antibiotic therapy. Less commonly, the cheek swelling persists. When this occurs, a biopsy of the glands is often done to determine the cause of the facial mass, largely to ensure it is not a tumor.

Parotitis (inflammation of the parotid gland or glands) is present in approximately 50% of children with Sjögren's. Some of these children, even though the swelling improves greatly, may have persistent parotid gland discomfort on a daily or nearly daily basis even between the episodes of more painful parotid gland swelling. Notably, the frequency with which children with Sjögren's have parotid gland swelling is another feature that differs from the presentation in adults, who are much less likely to have recurrent episodes of parotid gland swelling.

Joint Pain and Musculoskeletal Pain

Approximately 25% of children with Sjögren's will have arthritis (inflammation of the lining of their joints). The hallmark symptoms that suggest arthritis include swelling of joints and prolonged stiffness of joints after periods of inactivity (such as sleeping overnight or long car rides). Pain may occur but does not always occur with arthritis. Even more children (40–50%) will have pain in their joints without detectable arthritis. These children may even have some degree of stiffness in the morning similar to that seen with arthritis. It is not entirely clear if this latter pain reflects a degree of inflammation that is not easily detectable or, rather, dysregulated pain-sensing nerves (see next section).

Fibromyalgia-like Amplified Pain and Fatigue

Some children will develop progressively worsening pain despite no evidence of joint, muscle, or bone inflammation or damage. This pain, called amplified musculoskeletal pain, is similar to that in adults with fibromyalgia and is believed to result from dysregulation of the pain-sensing nerves; in other words, nerves that are supposed to sense pain when there is inflammation or damage continue to sense pain even after the inflammation or damage has resolved, or sometimes when no inflammation or damage is present. Notably, fibromyalgia is also more commonly diagnosed in adults with Sjögren's compared to the general population. The reasons for this association of amplified pain and Sjögren's is not entirely clear. This pain is real—in fact it is sometimes debilitating—but may not signify any damage or active inflammation. Also similar to adults, some children with Sjögren's develop profound fatigue, making their prior regular activity levels more challenging. This degree of pain and/or fatigue can be difficult to deal with, especially in a child who was previously active in sports, dance, or other physical activities.

Effects on Other Organ Systems

Similar to adults, Sjögren's in children may affect nearly any organ in the body. Lymphadenopathy (enlarged lymph nodes) may be apparent in 10% to 20% of children with Sjögren's. Low blood counts (white blood cells, platelets, and/or red blood cells or hemoglobin) occur in 15% of children with Sjögren's. Skin manifestations occur in 10% to 15% of children with Sjögren's and may manifest as different forms of rash, including circular ("annular") areas of redness with paler central redness, urticaria or hives, ulcerations, or vasculitis. Raynaud's phenomenon (discoloration of fingers and/or toes in response to cold exposure or stress) is not uncommon. Neurologic manifestations affecting the brain or spinal cord (central nervous system) or other nerves (peripheral nervous system) occur in up to 10% of children with Sjögren's. These nervous system manifestations may range from headaches to numbness/tingling to encephalopathy (inflammation of the brain). Sjögren's affects the kidneys in 5% to 10% of children; these changes range from abnormal urine tests without other signs of kidney damage to calcium deposits within the kidneys (nephrocalcinosis) to inflammation of different parts of the kidney (tubulointerstitial nephritis or glomerulonephritis). In some children, inflammation of the kidneys may manifest as paralysis due to low potassium levels that may occur when the damaged kidneys fail to reabsorb potassium before it is excreted in the urine. This is called renal tubular acidosis (RTA); while rare, this is one of the more severe manifestations of Sjögren's. Inflammation of the lungs (interstitial lung disease) or the muscles (myositis) is uncommon, occurring in fewer than 10% of children with Sjögren's. Other nonspecific symptoms, such as fevers or weight loss, occur in 5% to 10% of children with Sjögren's.

How Is Sjögren's Diagnosed in Children?

As with Sjögren's in adults and many other rheumatologic diseases in children and adults, there is no single test that will definitively diagnose Sjögren's in a child. Because of this, we rely on combinations of several tests, including blood tests, urine tests, tests of tears and saliva, eye examinations, imaging tests, and biopsies, to determine if a child likely has Sjögren's or not. The best way to diagnose Sjögren's in adults has been continually debated for decades. Some consensus criteria have been developed for use in research studies but may not be adequate for clinical practice. Several studies have demonstrated that these adult criteria for Sjögren's do not often work well in diagnosing Sjögren's in children. With that said, if a child meets the adult criteria with enough positive tests, then the diagnosis of Sjögren's should be made. However, many children will not meet these adult criteria, and no child-specific criteria for the diagnosis of Sjögren's have been established.

While work is under way to develop criteria to better diagnose Sjögren's in children, at present we rely on finding evidence of the three main areas involved in the development of Sjögren's: (1) inflammation of the saliva- or tear-producing glands, (2) autoantibodies (proteins in the blood that suggest the immune system is attacking one's own body), and (3) tests of gland dysfunction (decreased tears, decreased saliva, or evidence of damage to the surface of the eye).

Gland Inflammation

Inflammation of the glands can be detected by imaging techniques (ultrasound, magnetic resonance imaging [MRI], computed tomography [CT] scan); through special tests to measure saliva flow (including sialography or scintigraphy); or by evaluation of a biopsy of the glands. The biopsy is most often taken from the minor salivary glands in the inner lower lip. When done by an experienced oral medicine or otolaryngology (ear, nose, and throat) specialist, this procedure provides a wealth of information, typically with few side effects other than mild post-procedure pain.

Autoantibodies

Evidence of autoantibodies includes the antinuclear antibody (ANA), the Sjögren's Syndrome (SS)-A and SS-B antibodies (also known as Ro and La, respectively), rheumatoid factor (RF), or any of a number of newly discovered antibodies that may have utility in some patients. These tests are done on blood samples.

Gland Dysfunction

Measurements of saliva can be done in several ways but are not routinely done on children. Measurements of tears most commonly include the Schirmer test, which involves placing a small moisture-absorbing strip of paper or cotton between the eye and the lower eyelid to measure the amount of moisture that is absorbed over a brief period of time. This test can be done with or without first placing a few drops of a numbing medicine in the eyes. Less frequently done measurements of tears include tear osmolarity, which may give information regarding the quality of the tears, and tear break-up time, which involves placing a dye on the surface of the eye and watching how long it takes for the dye to disperse or break up. Staining of the ocular surface should be done with two different dyes: fluorescein to measure corneal damage and lissamine green to measure damage to the conjunctival surface of the eye (the surface over the white part of the eye around the cornea). These ocular staining tests are typically done by an experienced eye doctor.

Depending on the symptoms, additional testing may be performed to evaluate for evidence of effects on other organs that might be consistent with Sjögren's (or other similar rheumatologic diseases that share many features).

If a child has recurrent episodes of painful swelling of the major salivary glands (typically the parotid glands in the cheeks) and has positive Sjögren's antibodies (SS-A especially), then the diagnosis of Sjögren's is highly likely, though additional tests may be performed to confirm the diagnosis, including salivary gland ultrasound or other imaging and biopsy of the minor salivary glands of the lip. When parotid gland swelling occurs but autoantibody tests are negative/normal, then additional testing must be done to help determine if the swelling is due to Sjögren's or some other cause. In a child presenting without symptoms of parotid gland swelling, a high index of suspicion is needed to even consider Sjögren's. Often, abnormalities are noted on other routine lab work (such as urine tests or blood tests), prompting referral to a pediatric rheumatologist, at which time Sjögren's may be considered and additional testing done. Unfortunately, we suspect that many children with Sjögren's do not get diagnosed as children because their symptoms are vague and symptoms clearly affecting tear- and saliva-producing glands are lacking. In our opinion, a child requires at least either positive SS-A and/or SS-B antibodies or positive lip biopsy for a diagnosis of Sjögren's, but formal consensus on the minimum positive/abnormal tests required for diagnosis has not yet been established.

Importantly, other conditions that may cause similar symptoms should be considered during the work-up of Sjögren's. For example, other rheumatologic diseases (sarcoidosis, ANCA-associated vasculitis, IgG4-related disease, immune dysregulation associated with immune deficiency), infections (mumps, hepatitis C, human immunodeficiency virus [HIV], mycobacterial infections such as tuberculosis, or other bacterial or viral infections), or cancers may cause salivary gland or lacrimal gland swelling similar to that seen in Sjögren's. Biopsy of the minor salivary glands or, in cases of persistent swelling of the major salivary glands, biopsy of the major glands may help aid in making the diagnosis. Sjögren's may also occur in children with other autoimmune diseases. Thyroid autoimmunity is the most common autoimmune disease to occur with other autoimmune diseases and may also co-occur with Sjögren's.

How Is Sjögren's Treated in Children?

Similar to Sjögren's in adults, the treatment of Sjögren's in children depends largely on the specific symptoms and organs involved in Sjögren's in the individual.

Salivary Gland Swelling

During episodes of salivary gland swelling, oral steroids (such as prednisone) may help control the inflammation. However, before the diagnosis of Sjögren's has been established, the use of steroids may not be warranted until after tests for infection and cancer have been performed to ensure neither of these is the cause of the symptoms. Hydroxychloroquine has been used in many children to minimize the frequency and intensity of recurrent episodes of parotid gland inflammation, though formal study of its efficacy has not been performed. Additional medications may be warranted if hydroxychloroquine is not sufficient. These include abatacept, rituximab, methotrexate, mycophenolate mofetil, and many others, though, again, no formal consensus on the optimal treatments has been established.

Symptoms of Dryness

Initial treatment of eye and mouth dryness is similar to that in adults, with conservative methods including increased fluid intake, sugar-free sour candies, and vigilant dental care for dry mouth symptoms and artificial tear drops and protecting from desiccating environmental stressors (such as dryness associated with cold weather, allergens, or prolonged screen time) for dry eye symptoms. Frequent fluoride treatments and dental cleanings are very important to prevent tooth loss because the risk is increased over time as saliva quality and quantity will wane with disease progression. Similarly, regular eye exams are important to maintain appropriate ocular health and to monitor for ocular surface damage that would suggest medicated drops (such as cyclosporine drops or lifitegrast drops) are needed to control the inflammation at the ocular surface. Beyond these measures, some children remain quite dry and require therapies that stimulate production of saliva and tears (sialagogues). These include the same medications, pilocarpine and cevimeline, that are used in adults.

Besides eye and mouth dryness, some individuals experience dryness of other areas, including the skin, airways (causing dry cough), or vagina. These should be discussed and monitored, and referral to additional specialists (such as dermatologists, pulmonologists, and gynecologists) should be considered to help with management if necessary.

Nonspecific Musculoskeletal Pain and Fatigue

Pain should be evaluated to determine if it is due to inflammation (such as arthritis; see the next paragraph), but in many children no inflammatory causes will be ascertained definitively. For these cases, and for all cases of fatigue, discussion should focus on maintaining healthy nutrition, healthy sleep, and healthy exercise habits. These may help to combat these symptoms over time, though these are some of the most debilitating and most difficult-to-treat symptoms. Hydroxychloroquine may also help reduce pain, including that of arthritis.

Arthritis

Arthritis is inflammation of the lining of the joints and, if not treated, may affect growth or joint integrity. The best treatments for this are not well defined in Sjögren's, but abatacept is one treatment used for juvenile arthritis that has shown some promise in initial studies treating Sjögren's in adults. TNF inhibitor therapies have not shown benefit in Sjögren's in adults, but given their excellent benefits in juvenile arthritis (including the treatment of juvenile arthritis in children with Sjögren's), these medications (adalimumab, etanercept, infliximab) may be considered for difficult-to-treat or damaging/aggressive arthritis in children. As noted earlier, hydroxychloroquine may help control inflammation in the joints. Methotrexate is another medication that shows benefit in controlling arthritis in some children and may be worth considering in children with Sjögren's with arthritis; however, it is not clear if methotrexate will help modulate Sjögren's-related autoimmunity to prevent progression of tear and saliva dysfunction.

What Is the Long-Term Outcome of Children with Sjögren's?

Since no formal diagnostic criteria for Sjögren's in children have been established, there are no long-term studies in children to determine their outcome over time. We presume that Sjögren's in children is an early form of Sjögren's in adults and that these children will eventually develop tear and saliva deficits and dry eyes and mouth, and may progress to have effects in other organs. Because of this, we often recommend prophylactic treatment, such as hydroxychloroquine, in the hope that this will slow disease progression until more effective preventive therapies can be identified. Unfortunately, there is not much in the way of monitoring that will allow us to know whether the treatment is actually slowing the process. We do not routinely repeat biopsies to evaluate for inflammation. Periodic ultrasounds may be used to monitor for progression or regression of any changes associated with inflammation of salivary glands. While it is well known that adults with Sjögren's have a higher risk of developing cancer, we do not know if children with Sjögren's also have an increased risk. Reports of cancers in childhood Sjögren's are rare. However, whether children with Sjögren's have a greater risk of developing cancer later in life is not known. Therefore, periodic monitoring for cancer is warranted.

Summing Up

Sjögren's occurs in children, but the presentation may not include profound dry eyes or dry mouth. Parotid gland swelling is common, but any organ may be affected. Often a high index of suspicion is needed to make the diagnosis, which relies on a variety of tests. Treatments are similar to those in adults, but no specific treatments have been proven to prevent progression from early disease in childhood to the more profound manifestations often apparent in adulthood. Active research is being conducted to address some of the gaps in our knowledge and will hopefully lead to a better understanding of Sjögren's in children, including more effective treatments.

For Further Reading

de Souza TR, Silva IH, Carvalho AT, et al. Juvenile Sjögren syndrome: Distinctive age, unique findings. *Pediatr Dent.* 2012;34(5):427–430.

Houghton K, Malleson P, Cabral D, et al. Primary Sjögren's syndrome in children and adolescents: Are proposed diagnostic criteria applicable? *J Rheumatol.* 2005;32:2225–2232.

Lieberman SM, Mehta J. Childhood Sjögren's: Guide for parents and doctors. *The Moisture Seekers.* 2016;34(1):1–10. https://www.sjogrens.org/sites/default/files/inline-files/TMS2016-01.pdf

Means C, Aldape MA, King E. Pediatric primary Sjögren syndrome presenting with bilateral ranulas: A case report and systematic review of the literature. *Int J Pediatr Otorhinolaryngol.* 2017;101:11–19.

Mehta J, Lieberman SM. Patient Education Sheet: Pediatric Sjögren's. Sjögren's Foundation; 2016. https://www.sjogrens.org/sites/default/files/inline-files/Pediatric%20Sjogren%27s%20Patient%20Education%20Sheet.pdf

Schuetz C, Prieur AM, Quartier P. Sicca syndrome and salivary gland infiltration in children with autoimmune disorders: When can we diagnose Sjögren's syndrome? *Clin Exp Rheumatol.* 2010;28:434–439.

Virdee S, Greenan-Barrett J, Ciurtin C. A systematic review of primary Sjögren's syndrome in male and paediatric populations. *Clin Rheumatol.* 2017;36(10):2225–2236.

Yokogawa N, Lieberman SM, Sherry DD, Vivino FB. Features of childhood Sjögren syndrome in comparison to adult Sjögren syndrome: Considerations in establishing child-specific diagnostic criteria. *Clin Exp Rheumatol.* 2016;34(2):343–351.

PART V
MANAGING SJÖGREN'S

23

Management of Dry Eye in Sjögren's

Peter Donshik

The management of dry eye disease (DED) or dysfunctional tear syndrome, a condition that affects over 20 million individuals in the United States, is continuously evolving. The recent report from the Tear Film & Ocular Surface Society (TFOS) Dry Eye Workshop II (DEWS II) published in 2017 has redefined the definition of dry eye. The new definition is:

> Dry eye is a multifactorial disease of the ocular surface characterized by a loss of homeostasis of the tear film, and accompanied by ocular symptoms in which tear film instability and hyperosmolarity, ocular surface inflammation and damage, and neurosensory abnormalities play etiological roles.

The management of dry eye syndrome should address each of these factors.

Previous management strategies were based on whether the patient was experiencing aqueous-deficient or evaporative dry eye. Present strategies are based on the belief that rather than representing two distinct categories, most people with symptoms secondary to DED suffer from variable combinations of both abnormal meibomian gland physiology (resulting in evaporative dry eye disease [EVD]) and tear underproduction (resulting in aqueous-deficient dry eye disease [ADDE]).

This chapter focuses on DED management guidance provided by the 2017 TFOS DEWS II, but patients and clinicians should also be aware of the 2015 Sjögren's Foundation Clinical Practice Guidelines for ocular management in Sjögren's patients. These guidelines closely parallel the recommendations by TFOS DEWS II, are easily downloadable from the Sjögren's Foundation website (https://www.sjogrens.org/), and include screening questions and other supplementary information that is helpful.

The first management principle is to perform a complete eye examination. This will determine whether the patient is symptomatic or asymptomatic and whether signs of ocular surface disease are present or absent. Further evaluation of the patient will determine whether specific ocular surface disease

Peter Donshik, *Management of Dry Eye in Sjögren's* In: *The Sjögren's Book*. Edited by: Daniel J. Wallace, Oxford University Press. © Sjögren's Foundation 2022. DOI: 10.1093/oso/9780197502112.003.0023 conditions exist that are related to both signs and symptoms, whether the patient is asymptomatic with signs or is symptomatic without significant signs.

In general, the majority of patients with DED have evaporative EDE, with fewer having ADDE. A much smaller percentage of DED patients will have mucin deficiency, neuropathic pain, or any of the other subtypes associated with DED.

While it is important to try and determine the degree to which each of the subtypes of DED (evaporative, aqueous-deficient, and/or other ocular surface disease) are contributing to the patient's signs and symptoms and to treat this component, it is also important to understand that the common underlying problem that results from all subtypes of DED is the disruption of ocular surface homeostasis. The goal of effective management of DED is thus to restore the homeostasis of the ocular surface and tear film. The management of DED is more of an art than a rigid algorithm and has to be tailored to each individual patient. In determining the initial therapeutic regimen for the DED patient, it is important to identify to what degree that EDE, ADDE, or any other specific subtype is the primary etiologic factor. However, it is also important to understand that the various subtypes often overlap, so they also must be addressed.

In general, DED therapies begin with conventional, low-risk, and easily accessible patient-applied therapies, such as over-the-counter lubricants (preservative-free) for early-stage disease, and progress to more advanced therapies for more severe forms of DED. The DEWS II workshop recommended the following stepwise approach. As proposed in the TFOS DEWSII report, "Should patients not respond to a given level of management, or should they present with more severe DED, the next level of management is recommended, and in some cases, the previous therapy may be continued in addition to any new therapies."

Step 1

Education and Minimizing Aggravating Factors

It is important to educate patients with regard to their clinical condition, the various management and treatment options, and their prognosis.

Since symptoms of dry eye are often aggravated by certain environmental stresses as well as physical and/or visual activities, it is often helpful for patients to anticipate and avoid or limit those situations. Dehumidified environments or those with strong air currents increase evaporation of the tear film. This is very common on long airplane trips, so patients should be prepared to supplement their tears on such excursions. Use of a room humidifier or furnace humidifier can improve the home environment.

Prolonged visual tasks such as reading or using a computer also aggravate symptoms of dry eye because blinking is reduced during these activities. It is helpful in these situations to look away occasionally from the reading material to stimulate a blink or periodically to rest the eyes or even intentionally blink. Supplemental tears to stabilize the tear film or increase the volume of the tear film may be used during such periods of prolonged near work. Lowering computer terminal displays to below eye level can reduce the amount of the surface of the eye that is exposed to evaporation of tears.

Wearing contact lenses can increase tear evaporation. Using contact lens wetting drops and limiting the duration of lens wear can reduce the drying effect of the contact lens and prolong how long the lenses can be used for.

Modification/Elimination of Offending Systemic and Topical Medications

A careful history of systemic and topical medications should be conducted to identify those that may be aggravating the DED. Medications such as adrenergic agents, antihistamines, beta-blockers, phenothiazines, atropine, oral contraceptives, anxiolytics, antiparkinsonian agents, diuretics, anticholinergics, antiarrhythmics, antihypertensives, and antivirals can aggravate borderline DED. Topical medication such as miotics, mydriatics, and cycloplegics, prostaglandins, and nonsteroidal anti-inflammatory drugs may have an adverse effect on DED (Box 23.1).

Ocular Lubrication

Historically the mainstay of DED therapy has been tear replacement with topical ocular lubricants. The majority of the products available are over the counter and are often referred to as "artificial tears." Numerous topical formulations of ocular lubricants are available to supplement the tear film, and each category of drop has benefits and limitations. While they may help to replace or supplement the tear film, they do not target the underlying pathophysiology of DED. The majority of the products available have an aqueous base with a variety of pH, osmolarity, and viscosity-enhancing agents. These viscosity agents help to increase tear film thickness, protect

---

Box 23.1 Medications That May Cause or Aggravate DED

Antihistamines and decongestants
- Cold preparations/nasal decongestants

Antidepressants/antipsychotics/Parkinson medication
- Tricyclic antidepressants
- Anti-anxiety medication
- Phenothiazines
- Trihexyphenidyl

Dermatologic medications
- Anti-acne medications

Gastrointestinal medications
- Proton pump inhibitors
- H2 receptor antagonists

Hormones
- Hormonal replacement therapy
- Birth control agents

Hypertension agents
- Beta-blockers
- Thiazides/diuretics

---

against evaporation, aid in tear retention and in protecting the ocular surface, and relieve symptoms. In general, high-viscosity drops and ointments are recommended for nighttime use while low-viscosity drops are better tolerated during the day.

Some artificial tears are designed not just to increase the volume of the tears but also to provide specific protection for the surface of the eye. For example, TheraTears is a solution that mimics the salt content of the tear film but at a lower concentration. When applied to the eye, it reduces the concentration (osmolarity) of the tear film. Elevated tear osmolarity is associated with damage to the surface cells of the eye in addition to being a stimulator of inflammation. The goal of TheraTears, by decreasing tear film osmolarity, is to prevent the damage and decrease the stimulus to inflammation. A different strategy is used by the drop Optive, which includes specific molecules in a solution to protect the surface cells against the highly concentrated tears of dry eye. Lipid-containing formulations, either as additives (Freshkote) or emulsion (Soothe, Systane Balance), are very helpful in preventing evaporation of the tear film and can be particularly helpful in treating the evaporative component of dry eye. NanoTears, on the other hand, attempts to address both the aqueous and evaporative aspects of DED and uses patented nano-lipid technology to create a colloidal lipid solution that attempts to replicate the lipids produced by the meibomian glands, thus restoring the lipid layer in an effort to reduce tear evaporation; this will allow for proper aqueous build-up and decrease osmolarity.

In patients who require frequent application of artificial tears, small inserts of a dissolvable material that lubricates the surface of the eye can be placed behind the lower eyelid into the conjunctival cul-de-sac on a daily basis. Many patients find the convenience and effectiveness of these Lacriserts to be helpful in reducing the need for frequent topical artificial tears.

There are few clinically controlled trials that have revealed that one tear supplement is superior to another. Table 23.1 lists some of the available tear supplements and lubricants.

Treatment of Lid Disease

When evaporative dry eye is present, it is most often associated with eyelid margin disease, either anterior blepharitis or meibomian gland dysfunction (MGD). Anterior blepharitis, inflammation of the anterior aspect of the lid, may be treated with warm compresses and topical antibiotics with or without steroids. The meibomian glands are lipid-secreting glands in the eyelid that are responsible for providing the lipid layer of the tear film. When MGD is present, the glands are plugged and have abnormal secretions. The abnormal lipid layer of the tear film fails to provide adequate protection against evaporation of the tears from the ocular surface. Such eyelid margin disease can be treated with warm compresses, lid massage, and expression of the meibomian glands. In more severe cases of MGD, topical azithromycin or oral doxycycline or tetracycline can improve symptoms of both eyelid inflammation and evaporative dry eye. If these medications are used, at least a month of treatment is required.

Recently, the LipiFlow® thermal pulsation system (TearScience) has been marketed to treat MGD. This procedure applies heat to the eyelids while simultaneously applying pulsating pressure to the eyelids. By applying both heat and pressure to the eyelids, it attempts to melt the abnormal meibomian secretions and then open and express this material from the glands. While many clinicians have embraced this form of therapy, others feel that warm compresses and lid scrubs are just as effective and significantly less expensive.

Table 23.1 Some of the Available Over-the-Counter Tear Supplements and Lubricants

Major Component(s)	Strength	Trade Name	Preservative
Carboxymethylcellulose	0.5%	Refresh	Purite
	1.0%	Celluvisc	None
	0.25%	Theratears	None
Glycerin	0.3%	Moisture Eyes	Benzalkonium
Hydroxypropyl-methyl cellulose	0.2–0.3%	GenTeal	Perborate
		GenTeal Gel	Perborate
Hydroxypropyl-cellulose	5 mg/ insert	Lacriset	None
Hydroxypropyl-methylcellulose/ Dextran 70		Bion Tears	None
Hydroxypropyl-methylcellulose/glycerin		Clear Eyes	Sorbic acid/EDTA
Hydroxypropyl-methylcellulose/glycerin/ Dextran 70		Tears Naturale	Polyquad
		Tears Naturale free	None
Polyvinyl alcohol/Glycerin	1.4%	AKWA Tears	Benzalkonium
		Optive	Purite
		Optive free	None
Nano-sized lipids (NanoPids)		NanoTears MXP/ Forte	None
Glycerin/HP-Guar		Systane	Polyquad
		Systane PF	None
Drakeol Oil emulsion		Soothe XP	PHMB
		Soothe	None
Ointment/lanolin		Lacrilube	None

Intense pulsed light (IPL) has also recently been advocated for the treatment of moderate to severe MGD. Pulses of non-coherent light in the range of 500 to 1,200 nm are delivered to the lids, which is followed by meibomian gland expression. Limited studies have reported improvement in meibomian gland function and decrease in dry eye symptoms

Omega-3 Supplements

The American diet has become deficient in omega-3 fatty acids, which are not produced by the body and thus must be ingested in the diet. Since our diet is high in omega-6 essential fatty acids, it is necessary to include omega-3 dietary supplements to balance the levels of fatty acid that protect against or reduce inflammation. In addition, studies have shown that omega-3 fatty acids have cardiovascular, anticancer, and possibly cognitive benefits. Thus, many clinicians have been recommending omega-3 dietary supplementation as part of their DED treatment in an attempt to suppress the inflammation associated with DED. There is anecdotal evidence that adding omega-3 supplements helps to reduce the signs and symptoms of DED. A dose of 3,000 mg/day or four or more servings of fish per week has been recommended. Recently, a multicenter study funded by the National Eye Institute and National Institutes of Health, the Dry Eye Assessment and Management Study Research Group (DREAM study), reported that omega-3 was no better than olive oil (placebo used in the study) in the treatment of DED. The conclusion from this study was that the beneficial effect of omega-3 supplements for the treatment of moderate to severe DED was not supported. However, other clinicians reviewing the study concluded that while there was no statistical difference between the two groups, both groups did show improvement in the signs and symptoms of DED at 12 months compared to baseline. Their conclusion was that perhaps olive oil (which may also have anti-inflammatory and antioxidant properties) was as effective as omega-3 supplementation in the treatment of DED. Thus, the question of the efficacy of omega-3 dietary supplements is still unsettled.

Step 2

The Step 2 interventions are used if the Step 1 options prove inadequate.

Non-preserved Lubrication

If topical lubrication (artificial tears) is required more than four times per day, non-preserved lubricants should be used. Box 23.2 lists some of the non-preserved ocular lubricants available.

Gels are more viscous than solutions and provide a longer duration on the surface of the eye but can blur the vision and are therefore usually recommended for use at night. Ointments are even thicker than gels and consequently last longer on the surface but produce even more blur in vision; they are also used before sleep.

Box 23.2 Non-preserved Ocular Lubricants

- Bion tears
- Soothe
- Systane
- NanoTears MXP/TF Forte
- TheraTears
- Refresh Optive Advanced
- GenTeal Lubricant Eye

Topical Anti-inflammatory Therapy

It is well accepted that inflammation of the ocular surface and lacrimal gland is both an etiologic and an aggravating factor. Anti-inflammatory treatment options include topical steroids and drugs that block mediators of inflammation such as cyclosporine (Restasis, Cequa) and lifitegrast (Xiidra).

Topical steroids have been shown to be effective in decreasing anterior segment inflammation and improving DED signs and symptoms. For patients with moderate to severe disease that is not controlled with other therapies, repeated short-term pulse therapy of corticosteroids is a therapeutic option that can be considered. For example, the drug can be used four times per day for 2 weeks and then tapered, depending on the clinical response to the drug. Topical corticosteroid therapy should be used on an intermittent and short-term basis for flare-ups of signs and symptoms since long-term use is associated with ocular hypertension, cataracts, and secondary infection. Loteprednol and methylprednisolone may be associated with fewer potential complications than dexamethasone, prednisolone, or even fluorometholone (FML) ophthalmic suspension.

Topical cyclosporine A (Restasis, Allergan) was the first drug approved by the U.S. Food and Drug Administration (FDA) for the treatment of aqueous-deficient dry eye. It is an immunomodulator that inhibits the activation of T lymphocytes and decreases the production of inflammatory mediators. In patients with moderate to severe DED that has been unresponsive to artificial tears or other modalities outlined in Step 1, then Restasis, twice daily, can be started. The cyclosporine can take up to 2 months before clinical efficacy is achieved, and the peak effect of the medication may not be reached until 4 to 6 months of therapy. The drug has been shown to be safe for long-term usage, with the main side effect being stinging upon instillation (reported in 17%, with 3% not able to tolerate such stinging). Artificial tear supplements are usually needed in conjunction with Restasis therapy. In an attempt to improve the tolerance of this medication, many clinicians pretreat their patients with topical steroids for 2 to 3 weeks before starting Restasis. After Restasis has been added to the therapeutic regimen, the topical steroid is tapered over the next few weeks and then discontinued.

Cequa (Sun Pharmaceuticals) is a 0.09% cyclosporine A ophthalmic solution that has recently been approved by the FDA. The proprietary nano-micellar formulation of the drug allows it to be dispensed in a clear, preservative-free aqueous solution. The drug is dosed two times per day. In phase 2 and 3 clinical trials, Cequa demonstrated increased tear production and a decrease in ocular surface staining compared to vehicle. The most common adverse reactions were instillation site pain (22%) and conjunctival hyperemia (6%).

Lifitegrast 5% ophthalmic solution (Xiidra [Novartis]), works by blocking specific key mediators of inflammation (LFA-1 and I CAM1) and inhibits the recruitment and activation of T cells and the release of pro-inflammatory mediators. It has FDA approval and is dispensed as a single-dose unit, instilled two times per day (12 hours apart) for the treatment of DED signs and symptoms. The more common adverse reactions were instillation site irritation (5–25%), an altered or impaired sense of taste (5–25%), and reduced visual acuity (5–25%); conjunctival hyperemia and eye irritation (1–5%) were also reported.

Numerous additional prescription DED therapies are currently in clinical trials, and some of these are likely to come onto the market over the next few years. Watch the Sjögren's Foundation website for the most up-to-date information.

Tear Conservation

In patients with moderate to severe DED, tear conservation should be considered once the inflammation of the anterior segment has been addressed. Punctal occlusion or moisture chamber spectacles can accomplish this goal. The lacrimal puncta can be closed by a number of methods. Dissolvable inserts can be placed into the puncta that provide temporary closure of the ducts lasting 1 to 2 weeks. Permanent replaceable plugs can be inserted in the puncta that last until they are removed or fall out, which is usually months or years. Finally, closure of the puncta can be performed with laser or cautery. Such closure is usually permanent and reversal requires surgical intervention if tearing should occur as a complication. By decreasing the drainage of tears from the eye, the volume of tears that can be retained on the eye is increased. This is a helpful modality when combined with other DED treatment options.

Tear conservation can also be aided by moisture chamber goggles, which are specially designed eyeglasses that decrease evaporation from the ocular surface, decrease airflow over the surface, and provide a more humid ocular environment. Wraparound sunglasses, which are more readily available than moisture chamber glasses, can also aid in reducing evaporation and provide relief similar to that offered by the goggles. Panoptik and microenvironment glasses (MEG) are two commercially available products.

Step 3

Again, these options are used if those previously described are inadequate.

Oral Secretagogues

Oral secretagogues such as pilocarpine (Salagen) and cevimeline (Evoxac) are available for the treatment of both oral and ocular signs and symptoms in patients with Sjögren's. Studies have shown that both oral pilocarpine and cevimeline can have a beneficial effect on the signs and symptoms of DED. However, the efficacy of oral secretagogues seems to be greater in the treatment of oral dryness than ocular dryness. In addition, both drugs are associated with side effects, including sweating and gastrointestinal side effects that can limit their usefulness in DED.

Autologous Serum Eye Drops

The use of autologous serum drops was first reported in the 1970s and has recently been shown to be effective in the treatment of DED in patients with severe ocular surface disease. The proteins and growth factors that are present in the serum protect and stimulate the ocular surface and contain anti-inflammatory mediators. The patient's serum is obtained and diluted with artificial tears. Once the individual dropper bottles of serum tears are made (the product requires refrigeration), they should be replaced after 30 days. A risk of contamination is present, so care in storage and application of the eye drop is required. Usually the treatment is continued for several months to aid in healing the ocular surface. However, the ocular surface disease can recur once the autologous serum therapy is discontinued.

Therapeutic Contact Lenses

Since wearing contact lenses can aggravative symptoms of dryness, their use to correct refractive errors is usually contraindicated in patients with DED. However, they can be a useful modality in the management of moderate to severe DED due to their ability to protect and improve the ocular surface as well as reduce corneal desiccation. The risks and benefits have to be determined for each patient with the understanding that there is an increased risk of infection when compared to the use of contact lenses in healthy individuals, especially when prescribed for extended wear. Soft therapeutic contact lenses, especially silicone hydrogels with their high oxygen transmissibility, can be invaluable in the treatment of corneal epithelial abnormalities such as epithelial defects or filamentary keratitis. Rigid gas-permeable scleral contact lenses have been gaining popularity in the management of severe DED. They are able to provide a reservoir of tears between the lens and the cornea in addition to protecting the ocular surface and improving its refractive surface.

Step 4

Again, these options are used if those previously described are inadequate.

Amniotic Membrane Grafting

In DED patients who develop severe ocular surface disease such as persistent corneal epithelial defects or ulceration, which are resistant to other forms of therapy, amniotic membrane grafts can be considered. They can protect the ocular surface by acting as a therapeutic bandage and can act as a platform to aid in re-epithelialization of the cornea. In addition, the tissue has anti-inflammatory mediators, an anti-scarring substance, and growth factors that can aid in corneal wound healing and decrease corneal scarring.

Tarsorrhaphy

Tarsorrhaphy is a procedure where the eyelids are partially or totally closed either temporarily or permanently. This protects the ocular surface by decreasing ocular surface exposure and thus decreasing evaporation of the tear film and ocular surface drying. Permanent tarsorrhaphy, due to problems with the patient's acceptance of the resulting cosmetic appearance, is reserved as a late-stage treatment modality.

Other Step 4 surgical modalities, depending on the underlying condition, are correction of lid abnormalities, conjunctival flaps, and removal of excessive abnormal conjunctival tissue (symptomatic conjunctivochalasis).

Summing Up

There is no one treatment or algorithm for the treatment of DED. In the last 10 years the options available to manage patients with DED have significantly increased. While we have more options at our disposal, management is an art that should be based on the best scientific evidence available. The ultimate management goal, as stated in the DEWS II report, is "to restore and maintain homeostasis of the ocular surface." This often involves long-term management strategies. Box 23.3, the stepwise approach discussed in this chapter, is an attempt to offer a reasonable approach to the management of DED rather than a rigid cookbook management tool.

Box 23.3 Stepwise Management and Treatment Recommendations for DED

Step 1
- Education regarding the condition, its management, treatment, and prognosis
- Modification of local environment
- Education regarding potential dietary modifications (including oral essential fatty acid supplementation)
- Identification and potential modification/elimination of offending systemic and topical medications
- Ocular lubricants of various types (if MGD is present, then consider lipid-containing supplements)
- Lid hygiene and warm compresses of various types

Step 2

If above options are inadequate, consider:

- Non-preserved ocular lubricants to minimize preservative-induced toxicity
- Tea tree oil treatment for Demodex (if present)
- Tear conservation
- Punctal occlusion
- Moisture chamber spectacles/goggles
- Overnight treatments (such as ointment or moisture chamber devices)
- In-office physical heating and expression of the meibomian glands (including device-assisted therapies, such as LipiFlow)
- In-office intense pulsed light therapy for MGD
- Prescription drugs to manage DED
- Topical antibiotic or antibiotic/steroid combination applied to the lid margins for anterior blepharitis (if present)
- Topical corticosteroid (limited duration)
- Topical secretagogues
- Topical non-glucocorticoid immunomodulatory drugs (such as cyclosporine)
- Topical LFA-1 antagonist drugs (such as lifitegrast)
- Oral macrolide or tetracycline antibiotics

Step 3

If above options are inadequate, consider:

- Oral secretagogues
- Autologous/allogeneic serum eye drops
- Therapeutic contact lens options
- Soft bandage lenses
- Rigid scleral lenses

Step 4

If above options are inadequate, consider:

- Topical corticosteroid for longer duration
- Amniotic membrane grafts
- Surgical punctal occlusion
- Other surgical approaches

As presented in the DEWS II report.

Source: Craig JP, Nelson JD, Azar DT, et al. TFOS DEWS II Report Executive Summary. *Ocul Surf.* 2017 Oct;15(4):802-812. doi: 10.1016/j.jtos.2017.08.003. Epub 2017 Aug 8.

For Further Reading

Asbell PA, Maguire MG, Pistilli M, et al. Dry Eye Assessment and Management Study Research Group. Omega-3 fatty acid supplementation for the treatment of dry eye disease. *N Engl J Med*. 2018;1681–1690.

Craig JP, Nichols KK, Akpek EK, et al. TFOS International Dry Eye Workshop (DEWS II) definition and classification report. *Ocul Surf*. 2017;15:276–283.

Foulks GN, Forstot SL, Donshik PC, et al. Clinical guidelines for management of dry eye associated with Sjögren disease. *Ocul Surf*. 2015;13(2):118–132.

Jones L, Downie LE, Korb D, et al. TFOS International Dry Eye Workshop (DEWS II) management and therapy report. *Ocul Surf*. 2017;15:575–628.

Nichols KK, Foulks GN, Bron AJ, et al. The international workshop on meibomian gland dysfunction: Executive summary. *Invest Ophthalmol Vis Sci*. 2011;52:1922–1929.

24

Management of Dry Mouth in Sjögren's

Vidya Sankar

Salivary dysfunction and the feeling of dryness of the mouth (xerostomia) are common characteristics in patients with Sjögren's. Saliva's functions include enamel remineralization, lubrication, antimicrobial defense, and digestion. Reduction in salivary flow rates is associated with an increased risk of dental caries (tooth decay or cavities) as well as with a host of difficulties with protective features of the oral cavity. This chapter will review the role of saliva and will discuss the treatments currently available, giving readers practical advice on ways to maximize the potential benefit of products they are currently using or ones they may have given up on due to improper use or understanding of what it was intended to do.

Saliva

A healthy person secretes up to approximately 1.5 liters (6 cups) of saliva per day, luckily not all at once. The major salivary glands (pairs of parotid, sublingual, and submandibular glands; Figure 24.1) are responsible for the secretion of about 90% of all saliva; the minor salivary glands (MSGs), located in the labial (lip), buccal (inner cheeks), and palatal (roof of the mouth) mucosa account for the remaining 10%. Whole saliva is composed mostly of water as well as many organic and inorganic substances. Two defining constituents are amylase (a digestive enzyme that breaks down starches from the food you eat into maltose and smaller carbohydrates) and mucins (slimy, viscous material that lubricates the mouth, preventing tissue desiccation). The parotid glands secrete predominantly amylase-rich serous saliva and are most active when eating/chewing. The sublingual glands and MSGs secrete predominantly mucin-rich mucous saliva, and the submandibular glands secrete mixed seromucous saliva, which contributes most of the saliva produced between meals. The MSGs produce up to 70% of the mucin and, for the most part, maintain a constant rate of flow throughout the day—with the exception of

Vidya Sankar, *Management of Dry Mouth in Sjögren's* In: *The Sjögren's Book*. Edited by: Daniel J. Wallace, Oxford University Press. © Sjögren's Foundation 2022. DOI: 10.1093/oso/9780197502112.003.0024

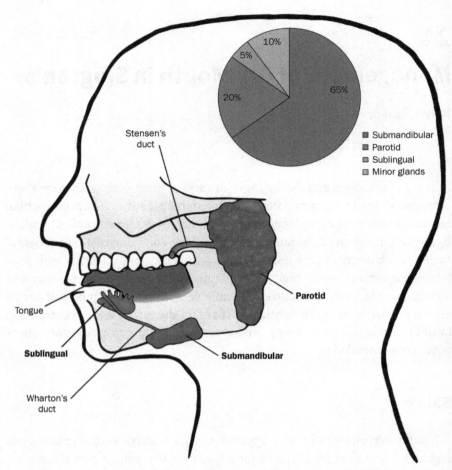

Figure 24.1 Anatomical location of human major salivary glands and their salivary contribution.
Minor salivary glands (not shown) also contribute approximately 10% of total salivary secretions. Salivary contributions in the pie chart are shown based on the resting state; differences in salivary contribution/gland may be observed when saliva is analyzed from stimulated states.

Source: Vila T, Rizk AM, Sultan AS, Jabra-Rizk MA (2019) The power of saliva: Antimicrobial and beyond. *PLoS Pathog* 15(11): e1008058. https://doi.org/10.1371/journal.ppat.1008058

the labial MSGs, which display a significant secretory circadian rhythm, with the highest rate in the evening.

Saliva provides a physical barrier against local irritants and promotes mucosal repair (epidermal growth factor); lubricates (mucin) and cleanses oral tissues; maintains a stable intraoral pH with its bicarbonate buffering system; and maintains electrolyte balance. Saliva prevents demineralization and contributes to the remineralization (providing proline-rich proteins) of dental hard tissues. Saliva contains antibacterial (lysozymes), antiviral (secretory leukocyte protease inhibitors), and antifungal (histatins) components, which help to maintain a favorable ecosystem for the normal oral flora. Finally, saliva has a salutary effect on the sense of taste, facilitates mastication, aids in formation of a bolus by adding mucin and water, aids in swallowing, and provides initial food processing (amylase).

Salivary dysfunction in Sjögren's can be characterized by decreased salivary output and/or a change in the consistency (quality) of saliva. A patient is considered to have reduced salivary flow if the unstimulated salivary flow rate measured for 5 to 15 minutes is 0.1 mL/min or less, or if the stimulated salivary flow rate measured for 5 minutes is 0.5 mL/min or less. As the disease progresses, there can be complete loss of the ability to produce saliva. To provide the best care to patients with salivary dysfunction, clinicians must determine if patients still maintain the ability to produce saliva. This information will help determine the most appropriate therapeutic interventions. For example, if a patient makes a moderate amount of saliva throughout the day, coating agents such as thicker gels and sprays will be washed away quickly, requiring frequent applications. For these individuals, sugar-free gums and candies may be more effective in managing dryness, as chewing and sucking on candies will stimulate the glands to produce saliva while the product is in the mouth. In patients who produce little to no saliva, gums and candies will have little effect; coating agents such as gels and sprays will remain in place for a longer period of time, offering a longer duration of benefit and decreasing the frequency of application.

Other Factors Contributing to Dryness

Concomitant medical diseases such as diabetes or sarcoidosis can cause decreased saliva production. Many medications used to treat common medical conditions (high blood pressure, depression/anxiety, allergies, bladder irritability, etc.) have drying side effects and can worsen xerostomia. Xerostomia is a common complication of both prescription and nonprescription drug therapy: More than 400 active medications have been implicated. The major classes of drugs causing xerostomia are listed in Box 24.1. Dryness increases if patients take multiple medications with xerostomic side effects.

Box 24.1 Major Drug Categories Causing Hyposalivation

- Anticholinergic agents
- Anticonvulsants
- Antidepressants
- Antiemetics
- Antihistamines
- Antihypertensive agents and diuretics
- Anti-inflammatory agents
- Antiparkinsonian drugs
- Antipsychotic agents
- Anxiolytic, sedative–hypnotic agents
- Cancer chemotherapeutic agents
- Muscle relaxants
- Opioids

Clinical Consequences of Hyposalivation

Qualitative and quantitative changes in saliva lead to reduced lubrication. Dryness affects taste and speech, mucosal tissues appear dry and atrophic, there can be abrasions and loss of mucosal integrity, and the tongue is often fissured. Hyposalivation alone may decrease the retention of even well-fitting prostheses, which in turn may lead to the development of traumatic ulcers. Impaired chewing and swallowing and/or the presence of dygeusia (altered taste), hypogeusia (decreased taste), or ageusia (inability to distinguish sweet, sour, salty, etc.) may cause patients to alter their diet and fluid intake, increasing the risk of malnutrition and weight loss and decreasing the potential social pleasure of meals.

Decreased saliva production can result in reduced production and subsequent activity of lysozymes, secretory leukocyte protease inhibitors, and histatins, which predisposes to bacterial, viral, and fungal infections. Reduction in salivary immunoglobulin levels leads to a highly cariogenic (tooth decay-producing) oral microflora (*Streptococcus mutans*, *Lactobacillus*, and *Actinomyces*). In addition, the lack of saliva reduces lavage and cleansing of oral tissues, promoting plaque accumulation, gingivitis, and dental caries. This prolongs the amount of time that sugars and other substrates essential for microbial survival remain on tooth surfaces. There is loss of salivary buffering capacity, leading to higher acidity in the mouth, which interferes with normal remineralization of teeth. As a consequence, a distinctive form of decay begins near the gum line on teeth as well as the cusp tips and incisal edges. This unusual pattern of decay should raise suspicion for Sjögren's. Tooth loss, a predictable sequela of advanced carious lesions, presents further difficulties for both the patient and clinician.

Reduced antibacterial and antifungal activity associated with hyposalivation also contributes to an increased risk of both acute and chronic infection by the fungal organisms, which under normal conditions are inhibited by a normal bacterial flora and salivary gland function. The lesions often appear as erythema (redness) of soft tissues and the corners of the mouth (angular cheilitis) more so than white, raised, or cottage cheese–like growths that can be scraped off. Patients will often feel symptoms of burning or soreness due to *Candida* infection. Bacterial infections, typically affecting the parotid glands, are more common, appearing as warm enlarged glands that are frequently painful.

Dental Implications

Caries Prevention

Dental decay is a potentially preventable disease. By modifying certain factors, one can delay or, in some cases, reverse the caries process. The tooth surface can be strengthened through the use of fluoride. The daily use of a fluoridated dentifrice (0.05% sodium fluoride) or the daily use of a prescription fluoride gel (1% sodium fluoride or 0.4% stannous fluoride) is recommended. In addition, the application of a 0.5% sodium fluoride varnish and regular preventive care (every 2–6 months, based on risk factors) should be implemented. The frequency and duration of exposure to fermentable dietary carbohydrates should be decreased. One option would be to eat and drink foods with less sugar or to limit the exposure time. Minimizing intake of sodas and "sugar-free" sodas is important. The sugar in soda allows the bacteria in the mouth to form acid, and diet or "sugar-free" soda contains acid that can weaken tooth enamel, leading to increased susceptibility to tooth decay.

Another option would be to introduce sugar substitutes, such as xylitol, that are not metabolized by decay-producing bacteria. Xylitol is found in many gums and mints that are readily available in grocery stores. Long-term use of xylitol encourages the growth of organisms with fewer adhesive properties, making it easier for plaque to be washed away by saliva. An additional bonus is that these gums and mints help to mechanically stimulate the salivary glands to produce more saliva, thus modifying the secondary factors involved with development of decay.

Patients with dry mouth have been reported to have more erosion, tooth wear, and sensitivity. There are agents on the market today that claim to aid in remineralization of teeth, such as MI Paste. To date, there is no evidence that this is actually capable of tooth remineralization; however, it may help to reduce sensitivity. And, of course, regular dental check-ups and cleanings are encouraged. The intervals should be determined by the dentist.

Candidiasis

Hyposalivation increases the risk of superinfection by several *Candida* species; under normal conditions, this overgrowth is inhibited by normal flora and salivary function. Topical antifungal agents such as the various nystatin formulations or clotrimazole troches may be prescribed. However, many of these agents contain sugar, which may add to the caries risk. A mucoadhesive disk that also delivers miconazole topically may contain less fermentable sugar, though a pharmacist may be able to prepare these formulations without sugar. Systemic antifungal agents, such as fluconazole, are systemic alternatives.

Treatments

Coping Mechanisms

It is important to maintain adequate hydration. Strive to drink several glasses of water throughout the day, and avoid caffeinated beverages, as caffeine is a diuretic (causes fluid loss). Remember that many soft drinks contain caffeine. Keep your mouth moist by sipping small amounts of water, because excessive sips of water can reduce the oral mucous film and increase symptoms. Avoid frequent intake of acidic beverages (such as most carbonated and sports replenishment drinks) as they may increase susceptibility to tooth decay. If you do drink these beverages, limit the number of beverages and length of time it stays in your mouth—meaning drink them quickly and brush your teeth afterward. If you are unable to brush, rinse your mouth with water to wash off the sugar.

For people who breathe through their mouths, room humidifiers are helpful to preserve moisture. Avoid ceiling fans. Chew and swallow carefully and take frequent sips of liquids to avoid choking and aspiration. Because desiccated oral tissues are friable and prone to irritation and ulceration, the following are recommended:

- Avoid products that irritate the oral soft tissues (such as alcohol and to-bacco; hot, spicy, and coarse foods; fruits and beverages with a high acid content).
- Refrain from wearing ill-fitting removable prostheses that may cause injury.
- Eat a soft diet.
- Frequently rinse with a sodium bicarbonate solution.

Mucosal lesions are susceptible to secondary infections by microorganisms of the normal flora that have become pathogenic and by transient organisms. Prompt treatment of such infections is mandatory. Retention of removable prostheses is frequently impaired and painful in the presence of desiccated oral mucosa tissues and the lack of adequate salivary output. Daily oral hygiene of dentures and prosthesis-bearing mucosal tissues is important, as is regular observation for *Candida* infections. Denture problems can be reduced with frequent dental examinations to identify sore spots and to enhance adhesion with soft- and hard-tissue relines.

Topical Treatments

A variety of over-the-counter saliva substitutes that aid in lubricating the oral tissues are available in stores as well as over the internet. Their viscosity, electrolyte concentrations, and flavorings vary greatly. Patient acceptance depends on effect, duration, viscosity, taste, delivery system, and cost. As mentioned earlier, the greater the patient's salivary flow, the faster these products are eliminated from the mouth, necessitating more frequent application. There are the mouthwashes that either soothe or help with remineralizing teeth. Check the alcohol content of these mouth rinses, as those with a higher alcohol content will tend to dry the mouth out more and be more caustic to the tissues. Dry, cracked lips may be soothed by oil-based balms placed over previously moistened lips. The use of vitamin E-containing ointments may also be helpful.

Masticatory and Gustatory Agents

Chewing gum and sucking on sugar-free candies provide mechanical stimulation of the salivary glands to produce more saliva.

Sialagogues

Pilocarpine hydrochloride (Salagen; Pharmacia, Saint Paul, MN) is a cholinergic agonist that stimulates the production of saliva from functioning salivary glands. It may take up to several weeks of treatment before achieving benefit from the drug. It enhances oral comfort, improves the ability to speak, and offers prolonged symptomatic relief. Pilocarpine hydrochloride is contraindicated in patients with uncontrolled asthma or narrow angle glaucoma and should be used with caution in patients with significant cardiovascular disease. Common dose-dependent side effects include sweating, nausea, rhinitis, flushing, and increased urinary frequency.

Another sialagogue, cevimeline hydrochloride (Evoxac; Daiichi Sankyo Inc., Tokyo, Japan) has been approved by the U.S. Food and Drug Administration (FDA) for the treatment of dry mouth in Sjögren's at a dosage of 30 mg three times daily. Like pilocarpine, it is a muscarinic agonist that increases production of saliva. Patients with uncontrolled asthma, significant cardiac disease, and narrow angle glaucoma should not take cevimeline. As with pilocarpine, it may take up to several weeks of treatment to achieve maximal benefit.

Saliva production onset is typically 20 minutes after administration and peaks at 1 to 2 hours after ingestion, which is why these may be taken several times throughout the day. Patients who have the most difficulty with eating/ chewing foods due to lack of saliva may benefit most from taking the medication about 30 minutes prior to a meal. Patients who have the most difficulty with dryness in between meals may benefit most by taking the product after meals. For patients whose most problematic time is dryness at night while sleeping, taking the product just prior to bed may provide additional moisture at the beginning of the night, allowing for a longer duration of sleep before having to wake up to sip on water. This may also decrease the amount of water consumed throughout the night, decreasing the need for frequent urination and ultimately decreasing fatigue levels the next day.

The best way to limit side effects of these medications is to begin with one tablet or capsule per day for several days before adding a second dose. Repeat this either up to the maximum dose prescribed or to the frequency where the side effects are tolerable.

Immunomodulatory Drugs

There are ongoing clinical trials in Sjögren's looking at new classes of drugs capable of decreasing systemic inflammation. In theory, if inflammation is decreased within the salivary glands, this may lead to an increase in salivary function or perhaps preservation of the current level of functioning. To date, no immunomodulatory drug has proved to be efficacious in the treatment of Sjögren's. Several studies have investigated the response to treatment with biologic agents. They showed improvement in various systemic features of the disease, such as pain, fatigue, vasculitis, and salivary gland enlargement, but there were conflicting reports of improvement of salivary flow or oral comfort levels.

Future Directions

There is a need for more therapeutic options with a low side-effect profile to increase salivary flow and maintain salivary gland function. Novel approaches can deliver currently available therapeutics in polymers and microfluid drug delivery systems, allowing for controlled drug release. Gene therapy has been investigated as a way to repair injured salivary glands. Salivary gland transplant to the eye has been conducted to replenish tears in patients with extreme dry eyes, and regenerative medicine strategies using stem cells to engineer artificial salivary tissues are currently under investigation. It is hoped that these approaches will yield more therapeutic options.

Summing Up

Symptomatic and supportive care of the xerostomic patient should include good oral hygiene, proper dietary control, and the use of saliva substitutes and/or a sialogogue. The substitutes should have a pleasant taste, should contain electrolytes in concentrations normally found in saliva, and should have an acceptable viscosity. The use of supplemental fluoride agents to promote enamel remineralization is recommended. Topical fluoride should be used in

Sjögren's patients with dry mouth, and fluoride-delivery systems that provide optimal protection are now available.

For Further Reading

Letaief H, Lukas C, Barnetche T, et al. Efficacy and safety of biological DMARDs modulating B cells in primary Sjögren's syndrome: Systematic review and meta-analysis. *Joint Bone Spine.* 2018;85(1):15–22. doi:10.1016/j.jbspin.2017.06.004

Mariette X, Criswell LA. Primary Sjögren's syndrome. *N Engl J Med.* 2018;379(1):97. doi:10.1056/NEJMc1804598

Ogawa M, Tsuji T. Functional salivary gland regeneration as the next generation of organ replacement regenerative therapy. *Odontology.* 2015;103(3):248–257. doi:10.1007/s10266-015-0210-9

Zero DT, Brennan MT, Daniels TE, et al. Clinical practice guidelines for oral management of Sjogren disease: Dental caries prevention. *J Am Dent Assoc.* 2016;147(4):295–305.

25

Management of Other Sicca Symptoms in Sjögren's

Dry Ears, Nose, and Sinuses

Soo Kim Abboud and Leila M. Haddad

Nasal Symptoms

Sjögren's patients often suffer from significant nasal dryness, which can lead to pain, crusting, epistaxis (bleeding), sinusitis (sinus infections), and even septal perforation (a hole in the cartilage and bone that separates the right from the left nasal passageway). Conservative treatment is typically effective at improving the majority of nasal symptoms and includes adequate humidification of the work and home environment, saline irrigation, and the avoidance of medications such as decongestants and antihistamines that can further dry the nasal passages and promote pain, crusting, and bleeding.

Epistaxis can occur due to significant dryness and usually originates from the front of the nose along the septum, where more than 90% of the blood vessels in the nose are located. Humidification, saline irrigation (with Simply Saline, Ocean Spray, or a neti pot, among many other brands), and moisturization of the anterior septum with a nasal gel, Vaseline, or an over-the-counter antibiotic ointment such as Neosporin or triple antibiotic ointment can significantly decrease the frequency and severity of nosebleeds. Regular use of secretagogues (pilocarpine, cevimeline) at moderate to high doses may also help, although they may cause other systemic side effects. If epistaxis persists despite these measures, silver nitrate cauterization of the offending blood vessels can be performed by an otolaryngologist (ENT) in the office. While this is a simple procedure to perform, the cautery is very superficial and generally does not provide longstanding relief.

Patients with Sjögren's are at increased risk of suffering from allergic rhinitis (itching, sneezing, and nasal congestion due to allergies) and can benefit from using a topical nasal steroid once or twice daily to decrease the inflammation.

Soo Kim Abboud and Leila M. Haddad, *Management of Other Sicca Symptoms in Sjögren's* In: *The Sjögren's Book*. Edited by: Daniel J. Wallace, Oxford University Press. © Sjögren's Foundation 2022. DOI: 10.1093/oso/9780197502112.003.0025

Care must be taken not to aim the nasal steroid spray toward the septum as this can increase septal dryness and bleeding. Nasal steroids can often reduce the inflammation from rhinitis and decrease the severity and frequency of sinusitis or sinus infections, which are more common in this population because the dryness, crusting, and swelling can trap bacteria. Antibiotics can cure bouts of sinusitis; oral steroids may be needed in refractory cases when the swelling is severe or in chronic cases.

Auditory Symptoms

Patients with Sjögren's are at increased risk of hearing loss, both conductive (hearing loss due to problems with the ear canal, eardrum, Eustachian tube, or ear bones) and sensorineural (nerve deafness) types. Autoimmune hearing loss can occur; this is a type of sensorineural hearing loss that results when a person's antibodies attacking the auditory nervous system. Treatment is similar to other forms of autoimmune hearing loss and centers on oral or intratympanic steroids and, at times, antivirals. Occasionally, other immunosuppressant drugs are used for steroid-sparing effects. Partial return of hearing can occur if treatment is prompt, although progressive deterioration is more common. Audiograms should be ordered in all Sjögren's patients who complain of hearing loss, and all other causes of hearing loss that are treatable must be excluded before the patient is diagnosed with Sjögren's-related autoimmune hearing loss.

Tinnitus, or ringing in the ears, also occurs more frequently in patients with Sjögren's. In patients with sensorineural hearing loss, tinnitus is often a byproduct of the nerve damage. However, even Sjögren's patients with normal hearing often complain of tinnitus for reasons that are unknown. Tinnitus occurs more often in patients with anxiety and depression; on many occasions, treating the anxiety and depression can improve the patient's subjective tinnitus. While most patients are able to live with the tinnitus, some patients suffer so greatly that more aggressive treatment such as tinnitus maskers (electronic hearing aids that emit sounds to mask the ringing caused by tinnitus), biofeedback, or medication such as antidepressants may be necessary. Acupuncture has also been found to be helpful in many patients.

Otalgia, or ear pain, can occur in as many as a quarter of Sjögren's patients. The origin of the ear pain is also largely unknown, although many suspect that the dryness in the upper airway can lead to Eustachian tube dysfunction. Because the Eustachian tube serves to equalize pressure within the middle ear, when the Eustachian tube is diseased or dry the middle ear develops negative pressure, which can lead to pain, hearing loss, fluid accumulation, and infection. The treatment of Eustachian tube dysfunction depends on the severity of the disease; avoiding decongestants and using a nasal steroid and nasal saline to improve function is usually all that is necessary. In severe cases of Eustachian tube dysfunction, patients may suffer from recurrent fluid build-up in the middle ear and middle ear infections. Patients with this level of disease may benefit from antibiotics or even a myringotomy tube (a tube placed in the eardrum to drain the middle ear). Dryness in the oropharynx due to Sjögren's can also potentially cause referred pain to the ears.

Ear pain, redness, and swelling may also occur due to relapsing polychondritis. This condition causes autoimmune inflammation of ear cartilage as well as other cartilaginous structures in the head and neck and may occur as an isolated condition or in association with other autoimmune diseases like Sjögren's. It is usually treated with high-dose oral steroids and other immunosuppressant drugs, and antibiotics for bacterial infections.

The Larynx

Patients with Sjögren's are at higher risk of suffering from laryngeal (voice box) symptoms due to salivary gland dysfunction and upper airway dryness. This can lead to hoarseness or laryngitis, dysphagia (difficulty swallowing), globus sensation (lump-in-the-throat sensation), dyspnea (difficulty breathing), coughing, or throat pain. Laryngeal dryness can be improved with humidification and adequate hydration. Secretagogues may also provide relief. When laryngeal dryness leads to thick mucus that is difficult to clear, a mucous thinner such as long-acting guaifenesin 600 mg up to several times daily can be used with some benefit.

While the exact causal relationship is unknown, many patients with Sjögren's suffer from gastroesophageal reflux disease (GERD). Patients with extra-esophageal manifestations of GERD commonly suffer from hoarseness, dysphagia, globus sensation, constant clearing of the throat with or without thick phlegm, cough, or recurrent sore throat. Many patients with these symptoms do not suffer from typical heartburn or indigestion and may be misdiagnosed. Symptoms often improve with medications that decrease the amount of acid produced in the stomach. These include over-the-counter H2 blockers like Tagamet and Zantac or proton pump inhibitors such as Prilosec, Prevacid, Aciphex, Protonix, Nexium, and Zegerid. These medications are taken for at least 2 months and may need to be taken long term. Because proton pump inhibitors cause side effects when taken long term, all patients taking these medications for a prolonged period of time need to be monitored carefully by their general practitioner or gastroenterologist. Dietary and lifestyle modifications are equally important for the successful treatment of GERD and extra-esophageal reflux.

Summing Up

The underlying cause of nasal, otologic, and oral symptoms of Sjögren's should first be ascertained. A general principle is to promote humidification measures, avoid drying agents (e.g., antihistamines), and use irrigation as needed (nasal saline, neti pot). Associated inflammatory conditions such as chondritis or vestibulitis respond to corticosteroids or other immunosuppressives, but these should be used sparingly due to their side effects. Ear pain can be relieved with a variety of approaches that decrease Eustachian tube dysfunction and improve moisturization of the nasal and oral cavity. Management of laryngeal involvement consists of anti-reflux measures such as proton pump inhibitors as well as mucolytic agents.

For Further Reading

American Academy of Otolaryngology—Head and Neck Surgery. Autoimmune inner ear disease. https://www.enthealth.org/conditions/autoimmune-inner-ear-disease/
American Academy of Otolaryngology—Head and Neck Surgery. GERD and LPR. https://www.enthealth.org/conditions/gerd-and-lpr/

26

Management of Vaginal Dryness in Sjögren's

Jolien F. van Nimwegen and Rita Melkonian

Vaginal dryness is a common yet under-recognized symptom in women with Sjögren's. Multiple studies have shown a higher prevalence of vaginal dryness in Sjögren's compared to respective controls. As a consequence, women with Sjögren's can experience discomfort in daily life and have an increased prevalence of dyspareunia (painful intercourse). Chronic dyspareunia can even be the presenting symptom of Sjögren's. Despite the vaginal dryness, the overall composition of the vaginal microbiome of Sjögren's patients was found to be similar to controls in studies to date.

As a result of vaginal dryness and dyspareunia, sexual function is often impaired in Sjögren's patients. Other symptoms of Sjögren's also negatively influence sexual function, such as fatigue, myalgia, and arthralgia. In one study, 62% of Sjögren's patients rated sexual activity as important and 68% reported that symptoms of Sjögren's affected their sexual ability, which shows that these symptoms should not be overlooked. Several other studies found that women with Sjögren's have impaired sexual functioning compared to other groups of women, as measured by the Female Sexual Function Index. Patients also experience more distress regarding their sexual functioning, as measured by the Female Sexual Distress Scale. Impaired sexual function is associated with anxiety, depression, relationship dissatisfaction, and lower quality of life. Sexual function is discussed in greater detail in Chapter 45.

Despite the major impact of vaginal dryness on sexual function and quality of life in Sjögren's, little is known about the pathogenesis of this symptom. In healthy individuals, the vaginal surface is lubricated by transudate from the rich vascular network in the lamina propria of the vaginal wall, as well as by mucus produced by the endocervical glandular epithelium. In healthy women, vaginal dryness is often caused by decreased estrogen levels after menopause, leading to vulvovaginal atrophy. In Sjögren's, however, vaginal dryness often occurs before menopause. One study comparing Sjögren's

Jolien F. van Nimwegen and Rita Melkonian, *Management of Vaginal Dryness in Sjögren's* In: *The Sjögren's Book*. Edited by: Daniel J. Wallace, Oxford University Press. © Sjögren's Foundation 2022. DOI: 10.1093/oso/9780197502112.003.0026 patients with healthy controls found a larger difference in premenopausal participants than in postmenopausal participants. The sexual dysfunction in premenopausal patients could not be explained by premature hormonal changes, as no macroscopic signs of vaginal atrophy were found. These results suggest that although menopause may worsen symptoms of vaginal dryness and sexual dysfunction in women with Sjögren's, other factors are likely to be more important in the pathogenesis of these symptoms.

Several manifestations of Sjögren's, such as the destruction of exocrine glandular tissue, interstitial nephritis, and interstitial lung disease, are caused by the presence of peri-epithelial lymphocytic infiltration. A similar pathogenetic mechanism may also play a role in vaginal dryness in Sjögren's. Several studies have described peri-epithelial lymphocytic infiltrates in the underlying stroma of the vaginal or vulvar epithelium of premenopausal Sjögren's patients with dyspareunia. Chronic cervicitis has been shown to be present in 48% of premenopausal and 33% of postmenopausal women with Sjögren's. In addition, a recent study quantitatively compared the presence of lymphocyte subsets in the vagina and endocervix of premenopausal women with Sjögren's compared to healthy controls, and a significantly higher number of infiltrating T cells were seen in the subepithelial layer of the vagina of Sjögren's. In the endocervix, the number of B cells was increased in Sjögren's patients.

It is currently unknown whether local inflammation in the vaginal and endocervical mucosa of women with Sjögren's indeed causes vaginal dryness, by impairing the production of transudate from vaginal blood vessels or mucus from the endocervical glandular mucosa, respectively. Interestingly, one study showed a decrease in the number of vascular smooth muscle cells in the connective tissue layer of the vaginal wall of Sjögren's patients. During sexual arousal, vascular smooth muscle cell relaxation in response to a sexual stimulus leads to vasodilatation, after which blood flow and production of transudate increases. Loss of vascular smooth muscle cells may therefore play a critical role in the development of vaginal dryness.

Lichen planus, lichen sclerosus, and yeast infections also can contribute to a burning sensation and itching of the skin and mucosal surfaces, including the genitalia, in Sjögren's and may be confused with and exacerbated by dryness. Lichen planus is an inflammatory condition that can involve mucosal surfaces. Lichen sclerosus is a chronic dermatologic condition associated with epithelial thinning, distinctive dermal changes, and inflammation. Diagnosis of the underlying cause or causes of a patient's symptoms is important to identifying the best treatment.

Management and Treatment

Treatment of vaginal dryness differs based on the patient's symptoms and impact of the symptoms on quality of life and patient goals (Box 26.1).

If menopause is contributing to the dryness, topical estrogens are often prescribed for treatment of vaginal dryness and dyspareunia when hormonal treatments are not contraindicated (e.g., those with estrogen receptor–positive breast cancer or history of uterine cancer). Topical estrogen treatments can be administered in various forms (Box 26.2).

Summing Up

Vaginal dryness is one of the most common manifestations in women with Sjögren's and has a direct impact on sexual function. Fortunately, successful management and treatment of vaginal dryness is possible, with options

---

Box 26.1 Treatments for Vaginal Dryness

Numerous non-hormonal over-the-counter products are available to provide hydration and lubrication. Examples include:

- FemmePharma products: lowest effective volume, made with concentrated hyaluronic acid, a natural hydrator and healer and vitamin E; Femmepharma intimate skin moisturizer, Femmepharma personal lubricant and vaginal moisturizer, and, coming soon, Mia Vita)
- Revaree (Bonafide): made from hyaluronic acid, a natural hydrator and healer; moisturizer and personal lubricant
- Luvena products (Laclede): a probiotic, restorative moisturizer and personal lubricant (Luvena vaginal moisturizer and lubricant, Luvena vaginal rinse, Luvena feminine wipes)
- Replens: bioadhesive, moisturizer and personal lubricant (Replens Moisture Restore External Comfort Gel, Long-Lasting Moisturizer, Lubricant)
- K-Y products: water-soluble lubricants that can be used during sexual activities (K-Y Ultragel, K-Y Liquid, K-Y Jelly, K-Y Liquibeads, K-Y True Feel, K-Y Warming Liquid, K-Y Warming Jelly)

Patients should ask their healthcare professional to instruct them on frequency and placement of these products.

Box 26.2 Topical Estrogen Treatments

Vaginal Estrogen Cream
- Premarin cream
- Estrace cream
- Compound vaginal estrogen

Vaginal Inserts (Estradiol)
- Vagifem, Yuvafem (10 mcg × 2 a week)
- Imvexxy inserts (4 mcg, 10 mcg; new vaginal insert, 2 weeks of daily loading dose, then twice a week)
- Intrarosa: Prasterone daily vaginal insert, 6.5 mg. Prasterone is a steroid product indicated for treatment of moderate to severe dyspareunia. Estrogen is a metabolite of prasterone. Prasterone converts into androgens and/or estrogens.

Estring
- A flexible vaginal ring that contains estrogen; lasts 3 months

---

including water-soluble lubricating products, probiotic and hyaluronic acid moisturizers, estrogen creams, estradiol-based vaginal inserts, and more.

For Further Reading

Al-Hashimi I, Khuder S, Haghighat N, Zipp M. Frequency and predictive value of the clinical manifestations in Sjögren's syndrome. *J Oral Pathol Med.* 2001;30:1–6.

Capriello P, Barale E, Cappelli N, Lupo S, Teti G. Sjögren's syndrome: Clinical, cytological, histological and colposcopic aspects in women. *Clin Exp Obstet Gynecol.* 1988;15:9–12.

Cirpan T, Guliyeva A, Onder G, et al. Comparison of human papillomavirus testing and cervical cytology with colposcopic examination and biopsy in cervical cancer screening in a cohort of patients with Sjögren's syndrome. *Eur J Gynaecol Oncol.* 2007;28:302–306.

Haga HJ, Gram Gsjesdal C, Irgens LM, et al. Reproduction and gynaecological manifestations in women with primary Sjögren's syndrome: A case-control study. *Scand J Rheumatol.* 2005;34:45–48.

Isik H, Isik M, Aynioglu O, et al. Are the women with Sjögren's syndrome satisfied with their sexual activity? *Rev Bras Reum [Engl Ed].* 2017;57:210–216.

Lehrer S, Bogursky E, Yemini M, et al. Gynecologic manifestations of Sjögren's syndrome. *Am J Obstet Gynecol.* 1994;170:835–837.

Maddali Bongi S, Del Rosso A, Orlandi M, Matucci-Cerinic M. Gynaecological symptoms and sexual disability in women with primary Sjögren's syndrome and sicca syndrome. *Clin Exp Rheumatol.* 2013;31:683–690.

Maddali Bongi S, Orlandi M, De Magnis A, et al. Women with primary Sjögren syndrome and with non-Sjögren sicca syndrome show similar vulvar histopathologic and immunohisto-chemical changes. *Int J Gynecol Pathol.* 2016;35:585–592.

Marchesoni D, Mozzanega B, Sandre P De, et al. Gynaecological aspects of primary Sjögren's syndrome. *Eur J Obstet Gynecol Reprod Biol.* 1995;63:49–53.

Mitsias DI, Kapsogeorgou EK, Moutsopoulos HM. Sjögren's syndrome: Why autoimmune epithelitis? *Oral Dis.* 2006;12:523–532.

Mulherin DM, Sheeran TP, Kumararatne DS, et al. Sjögren's syndrome in women presenting with chronic dyspareunia. *Br J Obstet Gynaecol.* 1997;104:1019–1023.

Priori R, Minniti A, Derme M, et al. Quality of sexual life in women with primary Sjögren syndrome. *J Rheumatol.* 2015;42:1427–1431.

Robboy SJ, Mutter GL, Prat J, et al., eds. *Robboy's Pathology of the Female Reproductive Tract* (2nd ed.). Elsevier Limited; 2009.

Sellier S, Courville P, Joly P. Dyspareunia and Sjögren's syndrome. *Ann Dermatol Venereol.* 2006;133:17–20.

Skopouli FN, Papanikolaou S, Malamoumitsi V, et al. Obstetric and gynaecological profile in patients with primary Sjögren's syndrome. *Ann Rheum Dis.* 1994;53:569–573.

Ugurlu GK, Erten S, Ugurlu M, et al. Sexual dysfunction in female patients with primary Sjögren's syndrome and effects of depression: Cross-sectional study. *Sex Disabil.* 2014;32:197–204.

van der Meulen TA, van Nimwegen JF, Harmsen HJM, et al. Normal vaginal microbiome in women with primary Sjögren's syndrome-associated vaginal dryness. *Ann Rheum Dis.* 2019;78:707–709.

van Nimwegen JF, Arends S, van Zuiden GS, et al. The impact of primary Sjögren's syndrome on female sexual function. *Rheumatology.* 2015;54:1286–1293.

van Nimwegen J, van der Tuuk K, Liefers S, et al. Pathogenesis of vaginal dryness in primary Sjögren's syndrome: a histopathological case-control study. *Rheumatology.* 2020;59(10):2806–2815.

27

Management of Chronic Musculoskeletal Pain in Sjögren's

Lan Chen

Chronic musculoskeletal pain is a frequent complaint among Sjögren's patients. The causes for pain include neuropathic, arthritic, para-articular (e.g., tendinitis, bursitis), and/or diffuse muscle pain such as fibromyalgia, which is one of the most common comorbidities in Sjögren's.

How Is Chronic Pain Evaluated?

The first step for management of chronic pain in Sjögren's patients is to identify the cause. As with any medical work-up, it begins with a thorough history and physical exam. Several questions can focus the evaluation: How did the pain begin? Where is it located? Is it localized or diffuse, inside or outside the joint? If nerve pain is suspected, does it occur in a dermatomal distribution (area of skin supplied by branches of a single spinal nerve) or a non-dermatomal distribution?

Second, physicians must keep in mind that the response to pain varies greatly from one individual to another one. A patient's culture, education, and psychological status can influence their pain expression. It is important to let the patient describe the pain using their own words. Uncovering emotional feelings in patients can be a helpful part of therapy.

Third, patients should be asked what improves the pain. Factors that improve patients' pain may prove helpful in directing the treatment. Determine what other types of therapy the patient has tried and what benefit, if any, they had. Inquire specifically about injections, surgery, medications (including past corticosteroid use), physical therapy, chiropractic, biobehavioral, and other complementary methods.

Fourth, inquire about how the symptoms have impacted the patient's life at home, with friends, and at work. In women, is the pain preventing her from

Lan Chen, *Management of Chronic Musculoskeletal Pain in Sjögren's* In: *The Sjögren's Book*. Edited by: Daniel J. Wallace, Oxford University Press. © Sjögren's Foundation 2022. DOI: 10.1093/oso/9780197502112.003.0027 caring for a child or a loved one, maintaining their job, or performing basic activities of daily living? Patients with pain that is severe or longstanding are vulnerable to physical or psychological dysfunction and job-related issues, such as disability, which all have an impact on pain management.

Finally, the presence of coexisting psychological disorders, such as depression, anxiety, or mood disorders, may add further complexity to the treatment of chronic pain, particularly when associated with drug or alcohol addiction. Additional therapy for these coexisting psychological disorders is always necessary for more effective pain management. However, these issues should not lead the clinician away from seeking a primary chronic pain diagnosis and treatment.

What Are the Available Pharmacological and Non-pharmacological Therapies for Chronic Pain?

Nonsteroidal Anti-inflammatory Drugs

The analgesic and anti-inflammatory effect of nonsteroidal anti-inflammatory drugs (NSAIDs) (e.g., Motrin, ibuprofen) play a central role in the management of many conditions. It is now known that NSAIDs also act centrally, at least in certain pain states. NSAIDs are primarily indicated for mild to moderate pain, particularly for arthritis, tendinitis, or bursitis. There are many NSAIDs from which to choose. Although their efficacy is similar, an individual's response to therapy can be highly variable; thus, a patient who does not tolerate or respond to a particular NSAID may do well on another.

The reluctance of many patients and physicians to use NSAIDs is in part due to the many side effects associated with these drugs. Most NSAIDs interfere with platelet aggregation and may cause bleeding. They produce adverse gastrointestinal side effects, including dyspepsia and gastric ulceration. There are also a variety of kidney side effects associated with their use, including salt and water retention and reversible renal insufficiency due to renal vasoconstriction, acute interstitial nephritis, or acute tubular necrosis. Therefore, NSAIDs should be prescribed with caution in patients with hypertension, preexisting renal insufficiency, or heart failure. Other side effects of NSAIDS include hepatic toxicity, confusion, an inability to concentrate, and allergic reactions. Under medical supervision NSAIDs can, however, be prescribed safely and effectively for management of short-term pain or for chronic therapy in selected patients, especially when used on an as-needed basis.

Disease-Modifying Therapies

Some patients with Sjögren's develop a rheumatoid-like arthritis with painful swelling of large and small joints. Others develop inflammatory joint pain (polyarthralgias) in the absence of obvious swelling. A wide variety of immunomodulating drugs and disease-modifying therapies such as hydroxychloroquine (Plaquenil) are available for treatment, following an approach similar to that used to treat true rheumatoid arthritis. Treatment decisions are based on the severity of arthritis, the patient's other health problems, and the patient's comfort level for certain side effects (e.g., infections, low blood counts).

Tricyclic Antidepressants

Amitriptyline (Elavil) has been the most widely studied tricyclic antidepressant (TCA) for use in chronic pain, although a number of others, including doxepin (Sinequan, Adapin), imipramine (Tofranil), nortriptyline (Pamelor), and desipramine (Norpramin) also have been used with success. TCAs are believed to have independent analgesic effects as well as an ability to relieve the depressive symptoms associated with chronic pain. The mechanism of their analgesic action has been theorized to relate to the analgesic properties associated with their properties as serotonin and norepinephrine reuptake inhibitors. There is also some evidence that TCAs potentiate the endogenous opioid system.

TCAs prescribed for chronic pain have typically been given to fibromyalgia patients at doses lower than those used in depression. TCAs can cause wide-ranging adverse effects. Aside from anticholinergic (drying) effects, most of the more troubling or serious side effects involve the gastrointestinal, cardiovascular, and neurologic systems. Physicians must explain to the patient why TCAs are used, how to take them, and what benefits and side effects might be expected. It is also important for Sjögren's patients to know of possible unpleasant side effects, such as dry mouth.

Anticonvulsants

A number of anticonvulsants are effective for chronic pain therapy, particularly for neuropathic pain. Phenytoin (Dilantin), carbamazepine (Tegretol), oxcarbazepine (Trileptal), valproic acid (Depakene), and clonazepam

(Klonopin), as well as the newer agents such as gabapentin (Neurontin) and pregabalin (Lyrica), have been used, frequently with reasonable results. Mechanisms of action for the anticonvulsants are different and not fully understood. Carbamazepine, which is pharmacologically related to the TCAs, prevents repeated discharges in neurons, an action that is consistent with its ability to relieve lancinating pain.

Pregabalin is similar in structure to gabapentin. Many physicians begin with gabapentin since it is inexpensive and well tolerated, even at high doses. Plasma levels do not need to be followed as they do with phenytoin and carbamazepine. Pregabalin can be given less frequently (twice daily) than gabapentin (usually three times daily) and may cause euphoria. It is a Schedule V controlled substance.

Opioids

The role of opioid (narcotic) therapy in the more severe forms of acute pain and in malignant pain is well established, but opioid administration in chronic nonmalignant pain remains controversial. For patients with chronic nonmalignant pain like most Sjögren's patients, the decision to begin long-term opioid therapy must be weighed carefully against the potential for side effects. Opioids are usually employed only after other therapies have failed. A psychological evaluation should take place initially, with an emphasis on uncovering comorbidity that may be interfering with current treatment strategies. Patients must continue to receive emotional support.

Opioid candidates should be evaluated and overseen by a pain management specialist experienced in prescribing these agents. Most such specialists have patients sign a "pain contract," which is in fact a detailed informed consent. Nearly 100,000 people die annually from complications of opioid abuse/overdose in the United States, so opioid use must be closely monitored by a specialist.

Patients may receive substantial relief of pain from opioid therapy. In short-term use, opioids are effective in relieving chronic neuropathic pain and can be prescribed safely without the development of tolerance or addiction. These problems, however, are likely to occur with chronic use. Patients should be closely monitored, especially after initiation of opioid therapy since the risk for an adverse event is greatest shortly after initiation. Additionally, patients receiving higher doses are at increased risk for overdose. The most profound analgesic effects of opioids are mediated by the μ receptors, which are found in large numbers in the central nervous system, such as midbrain periaqueductal gray and the substantia gelatinosa in the dorsal horn of the spinal cord. This explains why opioids induce intense analgesia and euphoria as well as other effects such as bradycardia, sedation, physical dependence, and respiratory depression. Opioids may also have anticholinergic effects. Patients should be continuously educated about side effects.

Medical Marijuana

There is some evidence for the use of low-dose medical marijuana in refractory neuropathic pain in conjunction with traditional analgesics. However, trials were limited by short duration, variability in the dosing and strength of delta-9-tetrahydrocannabinol used, and lack of functional outcomes. The long-term psychoactive and neurocognitive effects of medical marijuana remain unknown. Clinicians should exercise caution when prescribing medical marijuana for patients, especially in those with non-neuropathic chronic pain.

Tramadol

To some degree, Tramadol (Ultram) is a novel analgesic that has some activity at μ receptors. It also inhibits the reuptake of serotonin and norepinephrine and may provide analgesia through this mechanism. Its side-effect profile is similar to that of other weak opioids, although the incidence of gastric upset seems to be higher. Seizures are an additional risk, particularly in patients taking antidepressants, neuroleptics, or other drugs that decrease the seizure threshold. A systematic review found that tramadol was effective for relief of neuropathic pain. Another systematic review concluded that it improved functional outcomes and pain in patients with fibromyalgia; however, it did not find tramadol to be more effective than NSAIDs or nortriptyline for relief of other chronic pain.

Ubrogepant

The new migraine medication ubrogepant is an oral calcitonin gene-related peptide (CGRP) receptor antagonist. The drug represents a new mechanism of action for the acute treatment of migraine compared with currently used medications such as triptans, ergot, opioids, and ibuprofen. There are no publications about its use in Sjögren's patients with chronic pain. Only one article has been published on ubrogepant use in rheumatic disease (Breen et al., 2021). This retrospective cohort study was performed from May 18, 2018, to September 15, 2020, in Mayo Clinic Health System patients with Raynaud's phenomenon while undergoing CGRP antagonist therapy to treat migraine. The results of this study indicate that microvascular complications of CGRP antagonist use in patients with underlying Raynaud's are uncommon.

Topical Therapies

An attractive approach to pain control is to apply drugs locally to the peripheral site of pain. Topical applications include creams, lotions, gels, oils, aerosols, or patches to involved sites. These topical remedies concentrate a large amount of the medication at the site of the pain while producing lower or negligible systemic drug levels, thus causing fewer or no adverse drug effects. Other advantages of topical application are lack of drug interactions and the ease of use. Topical applications of NSAIDs (e.g., 1% diclofenac gel) are available for prescription use and help localized arthritic pain. Local anesthetic patches (e.g., 5% Lidoderm patch) or gels are also effective treatments for many painful conditions.

Capsaicin is a natural constituent of pungent red chili peppers. It can selectively activate, desensitize, or exert a neurotoxic effect on sensory neurons, depending on the concentration and the delivery mode. Topical capsaicin cream is an over-the-counter preparation that is available in two strengths (0.025% and 0.075%) and have approval from the U.S. Food and Drug Administration (FDA) for the treatment of osteoarthritis and rheumatoid arthritis. Interestingly, this extract from red chili peppers has long been used in traditional topical Chinese medication mixes for joint pain.

Non-pharmacological Therapies

Non-pharmacological therapies encompass a wide array of treatments that may be grouped into physical interventions (physical therapy, acupuncture, chiropractic manipulation, and massage) and psychoeducational interventions (cognitive–behavioral therapy, family therapy, patient education, and psychotherapy).

Box 27.1 Medications Used in Sjögren's Patients for Chronic Musculoskeletal Pain

---

A. Inflammatory pain
- NSAIDs or aspirin
- Disease-modifying agents
- Hydroxychloroquine (Plaquenil)
- Immune suppressants, including methotrexate, azathioprine (Imuran)
- Biologics, including rituximab (Rituxan)

B. Noninflammatory pain (e.g., deformities, fibromyalgia, mechanical, neuropathic pain)
- TCAs
- Anticonvulsants
- Tramadol (Ultram)
- Narcotic analgesics, including opioids

Summing Up

Chronic pain is a summation of physical and psychological derangements. For each individual patient, pain means the pain to the body and mind in a literal way, even though sometimes the pain is invisible to the physician in an objective anatomic way. We might not always be able to cure the pain, but we can always care and try to understand and use all the options to alleviate the pain and diminish it for our patients. Therefore, successful management requires addressing all of the various aspects of pain. A number of interventions can help (Box 27.1). The selection of therapies is based on the etiology of pain and the patient's other medical problems, including social and psychological aspects. Proper patient education is crucial to achieve optimal results. Most studies suggest that combinations of therapies are more effective than any single approach for maintaining long-term gains.

For Further Reading

Allegrante JP. The role of adjunctive therapy in the management of nonmalignant pain. *Am J Med*. 1996;101:33S.

Ballantyne JC, Mao J. Opioid therapy for chronic pain. *N Engl J Med*. 2003; 349:1943.

Breen ID, Brumfiel CM, Patel MH, et al. Evaluation of the safety of calcitonin gene-related peptide antagonists for migraine treatment among adults with Raynaud phenomenon. *JAMA Netw Open*. 2021;4(4):e217934.

Carsons SE, Vivino FB, Parke A, et al. Treatment guidelines for rheumatologic manifestations of Sjögren's syndrome: Use of biologic agents, management of fatigue, and inflammatory musculoskeletal pain. *Arthritis Care Res*. 2017;69(4):517–527.

Chen LX. Fibromyalgia: A commonly co-existing condition in Sjögren's patients. *Sjögren's Quarterly*. 2009;4(1):1.

Chen LX, Goldman J, Pullman-Mooar S. Local therapy for fibromyalgia and nonneuropathic pain. In Wallace D, Clauw D, eds. *Fibromyalgia and Other Central Pain Syndromes*. Lippincott Williams & Wilkins; 2005:353–368.

Dobscha SK, Corson K, Perrin NA, et al. Collaborative care for chronic pain in primary care: A cluster randomized trial. *JAMA*. 2009;301:1242.

Dühmke RM, Cornblath DD, Hollingshead JR. Tramadol for neuropathic pain. *Cochrane Database Syst Rev*. 2006;(3):CD003726.

Eisendrath SJ. Psychiatric aspects of chronic pain. *Neurology*. 1995;45:S26.

Fields HL. *Pain*. McGraw-Hill Information Services Company, Health Profession Division; 1987.

Holzer P. Capsaicin: Cellular targets, mechanisms of action, and selectivity for thin sensory neurons. *Pharmacol Rev*. 1991;43(2):143–201.

Jaeschke R, Adachi J, Guyatt G, et al. Clinical usefulness of amitriptyline in fibromyalgia: The results of 23 N-of-1 randomized controlled trials. *J Rheumatol*. 1991;18:447.

Joranson DE, Ryan KM, Gilson AM, Dahl JL. Trends in medical use and abuse of opioid analgesics. *JAMA*. 2000;283:1710.

McCormack K. Non-steroidal anti-inflammatory drugs and spinal nociceptive processing. *Pain*. 1994;59:9.

Mücke M, Phillips T, Radbruch L, et al. Cannabis-based medicines for chronic neuropathic pain in adults. *Cochrane Database Syst Rev*. 2018 Mar 7;3(3):CD012182.

Swerdlow M. Review: Anticonvulsant drugs and chronic pain. *Clin Neuropharmacol*. 1984;7:51.

28

Management of Pulmonary Complications in Sjögren's

Augustine S. Lee

What Are Common Symptoms to Indicate a Respiratory Complication of Sjögren's?

Pulmonary complications are likely the most common visceral organ complication of extraglandular Sjögren's. The frequency can vary widely from less than 10% to more than 70% of patients with Sjögren's. The variability is related significantly to the specific patient population being studied and how they were identified, as half the patients may be asymptomatic despite objective evidence of respiratory pathology.

The cardinal symptom indicating a respiratory disorder is dyspnea. This can be challenging to tease out from the fatigue and deconditioning that can complicate Sjögren's, but typically, the dyspnea is exacerbated by exertion for most of the obstructive and restrictive lung complications. Episodic non-exertional dyspnea would be atypical for most, but consideration should be given for asthma, thromboembolic disease, vocal cord dysfunction, or episodic arrhythmias. When dyspnea is aggravated in the supine position, this may indicate heart failure complicating pulmonary hypertension, respiratory muscle weakness, or upper airway disorders such as obstructive sleep apnea. Wheezing is characteristic of obstructive lung disease, including asthma, and is rarely a central airway problem.

Cough is also a common indicator of a respiratory problem, occurring in approximately half of patients with Sjögren's. An acute cough is typically an indicator of an infection, for which patients with Sjögren's are at a higher risk. Not unusually, the patient with a persisting chronic cough, with an otherwise negative work-up for a primary respiratory problem on objective testing, is often diagnosed as having xerotrachea. Unfortunately, this may be an over-attribution, as chronic cough is prevalent in the general population and is not uniquely a symptom related to a respiratory condition. For example, one of the leading causes of chronic cough is gastroesophageal reflux, for which

Augustine S. Lee, *Management of Pulmonary Complications in Sjögren's* In: *The Sjögren's Book*. Edited by: Daniel J. Wallace, Oxford University Press. © Sjögren's Foundation 2022. DOI: 10.1093/oso/9780197502112.003.0028

Sjögren's patients are at a higher risk, but also, for many, chronic cough may be rooted in a derangement in the cough nerve reflex, most likely a central sensitization process, most recently dubbed cough hypersensitivity syndrome.

In all, the best estimate of the frequency of respiratory symptoms comes from a study of 414 patients with Sjögren's, where approximately 20% had dyspnea and/or cough on systematic structured interviews. Not surprisingly, a third of these patients were felt to have "other" conditions that they could attribute the symptoms to, and after a complete work-up including lung function testing and computed tomography (CT) imaging, just about half the patients had normal studies. This acknowledges that dyspnea and cough are common symptoms of many other more common disorders, including both pulmonary and extrapulmonary conditions, that should be maintained in the differential before attribution to Sjögren's or a complication thereof.

What Are Some Pulmonary Complications of Sjögren's?

Depending on the series, the definitions used, and the manner of ascertainment of cases, airway disorders and interstitial lung disease appear to be the leading pulmonary manifestations of Sjögren's. However, as with symptoms, most of these complications, barring a few exceptions, are not unique to Sjögren's, and other etiologies are likely contributing to the overall reported frequencies. Table 28.1 summarizes some of the known pulmonary associations or complications of Sjögren's.

Airway disorders are often categorized as involvement of the central airways, including the trachea and the mainstems; the medium-sized airways, as in bronchiectasis; or the small airways and the bronchioles. More often, these conditions represent a spectrum, and, often radiographically, there will be features of airway involvement at multiple levels. The most common attribution of large airway disorders is xerotrachea, which can be considered essentially an extension of xerostomia, due to lack of hydration of the proximal airways. The primary manifestation is cough, and standard testing with CT imaging and pulmonary function tests (PFTs) will be negative. However, at least half may exhibit evidence of bronchial hyper-responsiveness, although it is not clear whether this is a result of xerotracheitis or a comorbid process such as asthma. Chronic obstructive pulmonary disease (COPD) as defined by PFTs appears to be more common in patients with Sjögren's than control cohorts. Further down the airways, high-resolution imaging may reveal abnormal, sometimes subtle, dilation of more distal airways, variably

Table 28.1 Respiratory Disorders Associated with Sjögren's

Upper airways	Xerotrachea
	Obstructive sleep apnea
Lower airways	Bronchiectasis
	Bronchiolitis and small airways disease
	Follicular bronchiolitis
	Asthma/bronchial hyper-responsiveness
	Chronic obstructive pulmonary disease
Parenchymal and interstitial lung disease	Lymphocytic interstitial pneumonia
	Nonspecific interstitial pneumonia
	Usual interstitial pneumonia
	Organizing pneumonia
Vascular	Pulmonary hypertension
	Venothromboembolic disease
	Vasculitis
Pleural	Pleural effusion
	Diaphragm dysfunction
Lymphoproliferative	Nodular lymphoid hyperplasia
	Follicular bronchiolitis
	Lymphocytic interstitial pneumonia
	Amyloidosis
	Light chain deposition disease
	Mucosa-associated lymphoid tissue (MALT)
	Other lymphomas

accompanied by wall thickening and mucous plugging, diagnostic of bronchiectasis (~44%). Bronchiectasis does increase the risk of pneumonia, but in Sjögren's, colonization with non-tuberculous mycobacterium does not appear common.

Finally, when there is involvement of the terminal bronchioles or alveolar ducts, the CT scan may show evidence of small airway disease or bronchiolitis with findings of "tree-in-bud" opacities, or centrilobular nodules. In some cases, where there is little mucous plugging or airway inflammation, air trapping can be seen revealing a lobular mosaic attenuation on CT imaging that is exaggerated by additional expiratory hold views. The clinical diagnoses involving these airways include bronchiolitis, including follicular bronchiolitis (which may additionally manifest with cystic lesions), and asthma. Finally, although localized above the trachea, it should be noted that obstructive sleep apnea is also more prevalent in Sjögren's patients, even considering the body-mass index, possibly related to the inflamed/dry mucosa disrupting airflow and causing the mucosa to become more easily adherent.

The small airways eventually lead to the alveoli, where gas exchange occurs across the interstitium (the connective tissue between the lungs and the body), and this is the location of the next most common and sometimes devastating complication of Sjögren's. A variety of interstitial lung diseases (ILDs) have been identified in the context of Sjögren's, including lymphocytic interstitial pneumonia (LIP), nonspecific interstitial pneumonia (NSIP), organizing pneumonia (OP), and less commonly usual interstitial pneumonia (UIP). They share a restrictive physiology on PFT and, even in moderate stages of disease, can be associated with exercise-induced hypoxia (low levels of oxygen causing shortness of breath). Although imaging can suggest these diagnoses and be diagnostic at least for UIP, they are all histopathologic diagnoses or patterns of injury that have been described in many other contexts. On CT, UIP will typically have little ground glass and manifest with basilar-predominant subpleural reticulations, honeycombing, and traction bronchiectasis. UIP is also the injury pattern observed in idiopathic pulmonary fibrosis (IPF), but it is notable that the prognosis of UIP related to Sjögren's is better than UIP of IPF. NSIP will also be basilar predominant, but ground glass dominates over reticular lesions, and there should be no or little honeycombing. OP has a variable manifestation, though ground glass frequently extending into consolidation is characteristic. However, nodules, in isolation or multiply, or masses can be the presenting appearance of OP. LIP suffers from changing definitions and descriptions over the literature. It shares features of follicular bronchiolitis in that they are both non-monoclonal lymphoplasmacytic infiltration of the lungs. If airway dominant, it may be described as follicular bronchiolitis, and if more diffuse and extending into the interstitium, it may be labeled as LIP. Radiographically, thus, it shares features of follicular bronchiolitis and NSIP, with some reticulation, ground glass, centrilobular nodules, and cystic lesions. Finally, other parenchymal lesions include nodular lymphoid hyperplasia; light chain deposition disease; nodular amyloidosis, often accompanied by cystic lesions and mucosa-associated lymphoid (MALT); and other lymphomas. Laboratory studies investigating for gammopathies and positron emission tomography/CT scans may be helpful, but a biopsy is required for a definitive diagnosis for most of these considerations.

Pulmonary hypertension (PH) is the third category of clinical importance that occurs at an increased frequency in patients with Sjögren's. PH can occur primarily in association with Sjögren's (World Health Organization [WHO] Group 1) or can be a secondary complication of underlying parenchymal lung disease (WHO Group 3). PH can be insidious and more difficult to diagnose, but as the disease advances, patients will manifest with typical signs of fluid retention and right heart failure, and sometimes with syncopal episodes that may herald sudden death. It may be suggested by an isolated or a disproportionately reduced diffusing capacity on lung function testing, but typically an echocardiogram is required as the screening test of choice. Ultimately, a right heart catheterization is required for confirmation and to guide therapy.

Finally, a few other respiratory complications have been noted in case series or with increased frequency compared to controls, including pleuritis with effusions, respiratory muscle weakness, and vasculitis (Table 28.1); however most notable among these is the apparent increase in venothromboembolism (VTE). When a patient with Sjögren's presents with acute dyspnea, chest pain, and/or hypoxia, this should be considered in the differential. Table 28.2 summarizes some of the diagnostic options available and their potential utility.

Table 28.2 Diagnostic Tests for Respiratory Complications

Test	Information Learned

Pulmonary function testing
  Methacholine
  Exhaled nitric oxide
	Evaluates for presence and severity of functional impairment in lung capacities
	Differentiates obstructive and restrictive disorders
	Can suggest pulmonary vascular disease (e.g., pulmonary hypertension)
	Helps to identify asthma or bronchial hyper-responsiveness
	Least invasive tool to monitor for progression of disease or response to therapies

Oximetry: rest, exercise, sleep	Identifies hypoxemia or potential for sleep disordered breathing
Ultrasonography	May be a sensitive and simple bedside tool to assess for interstitial lung disease complicating Sjögren's

CT chest
  High resolution
  +/- Expiratory views
  +/- PET imaging
	Anatomic assessment of parenchyma, airways, vessels, mediastinum, pleura
	Evaluates for interstitial lung disease, lymphoma, airway disease, pleural disease, pulmonary embolism, cystic lung disease

Echocardiography	Screening test for pulmonary hypertension Evaluates for other cardiac disorders, including ventricular function and valvular disease
Right heart catheterization	Definitive test to confirm and evaluate for causes of pulmonary hypertension
Polysomnography	Definitive testing to diagnose sleep apnea or other sleep disorders

Bronchoscopy
  Bronchoalveolar lavage
  Transbronchial biopsy
  Cryobiopsy
  Endobronchial ultrasound
	Fiberoptic endoscopic visualization of airways
	Identifies gross evidence of inflammation or central airway lesions
	Limited biopsies can be obtained of parenchyma.
	Mediastinal lymph nodes can be biopsied.
	Cultures can be obtained directly from area of concern.
	Identifies alveolar hemorrhage

Table 28.2 *Continued*

Test	Information Learned
Surgical lung biopsy Video-assisted thoracoscopy	Definitive histopathologic assessment
Upper airways	Xerotrachea Obstructive sleep apnea
Lower airways	Bronchiectasis Bronchiolitis & "Small airways disease" Follicular bronchiolitis Asthma / Bronchial hyper-responsiveness Chronic obstructive pulmonary disease
Parenchymal and Interstitial Lung Disease	Lymphocytic interstitial pneumonia Nonspecific interstitial pneumonia Usual interstitial pneumonia Organizing pneumonia
Vascular	Pulmonary hypertension Venothromboembolic disease Vasculitis
Pleural	Pleural effusion Diaphragm dysfunction
Lymphoproliferative	Nodular lymphoid hyperplasia Follicular bronchiolitis Lymphocytic interstitial pneumonia Amyloidosis Light chain deposition disease Mucosa associated lymphoid tissue (MALT) Other lymphomas

What Are Some Management Principles and Options for Patients with a Respiratory Complication of Sjögren's?

Unfortunately, there continues to be a paucity of rigorously tested interventions to guide clinicians and patients for most of the conditions described. This is largely due to the relative infrequency of these complications, the lack of standardized definitions, and limited funding resources to coordinate such studies across multiple centers. The typical clinical management is thus predominantly guided by an understanding of proposed biological mechanisms, observational data, clinical experience, and extrapolation from management strategies for these respiratory conditions seen in other contexts. This inherently implies the need for shared and informed decision-making between the clinician and the patient on the pros and cons of whatever intervention is being considered. For the clinician, it is also important that once a plan of management is decided, the respiratory condition being addressed is carefully and serially monitored to determine whether the intervention is achieving the desired benefit over any accumulating side effects.

The role of screening is unclear, but some observational reports indicate (for example, in the context of pulmonary hypertension, where effective treatment options are available) that diagnosis can be delayed and confer a worse prognosis. Thus, in the completely asymptomatic patient, as a personal preference, I recommend at least a complete set of PFTs and echocardiography at baseline. Many of the respiratory complications noted earlier are only appreciated radiographically (e.g., cystic lesions, micronodules, bronchiectasis, adenopathy, early ILD). It is reasonable to consider advanced imaging in any patient with respiratory or systemic symptoms (e.g., weight loss, fevers, night sweats) and in patients with abnormal lung function tests on screening, but not necessarily in asymptomatic patients. Ultrasonography appears to have potential as a bedside screening tool, at least in screening for ILD.

Monitoring is guided by the specific respiratory complication, but PFTs and oximetry are the least invasive methods for most airway or parenchymal lung disease. The simple 6-minute walk and the incremental shuttle walk tests provides a measure of functional status and can usually be implemented in most clinical settings. For pulmonary hypertension, echocardiography will be necessary. Advanced imaging, such as CT, should be used sparingly due to increased radiation exposures and should be used only if the results will have direct implications for management. It may be the only tool, however, to monitor certain complications such as nodular or cystic lesions.

In the initial assessment of the patient presenting with respiratory symptoms, the acuity should be considered. Acute presentations may herald acute cor pulmonale from progressive PH or acute VTE, exacerbation of the ILD, and infections complicating immunomodulator therapies or bronchiectasis. Because acutely or sub-acutely deteriorating patients are often challenged with corticosteroids, and because the radiographic lesions for some of the listed complications are indistinguishable from infections, a bronchoscopy and other assessment to rule out an infection should be considered before embarking on immune-suppressant therapies. Best supportive care for acute obstructive lung disease (asthma or COPD exacerbation), hypoxic respiratory failure, cor pulmonale, infections, and VTE is offered as per standard guidelines.

Similarly, a patient with evidence of bronchial hyper-responsiveness or fixed obstructive lung disease is treated as per asthma or COPD guidelines. The mainstay of asthma therapy is inhaled corticosteroids in addition to bronchodilators, while for COPD, first-line consideration goes to short and long-acting beta2-agonists or muscarinic antagonists. There have been recent exciting developments in the management of asthma for the "eosinophilic" asthma phenotype; however, if this is the case, there should be an investigation for a primary connective tissue disease other than Sjögren's, such as eosinophilic granulomatosis with polyangiitis.

Management of patients with bronchiectasis is challenging. These patients often have persistent refractory productive cough and are prone to infectious complications. Sputum or bronchoscopic samples should be obtained to assess for specific pathogens, such as *Pseudomonas* and *Mycobacterium avium* intracellular complex (MAC), that may imply specific antimicrobial strategies. However, an initial principle of management is summarized as "bronchial hygiene," where the goal is to facilitate the removal of excess secretion build-up to minimize colonization, infectious complications, and hopefully their symptoms. This typically entails oscillatory positive expiratory pressure devices, nebulization of hypertonic saline, bronchodilators, and/or high-frequency chest wall oscillation devices. Chronic and rotational antibiotics are also considered, with clinical trials supporting the potential role of macrolide therapies, but this should only be done after confident exclusion of MAC, which becomes easily resistant to single-agent therapies.

If the airway disease is more rooted in the small airways (i.e., bronchiolitis pattern), similar evaluation and management should be pursued as for bronchiectasis and COPD. However, in the context of Sjögren's, follicular bronchiolitis may be the fundamental diagnosis, especially if the classic bronchiolitis pattern (as suggested by CT imaging and PFTs) is accompanied by cystic lesions. In this case, a biopsy may be considered (although by some reports this is always necessary), followed by a trial of steroids, macrolides, or other immunomodulator therapy based on severity of symptoms and PFT limitations.

The patient who has developed chronic cough without an apparent respiratory process should also be approached as others with a refractory or chronic cough, with a thorough investigation or therapeutic trial for reflux-mediated cough and upper airway cough syndrome. Xerotrachea would be an appropriate diagnosis if all other pulmonary and extrapulmonary causes have been excluded in the context of Sjögren's. These patients may variably respond to a trial of sialogogue agents, airway hydration (nebulizer therapy), and anecdotally hydroxychloroquine. For most, this will be partially effective at best, and a trial of speech therapy with gabapentin (or pregabalin) is supported by the literature and guidelines for patients with refractory chronic cough.

Patients with PH are best referred to a center with expertise in its management. If it appears the basis of PH is (at least predominantly) WHO Group 1, therapeutic options are available, from multiple oral agents to the

"gold standard" infusion prostanoids that appear to produce improved survival in observational data from the U.S. REVEAL registry.

Other than for UIP associated with IPF, there are no therapies approved by
the U.S. Food and Drug Administration (FDA) for most ILDs. However, extrap-
olating from the literature, patients with connective tissue disease–associated
ILD, including Sjögren's, have a better prognosis, even when the underlying
histopathologic pattern appears to be UIP. Most of these patients in these favorable observational series have been treated with immunomodulators.
Unless severely affected, a period of observation is reasonable and/or a biopsy
before committing to a trial of immunomodulator therapy. Some clinicians
advocate a limited therapeutic trial with corticosteroids to understand the re-
sponsiveness or reversibility of the disease. This may be helpful particularly
for patterns that resemble OP, NSIP, and possibly LIP, but it is unlikely to demonstrate any short-term measurable benefit for the UIP pattern; historically,
these patients do not respond to steroids, and in the case of IPF, immunomodulator therapy may worsen their prognosis. When an immunomodulator agent is tried specifically targeting the ILD, mycophenolate is typically
used first, again based on supportive observational series. The role of the two
FDA-approved drugs for IPF, nintedanib and pirfenidone, for other non-IPF
ILDs is currently being investigated. Lung transplantation is the ultimate option for patients with chronic and progressive respiratory failure but is not
always a suitable or available option for many patients. Evolving biological
agents targeting the pathogenic pathways for Sjögren's will need to be separately tested for these respiratory complications.

Lymphoproliferative disorders range from non-neoplastic lesions (such as
nodular lymphoid hyperplasia, follicular bronchiolitis, and lymphocytic interstitial pneumonia) to frank evolution to lymphoma, sometimes in association with amyloid. Fortunately, most lymphomatous complications that occur
in the lung are of the MALT type, which tends to have a slower course. Close
collaboration with an oncologist is necessary to determine the timing of a biopsy and treatment.

Summing Up

There are many respiratory manifestations that may complicate Sjögren's, with
the potential to affect all compartments of the respiratory system, including
the airways, interstitium, lung parenchyma, vasculature, and the lymphatics.
Screening may be appropriate for the asymptomatic patient. Once a respiratory condition is suspected, there are a multitude of diagnostic tests available

to confirm the specific condition. Close collaboration is required between the rheumatologist and the pulmonologist, and often also a chest radiologist and pathologist, to identify the timing of any more invasive diagnostic procedures and interventions. At all levels, given the lack of proven management strategies, the informed patient must partake in all decisions. Much more work is required to understand best practice for such patients, from the difficult chronic cough to the management of advanced ILD complicating these cases. The first-ever clinical practice guidelines for pulmonary disease management in Sjögren's have recently been published (Lee et al., 2021).

For Further Reading

Lee AS, Scofield RH, Hammitt KM, et al. Consensus guidelines for evaluation and management of pulmonary disease in Sjögren's. *Chest*. 2021;159(2):683–698. doi:10.1016/j.chest.2020.10.011

29

Management of Peripheral Nervous System Complications in Sjögren's

Shalini Mahajan and Daniel J. Wallace

Sjögren's can affect the central nervous system (CNS), the peripheral nervous system (PNS), and the autonomic nervous system. The prevalence of PNS involvement is more common: About 16% of Sjögren's patients experience PNS involvement compared to about 3.6% with CNS involvement. Based on a large epidemiologic study in 2016, the disease burden in Sjögren's was higher in the group with neurologic manifestations. Furthermore, patients who suffered neurologic complications had a higher risk of developing new neurologic symptoms.

The CNS comprises the brain and the spinal cord. The PNS comprises the cell body (ganglion) in the spinal cord, where the nerve originates; the peripheral nerve; the neuromuscular junction; and the muscle. The autonomic nervous system, which is categorized medically under the PNS, controls the muscles of the internal organs without conscious control, such as those of the heart, digestive tract, and sweat glands. Symptoms involving the neurologic system can range from sensory symptoms such as numbness, tingling in the feet, painful sensations in the feet/hands, and gait ataxia (difficulty with balance) to motor symptoms such as limb weakness or to visual impairment/vision loss.

PNS Involvement

PNS involvement is more common than CNS involvement, and according to a recent, large epidemiologic study, PNS manifestations can be present in up to 16% of patients with Sjögren's. However, epidemiologic studies show a broad range of 20% to 70%. PNS involvement with Sjögren's can include sensory polyneuropathy, sensorimotor polyneuropathy, small fiber neuropathy, sensory ganglionopathy, or cranial neuropathies (involvement of the nerves originating from the brain). The most common PNS manifestation is that of

Shalini Mahajan and Daniel J. Wallace, *Management of Peripheral Nervous System Complications in Sjögren's*
In: *The Sjögren's Book*. Edited by: Daniel J. Wallace, Oxford University Press. © Sjögren's Foundation 2022.
DOI: 10.1093/oso/9780197502112.003.0029

Table 29.1   Treatment of Neurologic Complications Associated with Sjögren's

	Pathology	Treatment of Underlying Pathophysiology	Symptomatic Treatment	Supportive Treatment

Peripheral nervous system	• Small fiber neuropathy
	• Distal sensory
	• Sensorimotor
	• Polyneuropathy
	• Sensory ganglionopathy
	• Mononeuritis multiplex
	• Cranial neuropathies
	• Myalgia/myositis
		• Corticosteroids
		• Rituximab
		• Mycophenolate
		• Azathioprine
		• Cyclophosphamide
		• IVIG
			• Serotonin-norepinephrine reuptake inhibitors (duloxetine)
			• Tricyclic antidepressants
			  • Nortriptyline
			  • Amitriptyline
			• Antiepileptic agents
			  • Gabapentin
			  • Pregabalin
			  • Carbamazepine
				• Aggressive physical therapy
				• Assistive devices (ankle foot/knee braces)

Autonomic nervous system	• Sensory ganglionopathy	• Fludrocortisone • Midodrine • Droxidopa • IVIG		• Cognitive-behavioral therapy • Biofeedback

a pure sensory neuropathy (9.2%) followed by a sensorimotor neuropathy (5.3%).

Patients may be symptomatic or completely asymptomatic. Symptoms can include sensory symptoms, motor symptoms, and symptoms from autonomic dysfunction. Treatment of PNS complications is threefold: (1) treatment of underlying Sjögren's disease; (2) symptomatic treatment; and (3) supportive treatment. Table 29.1 provides a summary of current options and approaches for these three treatment areas.

Treatment of Distal Pure Sensory or Sensorimotor Polyneuropathy

Among the neuropathies, the most common involvement is that of the sensory nerves (nerves that supply the skin/sensation as well as the sense of position), causing a pure sensory neuropathy. However, motor (nerves that supply the muscles) involvement can also be seen, such as in sensorimotor polyneuropathy or chronic inflammatory demyelinating polyneuropathy.

Treatment of severe painful sensory neuropathy or motor involvement is directed toward the underlying pathophysiology of Sjögren's. Treatment includes corticosteroids as well as steroid-sparing immunosuppressive agents such as rituximab, mycophenolate (Cellcept), or azathioprine (Imuran).

Intravenous immunoglobulin (IVIG) is also helpful as an immunomodulatory therapeutic agent. Monotherapy or a combination of therapeutic agents can be used, based on the severity of symptoms and the clinical profile of the patient, taking into account comorbid and coexisting medical conditions. Supportive treatment with physical therapy to improve muscle strength, improve core balance, and avoid secondary disuse muscle atrophy is also helpful and recommended.

The treatment of pure sensory neuropathy or mild sensory symptoms can remain symptomatic. Symptomatic treatment includes serotonin–norepinephrine reuptake inhibitors (SNRIs) such as duloxetine, tricyclic antidepressants such as nortriptyline (Pamelor) and amitriptyline (Elavil), and antiepileptic agents such as gabapentin (Neurontin) and pregabalin (Lyrica).

Treatment of Multiple Mononeuropathies (Mononeuritis Multiplex)

When Sjögren's affects two or more individual peripheral nerves, asymmetrical involvement of the peripheral nerves can develop in different areas of the body (mononeuritis multiplex). Patients usually present with acute to subacute, asymmetrical sensory symptoms (pain, numbness, or tingling) along with muscle weakness in the distribution of the affected nerves.

The underlying pathophysiology of mononeuritis multiplex is usually vascular damage, secondary to inflammation of the blood vessels related to Sjögren's. Therefore, treatment is directed toward reducing the burden of vascular damage. This involves the use of one or more immune agents, including corticosteroids and other immunosuppressive agents such as rituximab, cyclophosphamide (Cytoxan), mycophenolate (Cellcept), hydroxychloroquine (Plaquenil), or azathioprine (Imuran).

Treatment of Small Fiber Neuropathies

Small fiber neuropathies occur in about 5% to 10% of patients. These involve the microscopic nerve endings that terminate within the skin (intra-epidermal nerve endings). Small fiber neuropathies manifest primarily as a slow, chronic onset of painful, burning sensations, or hypersensitivity to painful stimuli involving the feet and less commonly the hands. Occasionally they can also involve the trunk. The diagnosis is based on the absence of electrophysiologic abnormalities on nerve conduction studies and the presence of reduced small nerve fiber density on skin punch biopsy. The mainstay of treatment of small fiber neuropathies is symptomatic treatment with SNRIs such as duloxetine (Cymbalta), tricyclic antidepressants such as nortriptyline (Pamelor) and amitriptyline (Elavil), and antiepileptic agents such as gabapentin (Neurontin) and pregabalin (Lyrica).

Treatment of Sensory Ganglionopathy and Sensorimotor Radiculoplexopathy

In rare cases, the neuron cell body in the spinal cord (ganglion), where the nerve originates, can also be affected. This results in a sensory neuronopathy/ganglionopathy that manifests primarily as ataxia (difficulty with balance). Rarely, patients can also have a combination of sensory and motor symptoms, including numbness, tingling, or muscle weakness. Autonomic dysfunction can also be present, manifesting as orthostatic hypotension. Patients experience lightheadedness and dizziness on standing and episodes of presyncope or syncope (passing out). Other symptoms may include abnormal sweating, abdominal pain, and problems with bowel movements, such as diarrhea or constipation.

In the treatment of sensory ganglionopathy, there have also been some case reports of the use of IVIG and rituximab, but the benefit has not shown to be consistent. If there is autonomic dysfunction, medications to increase blood pressure such as fludrocortisone (Florinef), midodrine, and droxidopa (Northera) have been helpful. Physical therapy targeting core balance also helps to improve functional outcomes.

Treatment of Cranial Neuropathies

The cranial nerves originate from the lower part of the brain, the brainstem. The most common cranial nerve involved is CN-V (the trigeminal nerve); less commonly involved are CN-VIII (the vestibulocochlear/auditory nerve) and CN-III (the oculomotor nerve). Treatment is directed toward management of underlying Sjögren's. Symptomatic treatment with the use of antiepileptic medications such as carbamazepine (Tegretol), tricyclic antidepressants such as nortriptyline (Pamelor) and amitriptyline (Elavil), and antiepileptic agents such as gabapentin (Neurontin) and pregabalin (Lyrica) can help reduce the pain.

Muscle Involvement

Clinical manifestations involving the muscle itself can range from pain (myalgia) to inflammation of the muscles (myositis) that could result in limb weakness. Commonly involved are the proximal (upper) muscles of the upper and lower limbs. Not directly because of Sjögren's disease but in association with it, rare forms of muscle diseases, such as inclusion body myositis, have also been reported.

Symptoms from muscle involvement include muscle pain and weakness, difficulty swallowing, and rarely difficulty breathing. Treatment is directed toward reducing inflammation in the muscle with the use of immunosuppressants. Aggressive physical therapy to encourage muscle fiber regrowth and avoid muscle disuse atrophy is strongly recommended. Assistive devices such as orthotic shoe inserts, ankle–foot braces, or knee braces can help in ambulation.

Autonomic Nervous System Involvement

Autonomic dysfunction can be seen in almost 50% of patients with Sjögren's. As stated earlier in this chapter, patients experience lightheadedness and dizziness when they stand up due to drop in blood pressure (orthostatic hypotension) as well as presyncope or syncope (passing out) episodes. Other symptoms may include abnormal sweating, abdominal pain, and problems with bowel movements, such as diarrhea and constipation. For autonomic dysfunction, medications to increase blood pressure such as fludrocortisone (Florinef), midodrine, and droxidopa (Northera) can be helpful.

Summing Up

Sjögren's can affect the central, peripheral, and autonomic nervous systems. Peripheral neuropathy is more common than CNS complications and may include sensory polyneuropathy, sensorimotor polyneuropathy, small fiber neuropathy, sensory ganglionopathy, or cranial neuropathies. Autonomic dysfunction may be characterized by feelings of lightheadedness, dizziness, changes in blood pressure, sweating abnormalities, and more. When managing these conditions, a three-pronged approach may be considered that includes treating the underlying pathophysiology and providing symptomatic and supportive treatments.

For Further Reading

Alegria GC, Guellec D, Mariette X, et al. Epidemiology of neurological manifestations in Sjogren's syndrome: Data from the French ASSESS cohort. *RMD Open*. 2016;2(1):e000179.

Birnbaum J, Lalji A, Saed A, Baer AN. Biopsy-proven small-fiber neuropathy in primary Sjögren's syndrome: Neuropathic pain characteristics, autoantibody findings, and histopathological features. *Arthritis Care Res*. 2019;71(7):936–948.

Bougea A, Anagnostou E, Konstantinos G, et al. A systematic review of peripheral and central nervous system involvement of rheumatoid arthritis, systemic lupus erythematosus, primary Sjögren's syndrome and associated immunological profiles. *Int J Chronic Dis*. 2015;2015:910352.

Chai J, Logigian EL. Neurological manifestations of Sjögren's syndrome. *Curr Opin Neurol*. 2010;23:509–513.

Margaratten M. Neurologic manifestations of primary Sjögren's syndrome. *Rheum Dis Clin North Am*. 2017;43:519–529.

Mekinian A, Ravaud P, Hatron PY, et al. Efficacy of rituximab in primary Sjögren's syndrome with peripheral nervous system involvement: Results from the AIR registry. *Ann Rheum Dis*. 2012;71(1):84–87.

Mori K, Iijima M, Koike H, et al. The wide spectrum of clinical manifestations in Sjögren's syndrome-associated neuropathy. *Brain*. 2005;128(11):2518–2534.

Tobón GJ, Pers JO, Devauchelle-Pensec V, Youinou P. Neurological disorders in primary Sjögren's syndrome. *Autoimmune Dis*. 2012;2012:645967.

30

Management of Central Nervous System Complications in Sjögren's

Pantelis P. Pavlakis, Theresa Lawrence Ford, Janet Lewis,
Shalini Mahajan, Steven Mandel, and Daniel J. Wallace

Autoimmunity and Pathophysiology

The focus of this section will be to review the role of the immune system and mechanisms by which immune dysregulation leads to neurologic dysfunction in Sjögren's.

Autoimmunity

A basic understanding of immunology includes the concept that immune cells continuously communicate with chemical messages that either promote or inhibit their function and, as an end result, inflammation. To maintain our health, the organization of this conversation is regulated and highly co-ordinated. Host responses and defense mechanisms in response to immune challenges, such as infections, lead to inflammation. They are usually limited, maintaining a balance between resolving these immune challenges and avoiding excessive tissue damage, ultimately keeping us healthy.

Autoimmune disease involves the development of immune responses against our own tissue, cells, or cellular components. It is the result of a dysregulation of the immune system leading to a loss of immune tolerance to, and production of antibodies against, self (autoantibodies). Autoimmunity coupled with persistent and excessive inflammation can lead to chronic inflammatory-mediated tissue dysregulation, destruction, and disease.

Animal studies and clinical research indicate that complex interactions among genetic, environmental, hormonal, and neuropsychological factors may potentially trigger the autoimmune response. However, the exact roles

Pantelis P. Pavlakis, Theresa Lawrence Ford, Janet Lewis, Shalini Mahajan, Steven Mandel, and Daniel J. Wallace, *Management of Central Nervous System Complications in Sjögren's* In: *The Sjögren's Book*. Edited by: Daniel J. Wallace, Oxford University Press. © Sjögren's Foundation 2022. DOI: 10.1093/oso/9780197502112.003.0030 that different parts of the immune system play in initiating and maintaining this dysregulation remain unknown. In Sjögren's, these factors are thought to lead to abnormal activation of epithelial cells (a cell type commonly lining various organs, including the salivary glands).

Pathophysiology

The mechanisms responsible for most forms of central nervous system (CNS) manifestations of Sjögren's are generally unknown, but several hypotheses have been proposed. One hypothesis is that direct invasion of the CNS by immune cells causes neurologic disease. Normally the blood vessels and a type of brain cells called astrocytes form the blood–brain barrier, which prevents free movement of cells and molecules in and out of the CNS. Analysis of the cerebrospinal fluid (CSF) from patients with CNS disease reveals evidence of inflammation such as elevated protein levels and increased levels of antibodies (IgG) and oligoclonal bands (see the section on laboratory and imaging studies later in the chapter), suggesting a breach of the blood–brain barrier by inflammatory cells.

Similar to various other autoimmune diseases and the involvement of other organs in Sjögren's, autoantibodies are also considered a possible mediator of CNS disease. However, so far, there have been no specific autoantibodies identified directly causing neurologic complications. Animal studies show that antibodies against acetylcholine receptors can bind to brain tissue and cause inflammation. Although such antibodies have been found in patients with Sjögren's, they have not been found in patients with Sjögren's and neurologic disease. Apart from directly acting on nerve cells, another mechanism by which antibodies are thought to cause neurologic symptoms is by causing damage, dysfunction, or inflammation of the blood vessels supplying the CNS.

Altered levels or function of cytokines, the molecules with which different immune cells communicate with each other, play a role in autoimmune diseases, including Sjögren's. One key factor is type I interferon, which, apart from promoting a cascade of activation of other pro-inflammatory factors, can activate B cells, which in turn produce autoantibodies.

Much remains to be learned regarding autoimmunity and the underlying processes leading to neurologic disease in Sjögren's. Although there have been multiple studies addressing these issues, there are several factors limiting our ability to better study and understand this disease. Probably the most important factor is studying a well-defined patient population. That allows us to more accurately describe disease processes, compare different studies with each other, and generalize study results to a larger population of patients.

Another challenge is the fact that studies vary in terms of the frequency and definition of neurologic manifestations of Sjögren's. Although it is considered a common extraglandular manifestation, neurologic disease is the least commonly diagnosed. This has led to controversial opinions as to its existence, definition, and classification, particularly for CNS disease. Extensive evidence has accumulated over the past several decades that has supported and confirmed the fact that neurologic disease is a manifestation of the underlying systemic immune-mediated disorder rather than a distinct, coexisting, disorder. This evidence has been illustrated through animal and clinical studies indicating interactions among genetic, environmental, hormonal, and neuropsychological factors potentially triggering this autoimmune response.

Clinical Manifestations

As noted, the frequency of CNS involvement in Sjögren's varies among different studies. This is partly due to the fact that studies use different criteria for what this consists of in Sjögren's. In addition, different studies performed at neurologic or rheumatologic centers could be biased and result in neurologic involvement being over- or under-represented, respectively. Many of the studies reporting a high frequency of CNS involvement have included symptoms such as cognitive disturbance and depression as neurologic manifestations, which in some cases may not be directly attributable to Sjögren's. The incidence of more "severe" CNS involvement has been estimated at 2.5% to 5%.

Problems with attention, concentration, memory (often referred to as "brain fog"), and mood are often reported in people with Sjögren's. In general, these symptoms are quite common in the general population as well and occur at high rates in people with many types of chronic diseases. It is unclear if these manifestations are always a direct result of Sjögren's on the brain, or if they are secondary due to the sleep disturbances, pain, and depression that may be associated with chronic illness. In two small series that specifically examined cognitive function, a significant number of Sjögren's patients were noted to have signs of cognitive dysfunction. An increased incidence of depression, anxiety, and disturbed sleep has been noted in people with Sjögren's as well. Depression is reported in about 30% of patients with Sjögren's, and fatigue occurs in up to 67%.

The spectrum of CNS manifestations in Sjögren's is diverse and includes syndromes mimicking neuromyelitis optica (NMO) or multiple sclerosis (MS); however, these diseases may also coexist with Sjögren's, making their distinction difficult at times (see the following section on Sjögren's, MS, and NMO). CNS vasculitis is a result of inflammation of the blood vessels supplying the brain or spinal cord; it may present with different neurologic symptoms depending on the areas affected and is often accompanied by headache, confusion, or even seizures. Systemic symptoms such as fever, malaise, or joint pains are often present, as well as symptoms from vasculitis affecting organs outside of the nervous system, including the peripheral nerves.

Less common manifestations include aseptic meningitis (inflammation of the meninges, the tissue surrounding the brain, in the absence of infection) either as a result of vasculitis or as a primary event, presenting with headache, possible confusion, and other neurologic symptoms as a result of cranial nerve involvement; these can present with eye or face movement abnormalities, facial numbness, problems swallowing, or vertigo. Seizures can occur in Sjögren's but are also present in 1% of the general population as well. Dysfunction of the cerebellum has been reported in a few cases, presenting as clumsiness, balance problems, and problems with speech and swallowing.

A retrospective study of 82 patients with neurologic manifestations of Sjögren's included 12 with acute spinal cord disease, 16 with chronic spinal cord disease, one with motor neuron disease causing progressive weakness, 13 with optic neuropathy, 10 with relapsing–remitting MS-like disease, 10 with progressive MS-like disease, seven with seizures, nine with cognitive dysfunction, and two with encephalopathy (severe confusion). A second study of 93 patients with Sjögren's identified 14 with neurologic disease (including both peripheral and central nervous system disease), which included three patients with parkinsonian syndrome, two with epilepsy, two with headaches with abnormal brain magnetic resonance imaging (MRI), two with chronic progressive spinal cord disease, and one with aseptic meningitis. Both of these studies illustrate the diversity of CNS manifestations in Sjögren's as well as the difficulty of ascertaining the frequency of specific manifestations.

Sjögren's, NMO, and MS

Both NMO (also known as Devic's disease) and MS are autoimmune diseases, meaning that the immune system attacks parts of the patient's organs, in which case the CNS is involved (brain and spinal cord). However, nervous system involvement can also be part of Sjögren's. As there can be considerable overlap in the clinical presentation and laboratory test and imaging findings, distinguishing between these cases may be a complicated process at times. It is important to do so, however, not only to better characterize the disease process but also to make treatment decisions, as the treatment approaches may differ. While MS responds to a number of different medications, the most frequently used first-line treatment being interferon-1b, NMO responds to other immunosuppressive treatments better than interferon-1b. These include medications used commonly to treat other rheumatic diseases, including rituximab, or azathioprine.

NMO was initially considered a variant of MS, preferentially affecting the optic nerves and spinal cord and sparing the brain. It was previously called opticospinal MS but is now regarded as a separate disease. It typically presents with sudden attacks of inflammation of the optic nerve (optic neuritis) or spinal cord (synonyms include transverse myelitis, myelitis, or myelopathy). Optic neuritis may present as sudden vision loss or blurry vision in one eye, with or without eye pain. Myelitis may present with symptoms such as leg weakness, stiffness, incoordination, and loss of sensation, usually accompanied by bladder and bowel dysfunction (either in the form of retention [difficulty urinating or having a bowel movement] or incontinence). Less common presentations may include otherwise unexplained attacks of hiccups or vomiting, sleep attacks due to narcolepsy, or hormonal abnormalities, which represent NMO spectrum disorders (NMOSD). Rare cases of NMO presenting as a brain mass in Sjögren's patients have been described as well. After the discovery of an antibody unique to patients with NMOSD, it is now considered a separate disease with different courses and responses to treatments. Antibodies against a water channel, aquaporin-4, have been found in the blood of patients with NMO. The normal function of this water channel is to maintain balanced amounts of water molecules inside and outside different cell types, including CNS cells called astrocytes. The astrocytes surround and engulf the nerve cells (neurons) of the brain, protect them by forming the blood–brain barrier along with the endothelial cells that line the blood vessels, and control which substances can enter the brain. They also support neurons by producing useful molecules for their function and removing toxic ones.

To make the diagnosis of NMO, specific criteria should be met regarding the areas of the nervous system affected, the presence or absence of anti-aquaporin-4 antibodies, and specific MRI findings. In aggregate, NMO is considered to lead to greater disability than MS, but individual cases may vary significantly in terms of the frequency of attacks and final degree of disability.

NMO and systemic autoimmune diseases, including Sjögren's, have been known to coexist in both adults and children. Either one may precede the other, or at times they are both diagnosed simultaneously. Up to a third of NMO patients have been reported to have a coexisting systemic autoimmune disease, with Sjögren's and systemic lupus erythematosus being the most common ones found. Antibodies against aquaporin-4 are also often found in the blood of patients with Sjögren's and optic neuritis, or myelitis. In fact, it is not uncommon for such patients to meet criteria for diagnosis of both Sjögren's and NMO. Antibodies commonly found in the blood of Sjögren's patients and patients with other autoimmune diseases, such as antinuclear antibodies (ANA) or anti-Ro antibodies, have also been found in patients with NMO who do not otherwise have any symptoms or clinical features of Sjögren's. However, anti-aquaporin-4 antibodies are only present in patients who have NMOSD, with or without Sjögren's, and are not found in patients without neurologic disease.

Investigating whether distinct groups of patients, i.e. (1) those with both NMO and Sjögren's; (2) those with either soley NMO or Sjögren's; and (3) those with positive ANA or anti-Ro but not Sjögren's, have different clinical features, have produced conflicting results. Earlier studies suggested that NMO patients with systemic autoimmune diseases, such as Sjögren's, had a shorter life expectancy than patients with NMO and no other autoimmune diseases. However, later studies failed to reproduce these results, showing no difference between these two groups. Other studies of burden of brain abnormalities on MRI have also produced conflicting results. Despite the significant overlap in terms of clinical features, blood test results (including antibodies present), MRI findings, and the immunologic pathways involved, the current view on these conditions is that they are two separate diseases coexisting in the same patient rather than one being a manifestation of the other.

Multiple Sclerosis

MS is the most common autoimmune disease that primarily affects the CNS. The immune response is complex and the main target is myelin, a structure surrounding the nerve projections (axons) with an insulating function. There are specific criteria regarding the clinical features and MRI findings leading to its diagnosis, but for most cases two attacks involving different parts of the CNS occurring at two separate times are required, with all other possible causes being excluded. It usually presents with a sudden onset of neurologic symptoms, which can vary depending on the part of the CNS involved. These usually improve to different degrees after days to weeks, but there can be residual disability. In its most common form, the disease remains clinically silent between these attacks (relapsing-remitting course), while a fewer number of patients follow a progressive course, with worsening symptoms between relapses (progressive-relapsing). However, as the disease becomes more chronic, more patients with relapsing-remitting course eventually develop progressive symptoms (secondary-progressive). A few patients follow a chronic progressive course without relapses from the time of disease onset (primary-progressive). Similar to NMO, it is important to distinguish Sjögren's with neurologic involvement from MS, as the treatments can be different.

Earlier studies have described cases of Sjögren's that have overlapping features with MS. These include a series of patients who had all the typical features and a diagnosis of MS and who were reported to meet criteria for Sjögren's diagnosis as well. Since then, there have been a number of studies estimating the frequency of Sjögren's in patients with MS as between 0.9% and 3.3%, which is relatively close to the frequency of Sjögren's in the general population; a study of 192 patients with MS found none with Sjögren's. However, Sjögren's seems to be more frequently found among patients with primary-progressive MS, as one study reported that 10 of 60 MS patients also met criteria for Sjögren's. Similar to NMO, an increased frequency of the antibodies found in Sjögren's, such as ANA and anti-Ro, has also been found in the blood of MS patients who do not have symptoms of Sjögren's. MS patients who also carry a diagnosis of Sjögren's have been reported to have more severe disability and visual impairment than patients with MS without Sjögren's.

There are a few points that can make the interpretation of these studies' results more complicated. Most of them included patients diagnosed with MS prior to the time NMO was considered a separate disease; therefore, they may have included patients with NMO, whom we now know also often have coexisting autoimmune diseases such as Sjögren's and can have different features, disease course, and response to treatment. Chronic interferon-1b treatment, one of the most commonly used first-line treatments for MS, can cause the production of antibodies, such as ANA or anti-Ro, or even autoimmune diseases. Therefore, in an MS patient with such antibodies or symptoms of Sjögren's on interferon-1b treatment, it may be difficult to ascertain whether these are due to coexisting diseases or represent a side effect of this medication. Nevertheless, there have been cases of Sjögren's described in MS patients receiving interferon-1b both shortly after treatment initiation as well as after long-term treatment, suggesting that probably both cases may apply.

To complicate matters further, dysfunction of the autonomic nervous system has been described in MS patients, which seems to be more severe in patients with more aggressive disease. The autonomic nervous system is responsible for many involuntary body functions, including regulation of heart rate and blood pressure, bowel motility, and saliva and tear secretion. As both

Sjögren's and autonomic nervous system dysfunction can cause dry eye, these associations may be another source of potential bias when evaluating a patient with MS and possible Sjögren's.

Laboratory and Imaging Findings

In cases of possible neurologic involvement, blood tests frequently performed include markers of overall disease activity, such as C4 complement levels, erythrocyte sedimentation rate (ESR), and C-reactive protein (CRP). Antibodies associated with Sjögren's, such as ANA, anti-Ro, or anti-La, can also be present in neurologic diseases with similar presentation to Sjögren's-related CNS disease, such as NMO or MS. The interpretation of such blood tests requires caution and should always take into consideration the overall clinical picture, as isolated tests rarely have diagnostic value.

CSF testing can be useful in certain cases of neurologic involvement, particularly those with a sudden onset or rapid progression. The CSF surrounds the brain, spinal cord, and proximal nerve roots, and its chemical composition differs from that of the blood due to the presence of the blood–brain barrier, which prohibits the free flow of certain molecules from the blood to the CSF and vice versa. Therefore, sampling of CSF can provide information that cannot be obtained by blood testing. Elevated CSF protein and IgG index (which indicates antibody production within the CNS) are strong indicators of CNS inflammation but do not provide information regarding its underlying cause. The presence of oligoclonal bands, which implies a specific pattern of "a few" (=oligo) clones of B cells producing immunoglobulins, is a typical finding in CSF studies from MS patients, as well as Sjögren's patients with CNS involvement; thus, it cannot reliably distinguish between the two.

CSF is sampled via a lumbar puncture. During this procedure, after disinfecting the skin and administering local anesthesia, a needle is inserted through the back in the space between two vertebrae and fluid is collected. This procedure may be done at the bedside or under X-ray guidance. The most common complication is headache, which is typically exacerbated by standing and relieved by lying down. This is thought to be due to fluid balance and pressure changes after removing fluid, causing vein engorgement within the CNS. It usually resolves after 3 to 4 days. If it persists, it can be treated by a procedure called a blood patch, during which the patient's blood is injected in the epidural space (the space between the outer layer of connective tissue surrounding the spinal cord and the subarachnoid space in which the CSF is located). Rare complications include excessive bleeding and infection as well as brain herniation. The latter was seen prior to the advent of modern brain-imaging techniques, such as computed tomography (CT) and MRI, and was usually caused by pressure from tumors or mass lesions of the brain descending from the lower part of the skull into the spinal canal after CSF was removed from the lower spine.

Cryoglobulins are a specific pattern of antibody production. Their name comes from the observation that these antibodies would precipitate after blood samples were exposed to lower temperatures. They can be associated with more severe systemic disease and are found more frequently in some cases of peripheral neuropathies but are not typically a part of CNS disease in Sjögren's.

Abnormalities seen on brain MRI are common in Sjögren's. Abnormal imaging findings of the brain's white matter, the area corresponding to nerve cell projections connecting different areas of the brain (as opposed to the gray matter, which consists of the nerve cell bodies themselves), are common in patients with Sjögren's. Their etiology is not always known, but they are usually either the result of microscopic blood vessel occlusion (microvascular disease) or due to white matter inflammation; both processes eventually lead to scarring of the affected areas, which causes an abnormal signal visible on MRI. Apart from Sjögren's, microvascular disease, due to hypertension or high cholesterol; migraine headaches; and diseases such as multiple sclerosis, NMO, or other inflammatory CNS diseases can also cause such white matter lesions. Whether patients with Sjögren's and CNS disease or Sjögren's without neurologic symptoms have such lesions more frequently, or in greater numbers, is unclear, as studies focusing on these questions have yielded conflicting results. Their location may be of more diagnostic value, as white matter lesions in the corpus callosum (a midline structure of the brain through which projections connecting the two brain hemispheres traverse) are usually associated with MS, while gray matter lesions are usually due to Sjögren's-related CNS disease.

A more recent study reported that white matter lesions surrounding veins are more predictive of MS than other neurologic diseases, including CNS disease due to Sjögren's. MRI of the spinal cord is also recommended in suspected cases of myelitis (spinal cord inflammation), which can help distinguish whether this is due to an active process as well as the underlying cause. Myelitis spanning more than three consecutive vertebrae is typical of NMO, which can be confirmed by blood testing for antibodies against aquaporin-4. Blood and CSF tests are also usually done to establish the latter. In both brain and spinal cord disease, active inflammation can cause disruption of the blood–brain barrier. This can be assessed by administering intravenous contrast material, which in the case of MRI is gadolinium. This should normally not cross the blood–brain barrier and should not be detected in the CNS. However, in cases of active inflammation it can be detected within the CNS, causing hyperintense signal on specific MRI sequences. Therefore, gadolinium may be given to patients undergoing brain and spinal cord MRI if active disease is suspected.

Electroencephalography (EEG) can be useful in the evaluation of suspected seizures or atypical mental status changes such as prolonged confusion. This involves recording the brain's electrical activity via electrodes placed on the scalp. EEG can detect patterns of abnormal electrical activity related to seizures or overall slowing of brain activity in cases of confusion. It can also detect focal abnormalities of brain electrical activity if a certain area of the brain is affected as opposed to the brain as a whole. However, it is of low sensitivity, which means that a negative test does not rule out the abnormalities being sought. Brain MRI is also usually performed in patients with seizures or atypical mental status changes, while a lumbar puncture can be performed in atypical cases.

In cases of cognitive impairment, the initial testing aims at ruling out systemic medical conditions causing the symptoms, such as depression; kidney, liver, or thyroid dysfunction; or vitamin B_{12} deficiency. In rapidly progressing cases, MRI and CSF studies can be useful to further evaluate underlying causes. Other imaging techniques, such as the diffusor tensor imaging sequence (DTI) used in MRI or single photon emission computed tomography (SPECT), are used in research, but their clinical value is still under investigation.

Treatment Outcomes and Disability in Patients with Neurologic Complications and Sjögren's

It is important to determine whether a neurologic syndrome is due to Sjögren's or a separate, coexisting, neurologic problem, as the treatments may be very different. Treatments for CNS manifestations of Sjögren's can be divided into two broad categories:

- Immunomodulatory treatments, which modify or suppress the immune response, in cases where the underlying process is inflammatory, aiming to reduce inflammation in the brain and the spinal cord

- Symptomatic treatments, which treat the presenting symptoms but may not address the underlying cause.

Assessment of the disease burden and timely intervention are very important to prevent cell injury and permanent neurologic dysfunction in inflammatory disorders of the CNS.

Medications used in such cases include high-dose intravenous corticosteroids, rituximab, or cyclophosphamide. Corticosteroids are usually the preferred first treatment, as they have rapid action and cover a broad range of inflammatory conditions; however, their long-term use is problematic due to side effects. In most severe cases of CNS manifestations, an additional treatment is usually required. Rituximab is a more targeted therapy reducing the number of B cells, which produce autoantibodies, and has been used more often due to its more favorable side-effect profile. Cyclophosphamide, although one of the most effective immunosuppressants, is reserved for more severe or difficult-to-treat cases as it has the most serious side effects.

An important part of treatment, especially in patients with transverse myelitis, vasculitis, and NMO, is preventive, to reduce the risk of further attacks of inflammation causing CNS damage. This also reduces the overall burden of long-term disability. Immunosuppressants such as rituximab, mycophenolate, and azathioprine are often used for long-term preventive therapy to prevent repeat attacks.

Treatment of mood disorders may involve the use of antidepressants such as selective serotonin reuptake inhibitors (SSRIs) or serotonin–norepinephrine reuptake inhibitors (SNRIs), tricyclic antidepressants, or mood stabilizers. These are often used and effective at low doses and can be given in conjunction with other medications.

Physical therapy to optimize muscle strength and balance is a very important treatment in neurologic syndromes resulting in weakness or balance problems. Occupational therapy is also helpful in cases where hand function is affected. Botulinum toxin is a bacterial toxin that causes muscle weakness by blocking the communication of nerve and muscle cells; it is used to selectively weaken muscles that may be overactive. This reduces spasticity in the limbs, which often occurs due to transverse myelitis, and can help improve functional outcomes. Neuropathic pain can be treated with topical treatments (such as lidocaine or capsaicin) or oral medications (including gabapentin, pregabalin, or duloxetine). Amitriptyline and nortriptyline are part of another group of medications that are very helpful for neuropathic pain, but one of their side effects is dry mouth and dry eyes; thus, they may exacerbate the ocular and oral symptoms of Sjögren's.

Burden of Disability

Based on a large epidemiologic study in 2016, the burden of Sjögren's and inflammation was higher in the group with neurologic manifestations. Patients with neurologic complications also had a higher risk of developing new neurologic symptoms. Patients who had CNS involvement, especially transverse myelitis or NMO, had an overall higher degree of morbidity compared to those with peripheral nervous system involvement but not CNS involvement. Therefore, the burden of long-term disability in patients with neurologic complications is high. The key to preventing long-term disability is appropriate assessment and timely treatment with immune medications; this will not only reduce ongoing inflammation but also prevent further inflammation and relapses. Please also refer to Chapter 47 for a more detailed overview of the disability process.

Summing Up

Estimates of the frequency of CNS involvement in Sjögren's vary widely, but it is less common than peripheral nervous system involvement. Regardless, patients and medical professionals should be aware of potential CNS manifestations. Considerable overlap between autoimmune disorders can exist; thus, CNS involvement can include NMO or MS as part of a patient's Sjögren's, or they may be considered separate comorbidities. Cognitive dysfunction and mood disorders, including anxiety and depression, also can be rooted in CNS Sjögren's or appear as comorbidities.

For Further Reading

Annunziata P, De Santi L, Di Rezze S, et al. Clinical features of Sjogren's syndrome in patients with multiple sclerosis. *Acta Neurol Scand.* 2011;124(2):109–114.

Birnbaum J, Atri NM, Baer AN, et al. The relationship between the neuromyelitis optica spectrum disorder and Sjogren's syndrome: Central nervous system extraglandular disease or unrelated, co-occurring autoimmunity? *Arthritis Care Res.* 2017;69(10):10.

Delalande S, de Seze J, Fauchais AL, et al. Neurologic manifestations in primary Sjogren syndrome: A study of 82 patients. *Medicine.* 2004;83:280–291.

Moreira I, Teixeira F, Martins Silva A, et al. Frequent involvement of central nervous system in primary Sjogren's. *Rheumatol Int.* 2015;35:289–294.

Nocturne G, Mariette X. Advances in understanding the pathogenesis of primary Sjogren's syndrome. *Nat Rev Rheumatol.* 2013;9:544.

31

Management of Cognitive Dysfunction and Central Nervous System Involvement in Sjögren's

Edward Maitz and Stephen Maitz

Sjögren's is a systemic immune disorder known to target systems in the body affecting the eyes and mouth, as well as other areas such as the lungs, kidneys, joints, nerves, thyroid, liver, and skin. Perhaps less well recognized is that Sjögren's can also affect the central nervous system (CNS), which comprises the brain and the spinal cord (Figure 31.1).

The brain is of particular interest in understanding the wide-ranging effects of CNS Sjögren's, as it is responsible for regulating our basic and essential physiologic functions (e.g., appetite, sleep cycle, temperature, breathing); performing higher-level cognitive functions (e.g., executive and problem-solving skills, visual/perceptual skills, concentration, memory, language abilities); interpreting sensory input; coordinating motor output (i.e., the execution of movement); and regulating emotions. There is virtually nothing that we feel, think, or do that is not in some fashion mediated by the brain.

Whereas the brain is responsible for coordinating and regulating these bodily, cognitive, and psychological processes, the spinal cord is responsible for transmitting signals within the body. The spinal cord carries messages from the brain to the rest of the body, including what we refer to as the peripheral nervous system (i.e., nerves in the trunk, arms, legs, hands, and feet).

If this seems confusing or complicated, think of the brain as the command center for virtually all of our physical, thinking, and emotional responses and the spinal cord as the conduit through which all information travels to the brain from other parts of the body and from the brain to the rest of the body. This is admittedly a simplified model, as the spinal cord does have input into the messages being delivered, but it will suffice for this discussion, which will be limited primarily to the brain.

Edward Maitz and Stephen Maitz, *Management of Cognitive Dysfunction and Central Nervous System Involvement in Sjögren's* In: *The Sjögren's Book*. Edited by: Daniel J. Wallace, Oxford University Press. © Sjögren's Foundation 2022. DOI: 10.1093/oso/9780197502112.003.0031

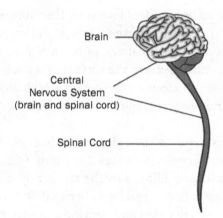

Figure 31.1 Organization of the central nervous system.
Source: https://commons.wikimedia.org/wiki/File:Central_nervous_system.
gif#filelinks

Organization of the Brain

The brain is organized into three parts: the cerebrum, the brain stem, and the cerebellum (Figure 31.2).

The cerebrum comprises four lobes: the frontal, parietal, temporal, and occipital lobes. A deep ridge running lengthwise, atop the cerebrum, effectively divides the brain into right and left hemispheres (though the hemispheres are

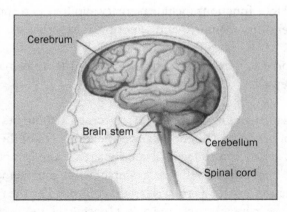

Figure 31.2 The major parts of the brain.
Source: National Cancer Institute

actually interconnected by bundles of nerves). Therefore, each lobe has both a left and right aspect (i.e., right/left frontal lobe, right/left parietal).

The surface, or cortex (gray matter), of the brain mediates certain brain functions, as do structures beneath the surface in the subcortical area (white matter). During most conscious tasks, there is a high amount of integration and coordination between brain regions and between the cortical and subcortical regions.

Certain functions tend to lateralize (i.e., left vs. right hemisphere). Specifically, for most people, language functions (e.g., vocabulary skills, verbal memory, reading, spelling, speech) are largely controlled by the left hemisphere of the brain. In contrast, visual-spatial skills (e.g., reading a map, putting puzzles together, drawing and copying a design, remembering visual information such as navigating familiar roads or where you parked your car) are largely controlled by the right hemisphere of the brain.

In addition to lateralization of brain functions, certain brain functions tend to localize to a specific area of the brain . Some functions localize more reliably than others:

- The frontal lobes are implicated in processes such as higher-order executive functioning (e.g., strategizing/planning, task initiation, alternating attention, self-monitoring, response inhibition, complex problem-solving); motoric output, including hand strength and manual dexterity; speech; personality; judgment; and behavior.
- Parietal lobe functions involve somatic sensation (i.e., touch, pain, temperature, body position in space), visuospatial interpretation, praxis (idea formation to guide sequencing of motor movement), and some language processing.
- Temporal lobe functions include primary auditory perception, language comprehension, memory, and emotional experiences, feelings, and reactions.
- The occipital lobe registers and integrates visual information received from the eyes.

It is important to remember that these complex thoughts, actions, and feelings do not originate and end in a specific focal area of the brain. While they might be *largely* controlled by a specific area, there is input from many other areas of the brain as well. For example, while our memory for visual spatial information, say for a cross, is largely controlled by the right temporal area, first we have to be able to see the object (occipital lobe), recognize visual-spatial configuration ("oh, it's a cross"; right parietal area), concentrate on the information in order to store it in memory (frontal lobe), then remember it (temporal lobe). Of course, if we are then asked to point to the cross, we have to hear and comprehend the request (left temporal lobe), and then perform the motoric action (frontal lobe). The left frontal lobe controls right-handed movements, and vice versa, because like other functions, motoric output is a process governed contralaterally (i.e., the opposite side of the brain controls whichever side of the body is being used). The entire process of responding to the request "point to the cross" happens in a matter of seconds, often without conscious thought. This is but one simple example of the complexity, organization, and integration of brain functions. It is also a testament to the exquisite efficiency of brain functioning and the complex and delicate processes involved in CNS (brain) functioning. Although we all become acutely aware of some mistake or impairment in normal brain functioning, we sometimes take for granted all of the things that go right in our day-to-day lives.

Given the topographical organization of the brain just described, it should be obvious that a lesion (an area of acute brain damage) will often produce a disruption in some specific brain ability or function. For example, a lesion in the left frontal lobe might result in impairment in motor functions in the contralateral (right) hand. A lesion in the occipital area might result in a visual field cut or even cortical blindness (a condition of vision loss owing to brain damage and not eye health). A lesion in the right parietal area might result in an inability to assemble a bicycle or piece of furniture. A lesion in the left temporal lobe might cause difficulty remembering conversations.

As we mentioned earlier, even basic thoughts, actions, and behaviors require communication and integration of information between the various areas of the brain. The brain structures that allow for this are located beneath the cortical surface of the cerebrum. These subcortical (white matter) structures are involved in a multitude of actions. Subcortical white matter tracts extend in all directions, acting as highways for neuronal communication between different brain regions. These myelinated axons have a fatty, insulating layer that facilitates more efficient neurotransmission. Lesions in the subcortical white matter (which are common in demyelinating conditions such as multiple sclerosis) result in a disruption in the communication between the various lobes of the brain and can result in impairment or disruption in normal brain functions, including motor impairment, cognitive impairment, and/or problems with psychological and/or emotional functioning.

The lower aspect of the brain, where the brain and spinal cord meet, is where the brain stem is located. The brain stem is implicated in the performance of vital, involuntary tasks related to breathing, cardiovascular functions, and sleep regulation, among others. Several cranial nerves, which facilitate sensory and motor functions of the head, face, neck, and trunk, are also present in this area. The brain stem interfaces with the cerebellum, a distinct structure that sits beneath the occipital lobes toward the back of the brain. Not to be confused with the cerebrum, the cerebellum incorporates a variety of information to regulate motor and cognitive activities, providing balance and smoothness in the execution of actions.

The CNS has several protective mechanisms. Thin membranes called the meninges form layers atop of one another and facilitate circulation of cerebrospinal fluid (CSF) surrounding the brain and spinal cord, while also protecting the vessels that supply blood to these areas. The meninges comprise the dura, arachnoid, and pia mater. Bony structures, namely the skull and vertebrae, offer further protection from harm. Despite these protective mechanisms, the CNS remains vulnerable to internal threats, including systemic illnesses such as Sjögren's as well as external threats such as trauma. An exhaustive review of the various neuropathologic conditions that can affect the brain is well beyond the scope of this chapter. The interested reader is referred to a basic neurology text for a more comprehensive review of various neurologic disorders.

Incidence and Prevalence

CNS involvement in Sjögren's is a relatively recent area of focus within Sjögren's research. As a result, incidence and prevalence rates of CNS Sjögren's vary significantly between studies. For instance, prevalence rates of CNS involvement have been characterized as nonexistent to very common. Some sources indicate that 20% of patients with Sjögren's develop neurologic involvement, with other sources indicating neurologic impairment in 2.5% to 60% of patients. It is reasonable to assert that the true incidence and prevalence of CNS Sjögren's cannot yet be determined reliably; however, this number is certainly not believed to be insignificant. One complicating factor is the fact that patients with Sjögren's sometimes have comorbid conditions such as multiple sclerosis or vascular disease that can also cause lesions and result in impaired brain functioning.

Pathophysiology of CNS Sjögren's

As previously stated, autoimmune disorders such as CNS Sjögren's can result in CNS lesions. Our understanding of the underlying cause or pathophysiology specific to CNS Sjögren's is not entirely clear. However, thanks to increasing awareness of CNS Sjögren's and advances in neuroimaging, the clinical picture is becoming clearer and better understood.

The pathophysiologic changes that may occur from CNS involvement in Sjögren's are numerous. One example is white matter changes, including demyelination, a process whereby the external fatty layer (myelin) of neurons deteriorates, compromising neurotransmission. A second type of pathophysiologic process includes inflammatory responses. Inflammation has been observed in the optic nerve (optic neuritis), meninges (meningitis), and spinal cord (transverse myelitis). Vascular changes represent another pathophysiologic change. Loss of brain volume, or atrophy, may also occur. Additional pathophysiologic changes include seizures, cerebellar syndrome, strokes, and other forms of encephalopathy (i.e., any brain disease or disruption of brain function).

Neuroimaging studies have revealed objective evidence of the pathophysiologic changes. Neuroimaging and monitoring techniques may include, among others, computed tomography (CT scanning), which in very simple terms is similar to an X-ray and shows a picture of the structures of the brain. Magnetic resonance imagining (MRI) is often more sensitive to CNS lesions and also captures a picture of the structure of the brain using a large magnetic field and radio waves to create images. With positron emission tomography (PET) and single photon emission computed tomography (SPECT) scanning, a radioactive isotope is injected into the bloodstream and acts as a dye, showing the uptake of blood to various regions of the brain and actually showing the brain working and functioning during various tasks. In diffusion tensor imaging (DTI), an evolution from conventional MRI, specific modeling of data provides information about the diffusion properties of water molecules among tissue. The process of capturing diffusion rates gives details about tissue properties such as integrity and architecture, among other variables, and provides an exquisite level of detail (e.g., integrity of white matter fibers), the likes of which was previously unknown. An electroencephalogram (EEG) measures the electrical activity in the brain. It is useful for identifying abnormal electrical activity as seen in seizures and generalized disruption in normal brain activity (due to a number of possible causes).

Several researchers have performed imaging studies specifically with patients with Sjögren's and other autoimmune disorders. White matter changes have been observed in nearly 50% of Sjögren's patients in some instances with variation among inflammatory/demyelinating findings, vascular lesions, and both focal and diffuse lesion findings; other researchers found white matter changes in 70% of patients. Microstructure alterations in the frontal area have been observed in Sjögren's patients evidencing mild cognitive impairment.

Volume loss or atrophy related to Sjögren's provides support for the organic etiology of cognitive and psychiatric dysfunction observed in Sjögren's, with evidence of even cerebellar atrophy related to Sjögren's.

In addition to the aforementioned studies that demonstrate the structural pathophysiologic changes that can occur in Sjögren's, there are also studies that actually show changes not just in the brain's structure but in brain activity as well. One study involving electrical activity monitoring found that 3% of patients with Sjögren's had seizure disorders. Visually evoked potentials were abnormal in 61% of the patients tested in one study, and electrophysiologic abnormalities on cognitive event-related potentials have also been associated with mild cognitive impairment in Sjögren's patients. Another class of imaging that demonstrated functional abnormalities involves cerebral blood flow studies. One study found that 56.3% of patients with Sjögren's who had a normal MRI showed hypoperfusion brain lesions on SPECT (mostly in the parietal lobes). Another study also demonstrated (left) parieto-temporal area abnormalities on MRI and SPECT that correlated with abnormalities on neuropsychological testing in a single-subject study. Research using SPECT revealed perfusion deficits in 80.9% of patients with Sjögren's, with vascular disease found in a small percentage (3%) of Sjögren's patients. This list is not intended to be an exhaustive review of the literature with respect to imaging studies of patients with CNS Sjögren's; rather, it aims to provide evidence that these disorders can result in objective, unequivocal evidence that Sjögren's can cause pathophysiologic changes in the brain. These techniques involve some sort of human–machine interface and vary considerably in application. In terms of their capacity for detail and image quality, these studies range from providing static (photograph-like) to functional (real-time monitoring) information about CNS networks and structures. In summary, the research literature using these imaging and electrophysiologic studies has revealed subcortical white matter abnormalities and changes, brain atrophy (volume loss), vasculitis, hypoperfusion (decreased blood flow), and electrophysiologic abnormalities (e.g., abnormal visual evoked potentials, seizures), among others.

Neuropsychological Symptoms and Functional Impairment in Patients with CNS Sjögren's

The information just presented has critical implications for researchers, clinicians, and, most importantly, Sjögren's patients:

1. While not all patients with Sjögren's have a compromised CNS, a subset of patients with Sjögren's will develop CNS Sjögren's with some degree of underlying neuropathology.
2. The neuropathologic changes can result in impairment in physical, cognitive, and/or psychological functioning.
3. The nature of functional impairment will depend largely upon the area of the brain that has been affected.

From a neuropsychological perspective, the question becomes, "How can we identify, evaluate, and treat the cognitive and psychological sequelae of CNS Sjögren's?" The answer comes from both patient reports and the research literature.

The disease onset and the course of symptoms associated with CNS Sjögren's are often slow and insidious, with a waxing-and-waning quality. As a result, they might not be immediately obvious to the patient or family member. In addition, the neuropsychological changes are sometimes misattributed to the normal aging process, psychological factors, and/or medication side effects. CNS Sjögren's often has an insidious course, with intermittent remitting and sometimes progressive evolution. One study found that *most* cases take an acute often recurrent course with spontaneous remission or only mild neurological impairment. According to another, CNS involvement is usually multifocal, additive, and progressive, with a clinical course of fixed and cumulative deficits or a relapsing-remitting course that may mimic multiple sclerosis. Echoing this outlook, another study reported that among patients with CNS disorders, 59% had disease that mimicked multiple sclerosis, with about half relapsing-remitting and half progressive. While changes in neuropsychological functioning can be due to a host of other factors, including aging, medication effects, stress, and lack of sleep, it is important to understand the underlying etiology of neuropsychological deficits in order to develop the most efficacious plan and to help the patient and family members better understand the nature and etiology of changes in neuropsychological functioning.

CNS Symptoms in Patients with Sjögren's

The symptoms of CNS Sjögren's include a variety of disturbances within physical, cognitive, and psychosocial domains. Physical symptoms can occur, some of which are relatively more common and others more rare. Physical symptoms may include headaches, such as migraines with or without aura, tension-type headaches, and medication-overuse headaches, all of which may present episodically or chronically. Pain, fatigue (physical, mental, and ocular), sleep disorders, dizziness, and vertigo have also been documented. Ophthalmologic disorders (e.g., optic neuritis) have been noted, and so too have voice, speech, and swallowing disorders (often implicating cranial nerve abnormalities). Balance disorders like cerebellar ataxia can also occur. Research demonstrates the range of physical problems, with the incidence of headaches ranging from nearly 50% of Sjögren's patients in some studies to 78% in others. Motor deficits have been observed. In one study, pure sensory neuropathy was reported as occurring in 9.2% of patients, with sensory/motor neuropathy occurring in 5.3% of patients with Sjögren's. Cognitive symptoms reported may include "brain fog," a general lack of clarity in cognitive actions or dulled cognitive proficiency. Changes in verbal abilities in the face of preserved perceptual abilities and full-scale IQ have been noted, along with verbal memory deficits. Individuals may also report problems with speed of information processing, higher-level executive abilities, and/or concentration. Difficulty understanding language may also occur. An evidentiary basis corroborates the many subjective accounts of CNS involvement in Sjögren's patients. One study found that among 72 Sjögren's patients, cognitive dysfunction was noted in 50%, while 60% to 70% of Sjögren's patients were found to have cognitive impairment(s). In another study among Sjögren's patients, 78% demonstrated impairments on measures of processing speed, attention, verbal learning and memory, and visual/spatial skills. Similar findings, with deficits observed in the same domains, reported that these effects were generally not mediated by depression. Among 120 patients with Sjögren's, cognitive impairment was found in 44.4% on measures of higher-level executive functioning and verbal memory.

Subtle impairments in verbal memory and cognitive efficiency have been noted in studies, with a reported correlation between self-report and objective testing with respect to verbal memory. Evidence of impairment on measures of verbal reasoning and psychomotor processing was also found in the same study. When corrected for depression, there was a group difference for verbal reasoning but not psychomotor processing. A separate study noted a trend of correlation on MRI findings in relation to the deficits observed in areas including processing speed, verbal memory, attention, and executive functioning, deficits that were found in 60% of the researchers' patients.

Psychosocial symptoms may relate to Sjögren's in a number of ways that need not be mutually exclusive. It could be helpful to consider the possibility of three distinct contributing factors in relation to psychosocial problems. First, there is some suggestion that physiologic changes in the brain may cause changes in mood and social interaction. Second, the disease burden associated with any chronic medical condition can result in psychological adjustment issues (we refer to this as an adjustment disorder in an otherwise well-adjusted individual). Third, here may be people who, prior to the onset of the illness, were already experiencing anxiety and/or depression. In these cases, the physical and cognitive symptoms associated with CNS Sjögren's may exacerbate the underlying psychological conditions. Dysphoric moods (e.g., anxiety, depression) or adjustment reactions may intensify during Sjögren's flares due to financial burden, social limitations, insufficient support(s), medication effects, or any number of possibilities implicated in the disease process. Concerns over one's mental well-being are often reported and may take several forms: Depression, apathy, anxiety, irritability, paranoia, obsessive–compulsive disorders, and atypical mood disorders, even psychosis, have been reported.

These subjective, anecdotal patient complaints have also been substantiated by objective research findings. A study of 120 patients with Sjögren's concluded that observed mood disorders were suggestive of an organic substrate. Research by Segal et al. (2009) indicated that 37% of the 277 patients studied were affected by depression, with a lower quality of life, owing to health, also reported. Lower quality of life related to pain and fatigue as well as elevated levels of depression has been observed in other research, and increased depression, fatigue, and deficits in activities of daily living are also represented in the research literature. A meta-analysis by Wan et al. (2016) demonstrated that the incidence of anxiety and depression was three times that of the normal control population. In a 2015 study, higher rates of depression, anxiety, and sleep disorders were found in Sjögren's patients relative to controls, with four possible mediating factors: preexisting personality traits and general psychological distress, physical discomfort, immune/inflammation dysfunction, and white matter lesions. Specific cases of anxiety and panic have also been reportedly related to possible autoimmune process(es). Affective disorders have also been noted, with the possibility that these could also be the result of immune-mediated brain dysfunction.

To be clear, many of these physical, cognitive, and psychosocial problems occur in patients who do not have Sjögren's or CNS Sjögren's. They can be due to the aging process, other physical factors described earlier (e.g., medication effects, pain, lack of sleep), and psychological factors (e.g., anxiety and depression). To further complicate matters, these physical, cognitive, and emotional factors are obviously not mutually exclusive. For example, a person might have some type of neurologic dysfunction in the left temporal area that impairs their ability to remember verbal information. As a result, they becomes anxious when speaking with others in a social situation, and their anxiety further compromises their memory skills, resulting in a self-perpetuating downward cycle and causing them to withdraw from family and friends.

Given the inherent difficulties in identifying (1) the functional neuropsychological sequelae of CNS Sjögren's and (2) the underlying etiology or etiologies, many patients are referred for a neuropsychological evaluation. The neuropsychologist typically reviews records and reports from other medical providers, interviews the patient, and administers a battery of neuropsychological tests. A neuropsychological evaluation involves the administration of a very comprehensive battery of tests designed to evaluate and map out brain functioning. Unlike imaging studies, it does not involve the use of leads, probes, or radioactive tracers or require confinement within enclosed spaces. Rather, it involves performance-based testing methods designed to assess the patient's sensory skills (tactile, auditory, and visual), motor skills (strength, speed, and dexterity), perceptual skills (visual and auditory), language skills, concentration (visual and auditory), overall intellectual and cognitive functioning, cognitive processing speed and efficiency, memory, and executive functioning (e.g., cognitive flexibility and higher-level problem-solving). Typically, a neuropsychologist will also administer some measures of psychological and emotional functioning. The goal is to identify any areas of impaired functioning and to identify the cause of the impairment (e.g., normal variation due to normal inter-individual differences; effects of normal aging; generalized or localized damage to the brain; interference from psychological or emotional factors; effects of other extraneous factors such as fatigue and medications). Not uncommonly, the observed deficits might be due to multiple causes. In addition, as with any medical test, the test findings might be very clear or they might be equivocal and inconclusive. Finally, based upon the test results, the neuropsychologist might recommend a referral to other medical specialists and provide specific treatment recommendations.

Prognosis

Prognosis depends on many factors, given that Sjögren's manifestations can vary markedly among individuals. In addition to variations between individuals, Sjögren's patients may experience differences across the lifetime of their own illness. Because symptoms may present for a relatively long period before formal diagnosis, as well as the unpredictability of symptom severity across flares (exacerbation of symptoms), many factors can be influential. For instance, disease progression, comorbid conditions, personality/emotionality characteristics, and declines associated with normal aging may all influence the short-term and long-term outlook. One study showed that most cases of CNS symptoms had an acute relapsing course. Another followed 12 patients with Sjögren's over 8 years and found mild decline in some areas and improvement in others not associated with progressive dementing disease.

Ancillary Services for Evaluation and Treatment

The diagnosis of Sjögren's is often initially made by a rheumatologist. However, particularly for those diagnosed with CNS Sjögren's, patients may be referred to a host of other medical specialists for evaluation or treatment or both.

- Patients will often be referred to a *neurologist*, whose role it is to examine and treat the overall issues related to the CNS and peripheral nervous system. The neurologist typically assesses the patient's sensory skills, motor skills, balance and coordination, and reflexes and might perform brief mental status testing. Based on the evaluation, the neurologist might refer the patient for an imaging study of the brain or a neuropsychological evaluation.
- Some patients are referred to a *physiatrist*, a physician who specializes in physical medicine and rehabilitation. Physiatrists are generalists who evaluate a patient, possibly prescribe medications, and coordinate an overall rehabilitation plan.
- Some patients are referred to a *neuro-ophthalmologist*, particularly if there is a question or concern regarding the patient's visual system. An ophthalmologist is a physician who specializes in the health of the eye. A neuro-ophthalmologist is a physician who specializes in the evaluation of the nerve fibers in the brain that carry the visual information from the eye to the occipital area of the brain.
- Some patients are referred to a *neuro-otologist*. A neuro-otologist is a physician who specializes in the nerve fibers and tracks in the brain that connect the ear to the areas of the brain that process auditory information.

Treatment of patients with Sjögren's can take many forms. Some patients are referred to an occupational therapist, who typically treats visual/motor problems, coordination problems, and vestibular problems (dizziness or disequilibrium). Other patients might be referred to a physical therapist to work on problems with gait or motor strength and might also treat vestibular disorders.

Patients who have documented cognitive deficits are sometimes referred to a cognitive rehabilitation specialist, typically a speech therapist or clinical neuropsychologist. These specialists will address the neurocognitive sequelae of the illness. This therapy typically takes one of two forms:

- One form of cognitive remediation therapy involves helping the patient develop strategies to help compensate for cognitive problems and minimize their impact in day-to-day functioning. This may involve developing a system of reminders, calendars, appointment books, or other strategies. It is not necessarily designed to remediate the problem or improve upon a specific skill deficit.
- Another form of cognitive remediation involves the use of specific cognitive exercises designed to work toward improving a skill or function as opposed to compensating for the deficit.

Some patients are referred to a psychiatrist or neuropsychiatrist if it is determined that they might benefit from psychopharmacological intervention for treatment of anxiety or depression, or both. Other patients are referred for individual psychotherapy to address the psychological and emotional sequelae of the illness. Family members are sometimes included in these sessions as well. Another adjunctive form of treatment to address psychological and emotional issues is the use of biofeedback or other strategies to reduce anxiety and stress.

Summing Up

Sjögren's is an autoimmune disorder that can affect virtually any area of the body. In some patients with Sjögren's, the CNS is compromised. The pathophysiologic changes in the brain have been documented in the medical literature using imaging studies as well as neuropsychological studies. Depending on the area of the brain that has been affected, pathophysiologic changes may affect physical functions, cognitive functions, and/or psychological functions. Since a multitude of factors, such as pain, fatigue, medication side effects, psychological factors, and normal aging, can mimic the deficits associated with brain damage, it is important that the patient undergo a comprehensive assessment in order to determine the exact underlying etiology of any neurologic or neuropsychological changes and to assist in the development of the most efficacious treatment program.

In our opinion, Sjögren's patients who present with cognitive problems and complaints should be referred for a neurologic evaluation, imaging studies, and a comprehensive neuropsychological evaluation. Although the treatment of the neurologic and neuropsychological sequelae of these disorders is still in the early stages, it is our experience that a well-informed treatment program can help to reverse some of the areas of impairment or at least help the patient better cope with the neuropsychological sequelae of the illness.

For Further Reading

Manzo C, Martinez-Suarez E, Kechida M, et al. Cognitive function in primary Sjögren's syndrome: A systematic review. *Brain Sci.* 2019;9(4):85. doi:10.3390/brainsci9040085

Indart S, Hugon J, Guillausseau PJ, et al. Impact of pain on cognitive functions in primary Sjögren syndrome with small fiber neuropathy: 10 cases and a literature review. *Medicine.* 2017;96(16):e6384. doi:10.1097/MD.0000000000006384

Riega-Torres JCL, Treviño-Castro MA, Hernandez-Galarza IJ, et al. Cognitive dysfunction in Sjögren's syndrome using the Montreal Cognitive Assessment Questionnaire and the Automated Neuropsychological Assessment Metrics: A cross-sectional study. *Int J Rheum Dis.* 2020;23(8):1019–1023. doi:10.1111/1756-185X.13889

Tezcan ME, Kocer EB, Haznedaroglu S, et al. Primary Sjögren's syndrome is associated with significant cognitive dysfunction. *Int J Rheum Dis.* 2016;19(10):981–988. doi:10.1111/1756-185X.12912

32

Management of Fatigue in Sjögren's

Nancy L. Carteron

According to the 2016 Sjögren's Foundation Patient Survey, fatigue is the third most common symptom experienced by Sjögren's patients at least weekly. This frequency of fatigue was reported by 80% of the survey group. Many patients describe the fatigue in Sjögren's as a lack of energy even when doing the easiest, most common tasks. Sleep, rest, or vacations do little to relieve this profound fatigue. In the survey, patients cited the need to make changes at home because of their fatigue, including decreasing housework and hiring service providers when financially feasible. Up to a third of patients stopped working due to Sjögren's, and many made changes in their work schedule and responsibilities. More than one-fourth of the patients made career changes or took less demanding jobs within their career path.

These major life changes contribute to the high disease and financial burden of Sjögren's. The causes of this type of severe fatigue remain largely unknown. However, research is beginning to grapple with the complexities of the fatigue and shed light on what goes awry.

Potential Causes of Sjögren's Fatigue

Inflammation and Autoimmunity

Some people with Sjögren's may have elevated markers of inflammation, such as erythrocyte sedimentation rate (ESR) or C-reactive protein (CRP). Elevated immunoglobulins, like IgG and IgM, in blood tests are indicators of B-cell immune activation. When inflammation improves, some of the fatigue can lift. Additionally, some of the protein molecules produced by immune cells, such as cytokines, may play a role in Sjögren's fatigue. Interferons are one group of these molecules that have been studied in Sjögren's, and there is supporting evidence that the "interferon signature" can correlate with some of the symptoms of Sjögren's and other autoimmune diseases. Immune cells of

Nancy L. Carteron, *Management of Fatigue in Sjögren's* In: *The Sjögren's Book*. Edited by: Daniel J. Wallace, Oxford University Press. © Sjögren's Foundation 2022. DOI: 10.1093/oso/9780197502112.003.0032 the central nervous system, such as microglia, may also play a role directly in the brain and lead to fatigue.

Neurogenic

The nervous system can be a target tissue in Sjögren's or can become dysregulated in the disease process. There is a wide spectrum of neurologic conditions that have been described in Sjögren's. Dysregulation of the autonomic nervous system can lead to internal organ malfunction. Automatic processes such as blood pressure and heart rate regulation misfire and can contribute to fatigue.

Poor Physical Conditioning

The body can become deconditioned in chronic illness due to the disease process and lack of physical activity, which is common in the setting of ongoing musculoskeletal pain. Aerobic exercise has been shown to decrease fatigue, and clinical guidelines for inflammatory musculoskeletal manifestations of Sjögren's strongly recommend using exercise to decrease fatigue in Sjögren's. Working with a physical therapist, personal trainer, and others with experience with autoimmune disease can be a good place to start.

Fibromyalgia

If present, the disease fibromyalgia may be a contributing factor to Sjögren's fatigue. Current thinking is that the chronic widespread pain results from dysregulation of pain-sensing signals primarily in the brain. The sensitivity to pain is abnormally increased and pain amplification occurs more easily. Peripheral inflammation is not a hallmark of fibromyalgia, nor is it an autoimmune process, as currently understood. Numerous studies over time have shown an increased association of fibromyalgia with Sjögren's and other autoimmune diseases. The reason for the link between autoimmune diseases and the chronic pain syndrome remains unclear. If fibromyalgia is present along with Sjögren's, management strategies including an exercise plan, and cognitive–behavioral therapy can help.

Depression

Fatigue is common with depression. Thus, if an individual with Sjögren's is also suffering with depression, effective treatment of the depression may lessen fatigue. One complication is that many of the medications available to treat depression cause dryness and worsen the sicca symptoms in Sjögren's. Thus, finding a balance between response to medications and unwanted side effects can take a while. Have patience!

Microbiome

The community of microorganisms that cohabitate with us on our skin and in our oral cavity and gastrointestinal tract can provide valuable nutrients but can also trigger autoimmune disease, which can lead to damage, such as dental decay. The exocrine gland dysfunction that occurs in Sjögren's can be widespread, resulting in ocular, oral, vaginal, respiratory, and gastrointestinal tract dryness. The decrease in epithelial cell barrier protection can increase susceptibility to infections and tissue dysfunction. Maintaining a healthy diet promotes a balanced microbiota, which may have an indirect effect on fatigue.

Other Causes of Fatigue

It is key to exclude other common causes of fatigue such as anemia, thyroid dysfunction, sleep apnea, and underlying health conditions (heart failure, chronic kidney disease). These can be excluded by a primary clinician. Some medications can be linked to fatigue, so it is important to review what you are taking and check online and with your clinician and pharmacist to see if any one medication or any combinations may be contributing to your low energy. A common cause of fatigue can be beta-blockers, which are used to treat heart conditions. Also, statin medications that manage high cholesterol can occasionally trigger muscle abnormalities, resulting in muscle aches and fatigue. Work with your prescribing clinicians to simplify the medications you are taking, and be sure to mention any supplements you are taking.

Research

A recent area of research has focused on pro-inflammatory cytokines and their relationship with disease activity and symptoms, such as fatigue in

Sjögren's. Analysis of Sjögren's patients from the Sjögren's International Collaborative Clinical Alliance (SICCA) registry were found to fall into a high interferon signature group or a low interferon signature group. Another research group using the United Kingdom Primary Sjögren's Registry found higher levels of 14 cytokines in Sjögren's patients. However, it was the low interferon-gamma group that had greater fatigue. These studies focused on cytokines in the blood, which may or may not correlate with cytokine levels in the brain. Further investigation is needed to better understand these initial findings.

Another interesting line of investigation involves modulating the vagus nerve, the 10th cranial nerve. The vagus nerve helps with control of the heart, lungs, and gastrointestinal tract. Both implantable and transcutaneous devices have been studied in the autoimmune diseases, rheumatoid arthritis, Crohn's disease, and lupus; an exploratory trial of 15 Sjögren's patients showed improved fatigue and lower inflammatory/autoimmune markers. Placebo-controlled studies are needed, but randomized controlled trials are challenging to design when using an external device.

Management Strategies

What strategies can Sjögren's patients use to improve the profound fatigue? The first step is to assess the patient's general health and exclude treatable causes of fatigue such as anemia, thyroid abnormalities, and possibly obstructive sleep apnea. Assessing the patient's new baseline after interventions can take several months. Once there is a sense of the new steady-state level of fatigue, discuss with your clinicians the additional interventions that could be considered. Options may include the following:

- Medications
  Low-dose naltrexone: not approved by the U.S. Food and Drug Administration (FDA); provided by compounding pharmacies
  Central nervous system stimulants (e.g., modafinil)
  Hydroxychloroquine: can improve fatigue and joint pain (arthralgia); potential clinical response is assessed with a 3-month trial

- Lifestyle shifts
  Diet: try a plant-based diet to see if this helps
  Movement: consider tai chi, qigong, and/or swimming
  Restorative sleep

Stress management
Meditation
Acupuncture

- Environmental adjustments
Create a healing space around you to conserve emotional energy
Spend time in nature
Decrease identifiable allergens; patients with frequent infections (sinus, respiratory) could explore why this is occurring with an allergist; an ear, nose, and throat doctor (ENT), or a pulmonologist
Spiritual exploration
Restorative boundaries ("no" is a complete sentence)
Volunteer (What are your passions? Where might you be uniquely called to serve?)

Summing Up

Sjögren's fatigue can be an added heavy burden to an already high-maintenance autoimmune illness. Understanding the components contributing to the fatigue, treating underlying causes, and exploring a range of management options can lessen fatigue. Education about Sjögren's in general allows patients some control and the ability to build more flexibility and balance into their life. A variety of clinicians and patient support groups can assist the individual on the journey to improved health.

For Further Reading

Carsons SE, Vivino FB, Parke A, et al. Treatment guidelines for rheumatologic manifestations of Sjögren's syndrome: Use of biologic agents, management of fatigue and inflammatory musculoskeletal pain. *Arthritis Care Res.* 2017;69(4):517–527. doi:1002/acr.22968

Carteron NL, Bootsma H, Kroese FGM, et al. Clinical aspects of Sjögren's. In Wallace D, Hahn BH, eds. *Dubois' Lupus Erythematous and Related Syndromes* (9th ed.) Elsevier; 2018:566–578.

Fremes R, Carteron N. *A Body Out of Balance: Understanding and Treating Sjögren's Syndrome.* Avery, Penguin Group Inc; 2003:95–100.

Lee AS, Scofield RH, Hammitt KM, et al. Consensus guidelines for evaluation and management of pulmonary disease in Sjögren's. *Chest.* 2021;159(2):683–698.

Living with Sjögren's Disease. https://healthpsychforliving.com

Masterson S. *You Mean It Isn't In My Head? What Sjögren's Syndrome Is and What You Can Do About It*. Independently published; 2021.

Sjögren's Advocate. https://www.sjogrensadvocate.com

SjogrensLife. https://sjogrenslife.com

Tarn J, Legg S, Mitchell S, et al. The effects of noninvasive vagus nerve stimulation on fatigue and immune responses in patients with primary Sjögren's syndrome. *Neuromodulation*. 2019;22(5):580–585. doi:10.1111/ner.12879

33

Management of Depression and Anxiety in Sjögren's

Valerie G. Loehr and E. Sherwood Brown

What Is Depression?

Many people with Sjögren's suffer from depressive symptoms. Prevalence estimates for depression in Sjögren's range between 8.33% and 75.56%, and a recent meta-analysis reveals that Sjögren's is associated with an increased prevalence of depression. Clinical depression (major depressive disorder) is a mood disorder that causes a persistent feeling of sadness or loss of interest for at least 2 weeks and differs from passing pangs of sadness. Clinical depression is often accompanied by weight gain or loss, insomnia or hypersomnia, psychomotor agitation or retardation, fatigue, feelings of worthlessness or guilt, and difficulty concentrating or indecisiveness. Some people who suffer from severe depression experience suicidal ideation. Depression can cause significant distress and negatively affect a person's personal, work, or school life. Depression is caused by a combination of genetic, environmental, and psychological factors. Risk factors include a family history of the condition, major life changes, certain medications, chronic health problems, and substance abuse.

What Is Anxiety?

Individuals with Sjögren's are more likely to have symptoms of an anxiety disorder than the general population. Anxiety and fear are normal human experiences to life-changing events or a reaction to danger or threatening situations. However, if anxiety becomes frequent, intense, or uncontrollable to the extent that it affects the person's ability to function, it may be indicative of an anxiety disorder or warrant treatment. Anxiety affects people physically, behaviorally, cognitively, and emotionally. Common physical symptoms

Valerie G. Loehr and E. Sherwood Brown, *Management of Depression and Anxiety in Sjögren's* In: *The Sjögren's Book*. Edited by: Daniel J. Wallace, Oxford University Press. © Sjögren's Foundation 2022. DOI: 10.1093/oso/9780197502112.003.0033 of anxiety include increased heart rate, sweating, shortness of breath, fatigue, dizziness, chest pain, gastrointestinal symptoms, and muscle tension/pain. People with anxiety generally engage in avoidance behaviors in an attempt to cope with anxiety-provoking situations or causes and may exhibit other behaviors such as restlessness, inability to sit and remain calm, difficulty sleeping, and social isolation. Cognitively, people may have difficulty concentrating, engage in catastrophizing, experience uncontrollable worry, or report "feeling crazy." Feelings of helplessness, panic, and irritability may affect a person's ability to function. Similar to depression, anxiety is caused by a combination of genetic, environmental, and psychological factors, and often occurs with depression. Without treatment, anxiety disorders tend to persist.

Symptom Overlap

Several symptoms of depression and anxiety, such as fatigue, trouble sleeping, and difficulty concentrating, overlap with symptoms of Sjögren's. Depression and anxiety can also be associated with a variety of physical symptoms, including aches and pains. Women with Sjögren's may experience vulvodynia, a chronic pain syndrome that affects the vulvar area. When accompanied by a depressed mood or loss of interest, it may be difficult to differentiate whether the fatigue, trouble sleeping, difficulty concentrating, and lack of interest in sex is caused only by Sjögren's, or whether depression or anxiety is exacerbating these symptoms. Individuals report that Sjögren's causes a significant negative impact on their ability to participate in hobbies, social activities, and extracurricular activities, which may lead to loss of interest in these activities. Regardless of whether Sjögren's or depression is the culprit, these symptoms lead to a significantly lower quality of life.

Other symptoms of depression and anxiety such as fatigue, altered sleep, appetite changes, and mood changes can be seen in medical conditions associated with Sjögren's, such as anemia, thyroid disease, and fibromyalgia. Certain medications for Sjögren's, including corticosteroids and other immunosuppressants, may increase symptoms of depression and anxiety. It is important to effectively treat comorbid conditions and to rule out effects of medication that may be causing or worsening depression or anxiety. At this time, there is no known biological mechanism or pathogenic process mediating the relationship between depression or anxiety and Sjögren's. Research from other chronic inflammatory diseases found that autoantibodies, genetic factors, interleukins, and side effects of medications contributed to depression. However, it is known that the effects Sjögren's has on people's lives and ability to function contribute to feelings of depression and anxiety.

Psychosocial Factors Contributing to Depression and Anxiety

Sjögren's is an untimely, unpredictable, and invisible chronic disease that can exhaust the patient's emotional resources. The average age of Sjögren's diagnosis is in the late 40s, when many individuals are managing family responsibilities along with a career. Many individuals with Sjögren's experience significant fatigue, pain, and a brain fog that limits their ability to function at home and in the workplace. Brain fog may include forgetfulness, spaciness, confusion, and difficulty paying attention or processing information. According to a Sjögren's Foundation survey, more than seven in 10 patients agreed that Sjögren's gets in the way of the things they need to do each day. The majority of patients reported cutting back or stopping housework. People may lose their jobs, work less, or take less demanding jobs due to these symptoms or due to medical and dental visits. Family relationships can be affected by the change in finances, physical abilities, and independence. Patients may feel guilty about how the illness is affecting their family. Patients may have difficulty coping with threats to their autonomy due to increased dependence on healthy family members. Family members may struggle with feelings of powerlessness when the patient is in pain or experiences pressure to be emotionally strong. Family roles and responsibilities may need to be restructured depending on the waxing and waning of symptoms. These changes can cause stress, anxiety, and anger for both the patient and family members. Individuals without family help may feel vulnerable and alone.

The average time from onset of symptoms to diagnosis of Sjögren's is around 3 years. During this time of uncertainty, patients may feel helpless, frustrated, and dismissed by the medical community. Once diagnosed with a chronic illness such as Sjögren's, people may temporarily feel relieved given that they finally have an explanation for their complaints. However, the distress often returns because the efficacy of current therapies is mild to moderate at best. Grief about having a chronic illness sets in, and patients and family members may experience various stages of grief, including denial, bargaining, anger, and sadness. The waxing and waning of symptoms may put the individual on an emotional roller coaster, which can add to confusion and denial.

Living with a chronic condition like Sjögren's can be frustrating, because the fatigue, pain, and other symptoms are not always visible from the outside. Individuals with Sjögren's may face skepticism from friends, family, coworkers, and strangers who don't understand or appreciate the severity of the illness. Doctors may focus on just the dryness and may not acknowledge other life-changing symptoms due to time constraints or lack of awareness. This may leave the individual feeling invisible or powerless.

Medication Treatment

The most common medications prescribed for depression and anxiety are called selective serotonin reuptake inhibitors (SSRIs). SSRIs increase the level of serotonin in the brain. It is important to take into consideration that these psychotropic medications do not work immediately: It may take up to 6 weeks to benefit from the medication. These medications are generally safe and effective but also have side effects. Depending on the severity of dryness or other comorbid disorders associated with Sjögren's (e.g., gastric reflux, irritable bowel syndrome, neuropathy, rheumatoid arthritis, fibromyalgia), the medication side effects may be intolerable for the patient. Side effects are generally the reason people choose to stop or change psychotropic medication.

Common side effects experienced when beginning an SSRI include eye and mouth dryness, headaches, joint pain, muscle aches, nausea, skin rashes, diarrhea, insomnia, and decreased sex drive. Unfortunately for patients with Sjögren's, they may not be able to tolerate these side effects as well as their friends and family members. Increased sleepiness, insomnia, and fatigue associated with psychotropic medications may further impact their ability to participate in daily and valued activities. Even if the patient does not suffer from other associated health conditions, antidepressants may cause an increase in the drying of mucous membranes, which could further aggravate symptoms of Sjögren's (dry eye/dry mouth). This alone may be reason to discontinue taking psychotropic medication and to seek non-psychotropic modalities to address depression and anxiety.

Other medications to assist with anxiety symptoms include benzodiazepines, buspirone, and hydroxyzine. Benzodiazepines work quickly, but because of their side effects and risk for addiction, many providers do not prescribe them or only prescribe them for very short periods of time. Side effects include increased drowsiness, memory impairment, nausea, vomiting, constipation, weight gain, reduced libido, and dry mouth. Because they work quickly, people build a tolerance and need higher doses. Buspirone and hydroxyzine, other medications to assist with anxiety management, have a low risk for addiction. Sjögren's patients should know that benzodiazepines, buspirone, and hydroxyzine all have the side effect of dry mouth.

SSRIs and benzodiazepines can cause serious withdrawal symptoms if stopped abruptly, so patients should inform their providers if they decide to discontinue any medication. As with all medications, the side effects and benefits should be weighed. For individuals who have severe depression or suicidal ideation, medication may be helpful, even life-saving. For individuals with mild to moderate symptoms of depression and anxiety, psychotherapy, exercise, or self-help strategies may work just as well or better, without un-pleasant side effects.

Behavioral and Psychological Modalities to Address Depression and Anxiety

Lifestyle changes, such as exercise, are simple but powerful tools to im-prove mood and well-being. Exercise has been shown to treat mild to mod-erate depression and anxiety as effectively as antidepressant medication. Regularly engaging in physical activity has been shown to enhance neural growth, reduce inflammation, and release endorphins, which trigger pos-itive feelings. Exercise also serves as a distraction from negative thoughts and stress from the day. However, many individuals with Sjögren's have flu-like malaise, fatigue, and pain, so beginning an exercise routine may appear daunting or counterintuitive. There is evidence that patients with Sjögren's benefit from exercise of moderate to high intensity, and comorbid medical conditions (e.g., rheumatoid arthritis) also benefit from regular physical ac-tivity. Patients should start slowly and gradually build up their stamina and endurance, especially if they are deconditioned or also have rheumatoid ar-thritis, osteoarthritis, or fibromyalgia, as incorrect forms of exercise may aggravate these illnesses.

Psychotherapy can assist with both symptoms of depression and anxiety and coping with the effects of Sjögren's. There are a variety of modalities to address mental health symptoms and difficulty coping with a chronic medical condition, such as cognitive–behavioral, interpersonal, and psychodynamic. Psychotherapy explores factors that contribute to depression and anxiety and helps the patient understand and cope with the psychological, behavioral, interpersonal, and situational causes. Therapy can focus on improving or building relationships to reduce isolation and increasing social support, set-ting healthy boundaries, and providing support in handling challenges and problems unique to Sjögren's. Skilled therapists assist patients in reframing negative thinking patterns that contribute to perpetuating anxiety or feelings of hopelessness, explore learned behaviors or thoughts that create problems, and help individuals regain a sense of control and pleasure in life.

Psychotherapy is offered in individual, group, and family/couples formats, and there are benefits to each. Individual psychotherapy offers individualized attention, and patients may feel more comfortable sharing sensitive information with one person rather than a group. Group therapy for anxiety or depression offers the ability to listen to peers going through similar struggles, which can validate the patient's experiences and build self-esteem. Attending group therapy can also increase the patient's social activities and broaden the patient's network. Family or couples therapy may be helpful in addressing changes in family members' roles, responsibilities, and boundaries. Family or couples therapy should be considered if Sjögren's, anxiety, or depression is affecting most or all family interactions; if a family member routinely withdraws into silence; when partners have different coping strategies and cannot find common ground regarding the demands of the illness; or when family is stuck in a crisis phase rather than adapting. Finding a therapist who is a "good fit" with the patient is important, as the therapist will be a caring and supportive partner in the patient's treatment and recovery.

Sjögren's support groups provide a resource that may fill a gap between medical treatment, psychotherapy, and need for additional emotional support. Doctors and family members may not fully understand the emotional, physical, and cognitive toll that Sjögren's takes. Group members often share similar feelings, worries, everyday problems, treatment decisions, or medication side effects. Attending a support group can help patients feel less isolated, lonely, or judged, which can in turn reduce depression, stress, and anxiety and increase hope and control. Group members are encouraged to talk openly and honestly about their experiences and feelings, share resources and coping strategies, and provide motivation for others to remain adherent to medical recommendations. Consequently, members may have improved understanding of Sjögren's and their experience of it, which can increase their feelings of self-efficacy and empowerment. Possible risks associated with support groups include disruptive group members, lack of confidentiality, conversations dominated by complaining, inappropriate or incorrect medical advice, and interpersonal group problems. An effective facilitator can address these problems as they arise. There are online and in-person support groups. The Sjögren's Foundation maintains a list of U.S. and international support groups.

Summing Up

Depression and anxiety, even when severe, are treatable. The earlier the symptoms of depression and anxiety are identified, the earlier treatment can begin and the more effective treatment is. Patients should first be evaluated by a physician to rule out effects of medications or medical conditions associated with Sjögren's. Once diagnosed, patients can be treated a number of ways, including psychotherapy and medication. Patients with Sjögren's need to weigh the benefits and disadvantages of taking psychotropic medication, as the side effects may be intolerable given that many medications worsen the symptoms inherent with Sjögren's. Lifestyle changes and joining support groups are additional methods to reduce symptoms of depression and anxiety and improve quality of life.

For Further Reading

Carsons SE, Vivino FB, Parke A, et al. Treatment guidelines for rheumatologic manifestations of Sjögren's syndrome: Use of biologic agents, management of fatigue, and inflammatory musculoskeletal pain. *Arthritis Care Res.* 2017;69(4):517–527.

Cui Y, Li L, Yin R, et al. Depression in primary Sjögren's syndrome: A systematic review and meta-analysis. *Psychol Health Med.* 2018;23(2):198–209.

Herman A, Taylor S, Noll J. Coping strategies and support networks for Sjögren's syndrome patients. *Oral Maxillofacial Surg Clin North Am.* 2014;26(1):111–115.

Lackner A, Ficjan A, Stradner MH, et al. It's more than dryness and fatigue: The patient perspective on health-related quality of life in primary Sjögren's syndrome—A qualitative study. *PLoS One.* 2017;12(2):1–12.

Lawrence E. The impact of chronic illness on the family. *IGLiving,* 2012:20–25. http://www.igliving.com/

Ramos-Casals M, Tzioufas AG, Stone JH, et al. Treatment of primary Sjögren syndrome: A systematic review. *JAMA.* 2010;304(4):452–460.

Segal BM, Pogatchnik B, Holker E, et al. Primary Sjögren's syndrome: Cognitive symptoms, mood, and cognitive performance. *Acta Neurol Scand.* 2012;125:272–278.

Sjögren's Syndrome Foundation. Living with Sjögren's: Summary of major findings. *The Moisture Seekers.* 2017;35(4):4–8. https://www.sjogrens.org/files/tms/TMS2017-04.pdf

Strömbeck BE, Theander E, Jacobsson LTH. Effects of exercise on aerobic capacity and fatigue in women with primary Sjögren's syndrome. *Rheumatology.* 2007;46(5):868–871.

Wong JKF, Nortley R, Andrews T, D'Cruz D. Psychiatric manifestations of primary Sjögren's syndrome: A case report and literature review. *BMJ Case Reports.* 2014;2014:bcr2012008038.

34

Management of Gastrointestinal Manifestations in Sjögren's

Katerina Shetler

Sjögren's is a chronic autoimmune process leading to diminished function of lacrimal glands (keratoconjunctivitis sicca) and salivary glands (xerostomia). Sjögren's is characterized by chronic inflammation of the exocrine glands and by serum autoantibodies that target the Ro/La ribonucleoprotein. Sjögren's can occur independently or in association with other autoimmune diseases such as rheumatoid arthritis, systemic lupus erythematosus, or scleroderma. It can involve other organs, including any part of the gastrointestinal (GI) tract, liver, or pancreas.

Pathophysiology

In genetically predisposed individuals, various environmental factors and viral infections lead to epithelial cell activation and a protracted inflammatory response, systemic autoimmunity, and exocrine dysfunction. GI motility and secretion are influenced by the autonomic nervous system (ANS), which is commonly altered in patients with Sjögren's and can lead to difficulty swallowing, abdominal pain, bloating, constipation, orthostatic dizziness, and postural hypotension.

Esophagus

The main function of the esophagus is to transport food and liquid into the stomach. Abnormal function of the esophageal muscles (dysmotility) may lead to failure of proper delivery of liquid or food from the mouth to the stomach. The lower esophageal sphincter (LES) acts as an anti-reflux barrier protecting the esophagus from the caustic gastric contents. Characteristic

Katerina Shetler, *Management of Gastrointestinal Manifestations in Sjögren's* In: *The Sjögren's Book.* Edited by:
Daniel J. Wallace, Oxford University Press. © Sjögren's Foundation 2022. DOI: 10.1093/oso/9780197502112.003.0034

esophageal involvement in patients with Sjögren's includes LES dysfunction, hypotension, and esophageal hypomotility. Upper endoscopy, esophageal manometry, and pH testing with a wireless pH capsule or a traditional pH/impedance probe are used to evaluate the esophageal symptoms.

Patients with Sjögren's commonly experience swallowing difficulty, heartburn, and acid regurgitation.

Swallowing Difficulty

Dysphagia (difficulty swallowing) affects 33% to 92% of patients with Sjögren's. The cause of swallowing difficulty is likely multifactorial—lack of saliva, esophageal dysmotility, esophageal webs, and/or low-grade myositis. Abnormality in esophageal function and motility is detected in up to 35% of patients with Sjögren's and no accompanying autoimmune disease. When compared to healthy controls, patients with Sjögren's may have a decreased LES pressure and prolongation of LES relaxation, which can predispose to reflux of gastric contents into the esophagus. Decreased esophageal peristaltic velocity and an increased duration of contractions with higher occurrence of simultaneous waves may impair bolus transfer into the stomach, resulting in difficulty swallowing. The severity of dysphagia, in general, is not related to any specific motility pattern. Only one study showed that the presence of simultaneous contraction in more than 30% of swallows was associated with severe dysphagia. The esophageal abnormalities did not correlate with disease duration, extraglandular manifestations, serologic markers (rheumatoid factor [RF], antinuclear antibody [ANA], anti-Ro, and anti-La), or the Saxon salivary test (a diagnostic method used to detect hyposalivation) in the majority of studies.

Gastroesophageal Reflux

Gastroesophageal reflux disease (GERD) develops when the gastric contents reflux into the esophagus, causing symptoms and complications. GERD can present as erosive esophagitis (characterized by endoscopically visible breaks in the mucosa with or without symptoms) or non-erosive reflux disease (characterized by the presence of symptoms of GERD without visible esophageal mucosal injury). In some cases, GERD can lead to Barrett's esophagus and esophageal adenocarcinoma. Up to 60% of patients with Sjögren's reported symptoms of gastroesophageal reflux compared to 23% of controls. Hiatal hernia can be identified in up to 25% of Sjögren's patients. A decrease in saliva production may result in decreased esophageal acid clearance and adversely affect the oral and pharyngoesophageal phase of swallowing. It can prevent the initiation of peristalsis and cause dysphagia in patients with normal peristalsis, but that requires further investigation.

Treatment of GERD includes lifestyle and dietary modifications. Lifestyle modifications include avoiding tobacco and alcohol; losing weight (for overweight patients); and elevating the head of the bed, which helps reduce nighttime symptoms of reflux. Mild and intermittent symptoms can be controlled with the help of antacids and histamine (H2) blockers. Antacids (aluminum hydroxide, calcium carbonate) neutralize gastric pH and provide relief within a few minutes but have a short duration of action (<60 minutes). Sucralfate (Carafate) and sodium alginate are beneficial, promoting mucosal healing and improving postprandial symptoms. H2 receptor agonists (Zantac and Pepcid) decrease the secretion of acid by inhibiting H2 receptors on gastric parietal cells.

Development of tachyphylaxis limits long-term use of these medications. Severe acid reflux is best managed with proton pump inhibitors (PPIs; omeprazole, lansoprazole, esomeprazole, dexlansoprazole, pantoprazole, rabeprazole), which effectively block gastric acid secretion by irreversibly inhibiting the hydrogen-potassium ATPase pump on the parietal cells. PPIs should be used at the lowest dose possible, once or twice daily. PPIs can lead to an increased risk of infections (*Clostridium difficile* and other enteric infections), contribute to the development of osteoporosis, and affect magnesium and vitamin B_{12} levels.

Stomach

Gastric function and motility can be affected by Sjögren's due to a combination of ANS disturbance and underlying inflammation.

Delay in gastric emptying occurs in up to 70% of patients with Sjögren's; of those, abnormalities in the autonomic nervous system were found in 16%. In another study, 29% of patients had delayed gastric emptying, and a significant correlation was found between a delayed lag phase at the beginning of the emptying process and increased levels of immunoglobulin G and the erythrocyte sedimentation rate (ESR), suggestive of underlying inflammation.

The presence of *Helicobacter pylori* infection should not be ignored in patients with Sjögren's. *H. pylori* is a prevalent chronic bacterial infection that is highly adapted to the gastric environment. It can be associated with chronic gastritis, peptic ulcer disease, gastric adenocarcinoma, and gastric mucosa-associated lymphoid tissue (MALT) lymphoma. Lymphoma development is a major long-term concern for patients with Sjögren's. Sjögren's is characterized by polyclonal B-cell activation as well as lymphocytic activation of the exocrine glands. Most lymphomas arise from a benign lymphoepithelial lesion. *H. pylori* can cause massive local expansion of a B-cell clonal population due to antigen stimulation, leading to gastric MALT lymphoma. Patients with Sjögren's should be checked and treated for *H. pylori* infection. Tests include urease breath test and stool antigen for *H. pylori*. For patients undergoing endoscopic evaluation, the gastric biopsy urease test and histology can establish the diagnosis.

There are few treatment regimens for *H. pylori* eradication. The choice of treatment depends on the patient's prior exposure to macrolide therapy and the presence of penicillin allergies. The first-line therapy is clarithromycin-based triple therapy with a PPI, clarithromycin, and amoxicillin. In patients with allergies to penicillin, metronidazole is used instead of amoxicillin. Bismuth quadruple therapy consists of bismuth subsalicylate, metronidazole, tetracycline, and PPIs. The duration of treatment is usually between 10 and 14 days. Due to the high resistance of *H. pylori* to antibiotics (there is a failure rate of ~20% after the initial course of treatment), alternative regimens may be used.

Small and Large Bowel

Ninety percent of patients with Sjögren's and systemic sclerosis (SSc) have GI complaints such as abdominal pain and bloating, constipation, and diarrhea. The causes include celiac disease, disturbances of small bowel motility, small intestinal bacterial overgrowth, and diet intolerances or hypersensitivities.

Celiac disease is a chronic small intestinal immune-mediated enteropathy precipitated by exposure to dietary gluten in genetically predisposed individuals. Patients with various autoimmune disorders are at higher risk for celiac disease. A coexisting diagnosis of celiac disease can be found in up to 12% of patients with Sjögren's, which warrants routine screening for celiac disease in this disorder. Celiac disease can be detected by serologic testing of celiac-specific antibodies. The diagnosis is confirmed by duodenal mucosal biopsies. Up to 60% of Sjögren's patients can have an HLA DQ2 and HLA DQ8 haplotype, demonstrating that celiac disease and Sjögren's share the same disease-susceptible genes.

Using the Rome III criteria, the prevalence of irritable bowel syndrome (IBS) is 39% in Sjögren's patients and the prevalence of functional dyspepsia is 65%. Sicca complex also has a higher prevalence in patients with IBS compared to healthy controls. Up to 70% of patients with IBS identify certain foods as symptom triggers. These trigger food groups include high-fiber foods, poorly absorbed carbohydrates (also known as fermentable oligosaccharides, disaccharides, monosaccharides, and polyols [FODMAPs]), gluten, dairy, fatty foods, spicy foods, caffeine, and alcohol. Avoidance of trigger foods may improve symptoms and quality of life.

Liver and Pancreas

Salivary glands and the pancreas have similar functions: secretion of fluid and electrolytes into the luminal space. The pancreas may be involved in patients with Sjögren's in the form of autoimmune pancreatitis, chronic pancreatitis, and exocrine pancreatic insufficiency. Candelli et al. studied 24 patients with Sjögren's and found that pancreatic impairment was more prevalent in Sjögren's than in controls (6/24 vs. 0/24). Patients with severe lacrimal dysfunction based on a lower Schirmer test score should be suspected of having impaired pancreatic exocrine function.

Autoimmune pancreatitis can have few distinct clinical features. It may present as a mild acute pancreatitis or biliary or pancreatic duct strictures, or can mimic pancreas tumors. A pancreas biopsy is usually required for definitive diagnosis. Other diagnostic criteria include an elevated level of IgG4 antibodies, characteristic radiographic findings, and response to corticosteroids.

Exocrine pancreatic insufficiency may cause abdominal pain, bloating, and steatorrhea and lead to weight loss and malabsorption of fat and protein. Diagnosis is established by a stool test for fecal elastase-1 or by an endoscopic secretin test. Fat malabsorption predisposes patients to deficiencies in fat-soluble vitamins A, D, E, and K. Treatment includes exogenous pancreatic enzyme replacement therapy and vitamin replacement.

Abnormalities in liver function tests occur in 49% of patients with Sjögren's. Twenty percent of these patients can have clinically noticeable liver involvement; the others are usually asymptomatic. Liver involvement in Sjögren's happens in the form of autoimmune hepatitis or primary biliary cholangitis (previously referred to as primary biliary cirrhosis) and presents in 5% to 26% of patients. Patients may be asymptomatic or present with jaundice (yellow discoloration of skin), pruritus, and fatigue. Diagnosis includes liver tests for anti-mitochondrial and anti-smooth muscle antibodies. Selected patients will require a liver biopsy to establish a correct diagnosis.

Summing Up

Sjögren's may involve the entire GI tract, liver, and pancreas. Symptoms may vary from mild to severe. Proper evaluation and diagnosis will prevent possible complications and significantly improve quality of life.

For Further Reading

Anselmino M, Zaninotto G, Costantini M, et al. Esophageal motor function in primary Sjögren's syndrome: Correlation with dysphagia and xerostomia. *Dig Dis Sci.* 1997;42(1):113–118.

Barton A, Pal B, Whorwell PJ, Marshall D. Increase prevalence of sicca complex and fibromyalgia in patients with irritable bowel syndrome. *Am J Gastroenterol.* 1999;94(7):1989–1901.

Bohn L, Storsrud S, Liljebo T, et al. Diet low in FODMAPs reduces symptoms of irritable bowel syndrome as well as traditional dietary advice: A randomized controlled trial. *Gastroenterology.* 2015;149:320–328.

Candelli M, Manganelli C, Celestino EC, et al. Exocrine pancreatic involvement in Primitive Syndrome of Sjogren. *Gastroenterology.* 2003;124(4) Supplement 1, A631.

De Vita S, Ferraccioli G, Avellini C, et al. Widespread clonal B cell disorder in Sjögren's syndrome predisposing to *Helicobacter pylori*-related gastric lymphoma. *Gastroenterology.* 1996;110:1969–1974.

Ebert EC. Gastrointestinal and hepatic manifestation of Sjogren syndrome. *J Clin Gastroenterol.* 2012;46(1):25–40.

Grande L, Lacima G, Ros E, et al. Esophageal motor function in primary Sjögren's syndrome. *Am J Gastroenterol.* 1993;88(3):378–381.

Hammar O, Ohlsson B, Wollmer P, Mandl T. Impaired gastric emptying in primary Sjögren's syndrome. *J Rheumatol.* 2010;37(11):2313–2318.

Kaplan MJ, Ike RW. The liver is a common non-exocrine target in primary Sjogren syndrome: A retrospective review. *BMC Gastroenterol.* 2002;2:21.

Kelly CP, Bai JC, Liu E, Leffler DA. Advances in diagnosis and management of celiac disease. *Gastroenterology.* 2015;148:1175–1186.

Kjellen G, Fransson SG, Lindstrom F, et al. Esophageal function, radiography, and dysphagia in Sjögren's syndrome. *Dig Dis Sci.* 1986;31(3):225–229.

Kovacs L, Papos M, Takacs R, et al. Autonomic nervous system dysfunction involving the gastrointestinal and the urinary tracts in primary Sjögren's syndrome. *Clin Exp Rheumatol.* 2003;21(6):697–703.

Liden M, Kristjansson G, Valtysdottir S, Hallgren R. Gluten sensitivity in patients with primary Sjögren's syndrome. *Scan J Gastroenterol.* 2007;42:962–967.

Mandl T, Bornmyr SV, Castenfors J, et al. Sympathetic dysfunction in patients with primary Sjögren's syndrome. *J Rheumatol.* 2001;28(2):296–301.

Mandl T, Ekberg O, Wollmer P, et al. Dysphagia and dysmotility of the pharynx and esophagus in patients with primary Sjögren's syndrome. *Scand J Rheumatol.* 2007;36:394–401.

Mandl T, Granberg V, Apelqvist J, et al. Autonomic nervous symptoms in primary Sjögren's syndrome. *Rheumatology*. 2008;47:914–919.

Mandl T, Wollmer P, Manthorpe R, Jacobsson LT. Autonomic and orthostatic dysfunction in primary Sjögren's syndrome. *J Rheumatol*. 2007;34(9):1869–1874.

Mariette X, Gottenberg JE. Pathogenesis of Sjögren's syndrome and therapeutic consequences. *Curr Opin Rheumatol*. 2010;22(5):471–477.

Nishimori Y, Morita M, Kino J, et al. Pancreatic ductal morphology and function in Sjögren's syndrome and primary biliary cirrhosis. *Int J Pancreatol*. 1995;17(1):47–54.

Ohlsson B, Scheja A, Janciauskiene S, Mandl T. Functional bowel symptoms and GnRH antibodies: Common findings in patients with primary Sjögren's syndrome but not in systemic sclerosis. *Scand J Rheumatol*. 2009;38(5):391–393.

Rubia-Tapia A, Hill ID, Kelly CP, et al. ACG clinical guidelines: Diagnosis and management of celiac disease. *Am J Gastroenterol*. 2013;108(5):656.

Szodoray P, Barta Z, Lakos G, et al. Coeliac disease in Sjögren's syndrome—a study of 111 Hungarian patients. *Rheumatol Int*. 2004;24(5):278–282.

Turk T, Pirildar T, Tunc E, et al. Manometric assessment of esophageal motility in patients with primary Sjögren's syndrome. *Rheumatol Int*. 2005;25:246–249.

Waterman SA, Gordon TP, Rischmueller M. Inhibitory effects of muscarinic receptor auto-antibodies on parasympathetic neurotransmission in Sjögren's syndrome. *Arthritis Rheum*. 2000;43(7):1647–1654.

35

Management of Gynecologic and Urologic Aspects of Sjögren's

Rita Melkonian

Sjögren's is often defined as a chronic inflammatory disease of the exocrine glands (salivary, lacrimal, and other moisture-producing glands) due to infiltration of these glands by lymphocytes and plasma cells for unknown reasons. The process progressively causes functional impairment of these glands and leads to a reduced or absent glandular secretion along with mucosal dryness.

Many women have symptoms of decreased lacrimal and salivary gland function that precedes the recognition of involvement of other exocrine glands, such as the upper airway (oral and tracheal mucositis, loss of teeth, and upper airway infection such as bronchitis), the gastrointestinal tract (atrophic gastritis, pancreatitis), and the external genitalia (painful intercourse [dyspareunia]). However, those with Sjögren's can present with any of these symptoms, including vaginal dryness and dyspareunia.

Since primary care physicians and obstetrician/gynecologists are often the first healthcare providers to address vaginal symptoms, these physicians are essential for the timely diagnosis and care of Sjögren's. Despite the high prevalence of Sjögren's in women, medical journals and textbooks in primary care and especially in obstetrics and gynecology may only briefly, if at all, discuss Sjögren's.

Gynecologic symptoms, especially vaginal dryness, dyspareunia, and itching (pruritus), are often reported in females with Sjögren's. Since Sjögren's most often is diagnosed in females in their 40s and 50s, many of these patients visit their gynecologists for premenopausal and menopausal symptoms, and some of the symptoms experienced can have significant overlap, such as hot flashes, vaginal dryness and dyspareunia, fatigue, sleep disorders, and depression. As a result, the possibility of Sjögren's is often overlooked.

Sjögren's can affect the bladder in the form of interstitial cystitis (IC) and cause symptoms of pelvic pain, frequency of urination, and the need to pass urine at night (nocturia). Additionally, Sjögren's can affect pregnancy. Of

Rita Melkonian, *Management of Gynecologic and Urologic Aspects of Sjögren's* In: *The Sjögren's Book*. Edited by: Daniel J. Wallace, Oxford University Press. © Sjögren's Foundation 2022. DOI: 10.1093/oso/9780197502112.003.0035 greatest concern is the development of fetal heart block in mothers who are positive for anti-Ro/SSA and/or anti-La/SSB. Fetal loss is frequently associated with systemic lupus erythematosus (SLE) and antiphospholipid syndrome. Blood clots (venous thrombosis), primarily in the lower extremities and less frequently in the lungs (pulmonary embolism), can occur more frequently in patients with Sjögren's who also have SLE and/or antiphospholipid syndrome.

In this chapter we will discuss the following gynecologic and urologic aspects of Sjögren's: (1) vulvovaginal manifestations, vaginal dryness, and lichen sclerosus; (2) IC and urinary tract infections; (3) cervical manifestations of Sjögren's and human papillomavirus; (4) the impact of Sjögren's on female sexual function; (5) endometriosis in Sjögren's; (6) reproductive manifestations and premature ovarian failure; (7) amyloid deposition in Sjögren's; and (8) pregnancy outcome in patients with Sjögren's.

Vulvovaginal Manifestations, Vaginal Dryness, and Lichen Sclerosus

Reports in the literature are available that examine the clinical and histologic consequences of Sjögren's in the female genital tract. As far back as 1922, Bloch et al. described dyspareunia, vulvar pruritus, and vaginal dystrophy in most cases from a cohort of 62 women with Sjögren's. The authors identified vaginal erythema and irritation on gynecologic examination and suggested that these features might reflect impaired function of the vaginal and vulvar exocrine glands due to Sjögren's.

Vaginal dryness is a common problem among women, especially after menopause, and can occur with even greater frequency and severity in patients with Sjögren's. The vagina is lined by a deep layer of nonkeratinized squamous epithelium overlying a lamina propria of dense connective tissue, with numerous elastic fibers, polymorphonuclear leukocytes, lymphocytes, and lymphoid nodules.

There are a variety of physiologic mechanisms of vaginal lubrication, and while there are no secretory glands in the vagina, a fluid exudate seeps through the vaginal wall from the underlying richly vascular stroma during sexual stimulation and is an important contributor to vaginal lubrication. In addition, the vaginal epithelium is rich in glycogen stores during the reproductive years, and it undergoes a process of continuous desquamation, also making an important contribution to vaginal lubrication. Finally, the cervical glands are another important source of vaginal secretions.

Symptoms of dryness in Sjögren's patients were thought to be mainly caused by inflammation (lymphocyte-mediated infiltration) and atrophy of vestibular glands that secrete a viscous fluid that serves as a lubricant during sexual excitation. However, vaginal dryness in many Sjögren's patients is likely attributed to multiple factors such as desiccation of the vaginal mucosa and cervix in addition to vestibular gland atrophy as well as action on the parasympathetic nervous system (specifically, muscarinic receptors).

It has been suggested that the histologic changes described in the vagina and cervix likely reflect pathologic processes similar to those seen in the salivary and lacrimal glands. A 1997 study by Mulherin et al. in the United Kingdom showed that many Sjögren's patients had longstanding symptoms of vaginal dryness and dyspareunia, which in most cases preceded the onset of symptoms of ocular and oral dryness, often by many years.

Vaginal dryness as a presenting feature of Sjögren's has been highlighted previously (e.g., Mulherin et al., 1997; Tayal, 1996) and as a major symptom in Sjögren's since the 1960s. However, vaginal dryness has not received the focus that ocular and oral dryness has in research studies or in clinical management. The lack of recognition that vaginal dryness is potentially connected with Sjögren's has contributed to the difficulties in diagnosing women with Sjögren's, particularly if ocular or oral dryness is not prominent.

During menopause, the dramatic reduction in estrogen levels due to cessation of estrogen production by the ovaries causes vaginal atrophy and dryness. Therefore, vaginal dryness and dyspareunia in older Sjögren's patients are more severe than the general population due to lack of estrogen in addition to the desiccation of the vaginal mucosa.

Diagnosis and Symptoms

The diagnosis of atrophic vaginitis is clinical and based on characteristic symptoms and physical findings. Women complaining of vaginal dryness may also experience symptoms of vaginal burning, dyspareunia, vaginal itching, a white or yellowish discharge, and vaginal spotting or bleeding. Typical physical examination findings of vaginal atrophy include narrowing of the vaginal introitus, petechiae (small hemorrhage) of vaginal tissue, loss of rugae (vaginal folds), fusion of the labia minora, and decreased vaginal moisture. A wet mount should be performed whenever a vaginal discharge is present to determine the cause of the discharge.

Treatment of Vaginal Dryness

Treatment of vaginal dryness differs based on the patient's symptoms, their impact on her quality of life, and her goals. Topical estrogen products, which can be administered in various forms, may be used in the treatment of postmenopausal patients with vaginal dryness and dyspareunia if hormonal treatments are not contraindicated (e.g., those with estrogen receptor–positive breast cancer or a history of uterine cancer). In addition, numerous non-hormonal products are available to supplement or use in place of estrogen products. Please see Chapter 26 on vaginal dryness for detailed treatment options.

Lichen Sclerosus

Patients with Sjögren's may also present with a vulvar condition known as lichen sclerosus, a vulvar dystrophy with unknown etiology and the most common of the vulvar white lesions. Lichen sclerosus can occur at any age and is not related to estrogen cessation. Autoimmune disorders, including Sjögren's, have been found in studies of series of patients with lichen sclerosus.

In lichen sclerosus, the vulvar architecture is progressively destroyed, as the labia minora become adherent to the adjacent labia majora prior to their eventual dissolution. Edema, scarring, and agglutination of the prepuce and frenulum gradually bury the glans of the clitoris in an amorphous mass of pale tissue. The diameter of the vaginal opening may shrink and result in true kraurosis or contraction of the introitus and dyspareunia. If untreated, reactive hyperplastic change can develop, which may be accompanied by atypia. The untreated atypia may lead to vulvar carcinoma.

Symptoms of lichen sclerosus are pruritus, vulvar burning, and dryness, and the structural alterations described in the previous paragraph are clinical hallmarks of lichen sclerosus. Treatment of lichen sclerosus is challenging as there are not many options. It can be treated with topical steroid ointments such as clobetasol 0.05% ointment or testosterone propionate 2%. A surgical approach is laser treatment or vulvectomy, but these are rarely considered.

Interstitial Cystitis and Urinary Tract Infections

Nearly 61% of patients with Sjögren's report significant urinary symptoms. Recurrent urinary tract infections (UTIs), leukocyturia, and IC occur frequently in association with Sjögren's. Of note, these features also have been reported in patients with rheumatoid arthritis (RA) who also have Sjögren's and much more significantly than RA patients without Sjögren's. In addition, studies have shown that patients with Sjögren's or SLE have significantly more urinary complaints overall, especially irritative bladder symptoms. Whether the dryness of the mucosal membrane or a local immune mechanism in these patients is the cause for frequent UTIs is unknown.

Both Sjögren's and SLE patients with urinary complaints reported mostly urinary frequency (27% and 62%) and suprapubic pain (36% and 34%). In a study by Haarala et al., many Sjögren's and SLE patients reported urinary symptoms typical of IC such as suprapubic pain relieved by voiding, urgency, dysuria, and nocturia. This was not an unexpected finding, because there are also several other similar clinical features in Sjögren's and IC patients., including unknown etiology, female preponderance, and a chronic course with exacerbation and remission.

IC accompanying Sjögren's was first reported by Van De Merwe et al. in 1993. They reported that as many as 28% of patients presenting with IC may have underlying Sjögren's; indeed, IC may be the initial presenting complication leading to the diagnosis of Sjögren's. As many as 10% of those with Sjögren's have a diagnosis of IC. Patients usually present with irritation of the urinary tract or suprapubic pain, urinary frequency, and nocturia with no sign of infection (negative urine culture and absent organism in the culture). In some cases, bladder capacity is reduced due to the chronic inflammation and scarring.

IC is a chronic inflammatory urologic condition, simulating cystitis, with a prevalence of about 1% in the general population and mainly affecting women. The most widely accepted theories regarding its etiology are increased permeability of the bladder epithelium due to a deficient glycosaminoglycan layer. The damaged bladder lining allows toxic substances in urine to cause inflammation and production of inflammatory mediators as a result of activation of mast cells. Infiltration of Th2 lymphocytes, eosinophils, and mast cells into the mucous membrane of the urinary bladder and coexistence of anti-bladder antibodies can implicate an autoimmune mechanism as one cause of IC. However, the etiology and pathogenesis of IC remain unclear. Although the cause of the disease has not been fully elucidated, it is known to accompany Sjögren's, thyroid disease, SLE, ulcerative colitis, and Crohn's disease.

The strongest link between Sjögren's and IC is the prevalence of autoantibodies to type 3 muscarinic acetylcholine receptors (M3R) in both conditions. Recent studies suggest that these autoantibodies may contribute to urinary symptoms shared by each. The presence of these antibodies in the urinary detrusor musculature plays a major pathologic role in the progression of IC in patients with Sjögren's. The autoantibodies to M3R may also cause secretory dysfunction that leads to dry mouth in Sjögren's patients. No studies have been done to determine whether muscarinic agonists, which are parasympathomimetic drugs and include sialogogues (pilocarpine and cevimeline) used to treat oral and ocular dryness in Sjögren's, might be an effective treatment for IC, but mucosal muscarinic receptors have been shown to enhance bladder activity, and an indication for use in urinary retention has recently been highlighted (Bui & Duong, 2021). Further studies are needed.

Histopathologic study of the bladder shows mucosal edema and mononuclear cell and mast cell infiltration of the interstitium. Cystoscopic examination shows specific IC changes of increased vascularity or typical Hunner's ulcers. Serologic testing for anti-La/SSB antibodies is usually positive in IC patients who have Sjögren's. Hydroureteronephrosis may rarely complicate the course of IC in patients with Sjögren's, and acute renal failure may rarely develop in these patients. Severe cases with obstructive uropathy have not been reported in Sjögren's patients.

IC can be easily confused with many different bladder conditions, and some patients with IC cannot get appropriate treatment because of misdiagnosis. It is prudent to consider the diagnosis of IC in patients with Sjögren's who complain of urinary frequency, urgency, nocturia, and suprapubic pain but have a negative urine culture.

Although the treatment of IC is complex and requires special coordinated multilevel treatment, in cases of IC associated with Sjögren's, a therapeutic trial of corticosteroids and immunosuppressives may be considered in addition to the traditional IC treatment. Patients with IC have multiple interventions such as a special diet and medications for frequency and urgency, such as anticholinergics and beta-3 adrenergic agonists. A tricyclic antidepressant such as amitriptyline (Elavil) and a selective serotonin–norepinephrine reuptake inhibitor like duloxetine (Cymbalta) could be beneficial in the treatment of IC.

One of the medications that has been specifically used for treatment of IC is pentosan polysulfate sodium (Elmiron). Elmiron is a semi-synthetically produced heparin-like macromolecular carbohydrate derivative that adheres to the bladder's mucosal lining, preventing potentially irritating solutes in the urine from reaching the bladder wall. Patients are also referred for pelvic floor physical therapy as a complementary treatment to the medical therapy.

In severe cases of IC when patients do not respond to medical treatment, bladder hydrodistension may be beneficial. Dimethyl sulfoxide (DMSO) bladder infusion has been used in the past for treatment of IC. Cervical precancerous lesions, particularly high-grade squamous intraepithelial lesions, may lead to invasive cervical cancer after 10 to 15 years or, in some cases, may spontaneously regress.

Cervical Manifestations of Sjögren's and Human Papillomavirus

Human papillomavirus (HPV) is the most common sexually transmitted infection (STI) and is thought to be the principal causal agent for cervical cancer worldwide and responsible for the largest cause of mortality in women due to cancer in most developing countries. Smoking, younger age at first intercourse, high number of sexual partners, history of STIs, and use of hormonal contraceptives are risk factors for cervical HPV infection. The majority of HPV infections are transient and spontaneously resolve in less than 1 year, but persistence of the virus in the cervix and high-risk HPV types such as 16 and 18 are associated with progression of cervical dysplastic lesions. Persistent HPV infection is related to older age, HPV genotype, coexisting infections, immunosuppression, and inflammation.

In rheumatic populations, immunosuppressive treatments and the rheumatic disease itself, especially Sjögren's, can play a role in the development of premalignant and malignant conditions. Autoimmune disorders are associated with the activation of autoreactive T and B lymphocytes and with the release of pro-inflammatory cytokines that can possibly increase the risk of cancer. The lymphocytic infiltration that occurs in Sjögren's can progress from a benign to a malignant process. Moreover, the immunosuppressive drugs commonly used in these conditions can reduce the host's immune surveillance against malignancy and increase infection risk in these patients.

In a previous systematic review, the frequency of cervical cancer in SLE was not different from the that in the general population. However, in recent studies with larger cohorts and a long-term follow-up, Raposo et al. showed an increased incidence of cervical cancer in SLE patients and in Sjögren's patients with SLE. SLE patients have an increased susceptibility to HPV infection, HR HPV types, and multiple infections that can develop precancerous lesions over time. The presence of the disease itself was found to be an independent predictor for HPV infection and an abnormal Papanicolaou (Pap) smear. The studies also provide evidence that exposure to prednisone and long-term immunosuppressives (in particular cyclophosphamide) increases the risk of premalignant lesions compared to the general population.

Colposcopic inspection has revealed dystrophic processes resulting in the atrophy of the cervicovaginal mucosa in 50% of cases. However, no alterations distinctive enough to be indicative of dystrophic Sjögren's have been found. The histologic findings of the cervical biopsies showed chronic cervicitis in 10% of the cases.

In conclusion, studies have shown an increased prevalence of cervical dysplasia and cancer, with HPV infection being an important associated factor, especially in SLE patients. Information regarding rheumatic disease and cervical pathology is scarce, and more studies should be performed.

Pap smear screening is recommended in rheumatic patients according to national guidelines and screening programs for the general population. The American College of Obstetrics and Gynecology (ACOG) guidelines recommend that any low-risk woman aged 30 years or older who has a negative Pap test on cytology and HPV DNA testing should be re-examined no sooner than 3 years. A strict follow-up should be performed in HPV-positive women. Despite the increased risk, no specific recommendations have been developed for patients with systemic autoimmune disease who are negative for HPV. Early detection of premalignant lesions has decreased morbidity and mortality in the general population, and population-based screening programs have significantly contributed to early recognition and treatment.

Although HPV vaccination, an emerging issue in young women, is safe and immunogenic, there is little evidence on the safety and immunogenicity of HPV vaccines in immunocompromised patients.

Impact of Sjögren's on Female Sexual Function

Sexual health is considered an important aspect of physical and mental health and is associated with general well-being and satisfaction with life. Sexual function is influenced by physical as well as psychological consequences of rheumatic disease, such as pain, fatigue, stiffness, functional impairment, depression, anxiety, negative body image, dyspareunia, reduced libido, hormonal imbalance, and side effects from treatment. Women with Sjögren's have impaired sexual function and more sexual distress compared with the healthy population. Sexual function and distress are influenced by vaginal dryness and dyspareunia that decrease enjoyment of sexual activity.

There is little information on sexual function in females with Sjögren's. Some studies have reported sexual dysfunction in 24% to 74% of women with rheumatic disorders. Previous studies have focused on the prevalence of vaginal symptoms and dyspareunia or frequency of intercourse rather than on the whole concept of sexual function.

A study by Van Nimwegen et al. demonstrated that females with Sjögren's have significantly more sexual dysfunction in the domain of desire, arousal, orgasm, lubrication, and pain compared with healthy controls. The Female Sexual Function Index (FSFI) measures sexual function in six subdomains: desire, arousal, orgasm, lubrication, satisfaction, and pain. Of all these domains, lubrication showed the greatest difference in Sjögren's patients. Vaginal dryness leading to dyspareunia can play a major role in sexual dysfunction.

Besides vaginal dryness, the study showed that a variety of physical and psychological consequences of Sjögren's are linked to sexual dysfunction, including fatigue, symptoms of depression, relationship dissatisfaction, and lower mental quality of life. Depression is known to contribute to sexual dysfunction, either directly or due to the effect of antidepressants.

The sexual health of patients with rheumatic diseases is often neglected as both patients and physicians may find it difficult to address sexual complaints. By simply acknowledging and discussing these complaints, rheumatologists can help patients cope with sexual problems and refer them to a gynecologist or sexologist. Use of products containing testosterone, such as 2% cream or testosterone orally, could be beneficial in patients with low libido. K-Y also has new products that can be used as stimulants during sexual activities, such as K-Y Touch, K-Y Intense, K-Y Yours+Mine, and K-Y Love.

In conclusion, women with Sjögren's experience significantly more sexual dysfunction and distress than the healthy population. Chapter 45 provides more information on sex and Sjögren's.

Endometriosis in Sjögren's

Endometriosis is an estrogen-dependent inflammatory disorder affecting 5% to 10% of females during their reproductive years. The disorder is caused by the implantation of endometrial tissue outside of the uterus, a phenomenon believed to be the result of retrograde menstruation (Sampson's theory) in combination with a defect in immune surveillance that would have otherwise eliminated the ectopic endometrium. Although Sampson's theory of retrograde menstruation is the most commonly accepted, since retrograde menstruation occurs very often during reproductive life, a much lower prevalence of endometriosis suggests that additional factors determine susceptibility to endometriosis.

The hypothesis that endometriosis may represent an autoimmune disease was first proposed in 1980. A number of immunologic dysfunctions have been reported among patients with endometriosis, such as an increased number and activation of peritoneal macrophages, high T- and B-lymphocyte counts, decreased T-cell reactivity and natural killer cell cytotoxicity, increased circulating antibodies, anti-endometrial antibodies, and changes in the cytokine network. It is unclear if the immunologic alterations induce endometriosis or if they are a consequence of the endometriosis. However, they appear to play an important role in allowing endometriosis implants to persist and progress and contribute to the development of infertility and pelvic pain.

A higher prevalence of autoimmune disease has been found among endometriosis patients who were members of the Endometriosis Association when compared with the estimated prevalence in the general U.S. population. Among those autoimmune diseases, Sjögren's and SLE had a very high prevalence. Sinai et al. reported 7-fold to 24-fold increased risks of Sjögren's, multiple sclerosis (MS), and SLE among U.S. women with endometriosis. However, these findings were based on self-reports obtained on a questionnaire without appropriate controls for major confounding factors. Matorras et al. and Nielsen et al. conducted studies that were among the largest epidemiologic studies on the possible association of endometriosis with autoimmune disease but failed to find support for claims of markedly increased risks of endometriosis in SLE and Sjögren's patients. Due to the conflicting reports in the literature, there is a need for large-scale, prospective studies to clarify the increased risk of endometriosis in patients with autoimmune diseases.

Reproductive Manifestations and Premature Ovarian Failure

A few studies have addressed infertility in Sjögren's compared to other connective tissue diseases such as SLE. Most of these studies did not show an increased rate of infertility in Sjögren's patients. Some studies have reported a higher serum level of the pituitary hormone prolactin, which can often be associated with menstrual cycle irregularities due to ovarian dysfunction.

Premature ovarian failure (POP) has previously been reported with hypothyroidism and sicca syndrome (which may or may not have included Sjögren's patients). POP, clinically defined by failure of the ovary before the age of 40, affects almost 1% of the Western female population. It is characterized by primary or secondary amenorrhea, hypoestrogenism, and elevated gonadotropin serum levels; in most cases, no precise cause can be identified and it is known as idiopathic. The observed association of several POP cases with a variety of autoimmune disorders, such as thyroiditis, Addison's disease, Graves disease, insulin-dependent diabetes, and hypothyroidism, along with the finding of circulating antibodies to normal ovarian tissues and anti-ovarian antibodies (AOAs) in patients' serum, suggests an autoimmune mechanism in the pathophysiology of the disease.

AOAs were detected in a significant percentage of patients with Sjögren's; however, a pathogenic role in the induction of POP could not be attributed to the AOAs. Their presence may be an inductor of autoimmune oophoritis, either clinical or subclinical. It is known that the antibodies may be simple epiphenomena in several autoimmune processes.

Amyloid Deposition in Sjögren's

Amyloidosis is the deposition of amyloid fibrils in the extracellular spaces of tissues and organs. Amyloid fibrils consist of low-molecular-weight proteins, and immunoglobulin components are often the major source of the amyloid protein. Their localization is limited to dermis, lung, or tongue and rarely the breast. Amyloidosis can be subdivided into systemic and localized forms as well as into different types, including primary, secondary, hereditary-familial, endocrine, and senile amyloidosis.

The coexistence of primary amyloidosis and Sjögren's is rare. Only eight cases of amyloidosis have been reported in Sjögren's patients, and only one of the patients had breast amyloidosis. Breast amyloidosis can present as a focal density containing microcalcifications or diffuse infiltration of the mammary gland with skin thickening, mimicking an inflammatory carcinoma. The radiologic picture may be indistinguishable from invasive carcinoma; therefore, these patients should be managed like all other cases of suspicious breast malignancies. While breast amyloidosis is rare in Sjögren's patients, it should not be ignored and should be managed accordingly. See Chapter 28 on the occurrence of amyloidosis in the lungs of Sjögren's patients.

Pregnancy Outcome in Patients with Sjögren's

Women with Sjögren's are at increased risk for both maternal complications and adverse neonatal outcomes. Adverse neonatal outcomes may occur from the disease itself, maternal complications and pregnancy-related disease flares, and teratogenic risk from medications used to treat Sjögren's. Infants of women with Sjögren's are at increased risk of preterm birth, admission to the neonatal intensive care unit, severe neonatal morbidity, and perinatal death. Among the neonatal anomalies, congenital heart disorders are the most common and are a major cause for concern. Anti-Ro/SSA and/or anti-La/SSB autoantibodies are associated with congenital heart block (CHB) in infants and mediate damage to the atrioventricular node. CHB is estimated to occur in approximately 2% of infants born to women with anti-Ro/SSA and 3% of infants born to women with anti-La/SSB. The recurrence rate of CHB in a subsequent pregnancy, once a mother has had a child with fetal heart block, jumps to nearly 20%. Autoantibody-associated CHB carries a substantial morbidity and mortality. CHB mortality varies from 12% to 43% in the literature, and it increases when the disease is associated with endocardial fibroelastosis or cardiomyopathy.

When CHB is diagnosed, intrauterine therapy is possible to increase the atrioventricular conduction speed and improve fetal outcome. Maternal treatment with fluorinated steroids, dexamethasone or betamethasone, can reduce the antibody-mediated inflammatory damage of nodal tissue and potentially reverse fetal heart block. These mothers will continue to require steroids for the remainder of their pregnancy. However, complete third-degree heart block often will not respond to steroids, and they will be discontinued after a 6-month trial. These newborns most likely will need a pacemaker upon birth. Alternative/additional therapies have included plasmapheresis, intravenous immunoglobulins, and beta-sympathomimetics.

CHB is a manifestation of what is termed "neonatal lupus," as the Sjögren's autoantibodies anti-Ro/SSA and/or anti-La/SSB can cross the placenta from mother to baby and cause this condition in newborns in either Sjögren's or lupus. Neonatal lupus can appear as a characteristic red rash and sometimes can also cause liver abnormalities or low blood cell counts. These manifestations are almost always transient. However, their appearance should lead the gynecologist to suspect Sjögren's or lupus in the mother and should be investigated further.

Women with connective tissue diseases in general have higher rates of preeclampsia, premature delivery, and cesarean section as well as a significantly increased relative risk of having a child who is small for gestational age. A high rate of pregnancy loss is often associated with antiphospholipid syndrome, which can occur in Sjögren's, and adverse events may precede the clinical onset of connective tissue diseases or indicate the presence of an underlying autoimmune disease such as Sjögren's.

Women with SLE may experience recurrent pregnancy loss and 50% may have disease flares during pregnancy, with potential negative impacts on pregnancy outcomes. In contrast, women with RA generally have reduced disease activity during pregnancy. They have good overall outcomes, if potentially teratogenic drugs such as methotrexate are not used at the time of conception or during the pregnancy.

A study by Chen et al. showed that women with Sjögren's had less desirable pregnancy outcomes compared to a general obstetric population. They were at increased risk of hypertensive disorders, hemorrhage, cesarean section, preterm birth resulting in low birth weight, and severe maternal morbidity. The low birth weight in women with Sjögren's could be due to underlying placental insufficiency or to immunologic mechanisms. These women showed a higher incidence of miscarriage (or spontaneous abortions) than the normal population. The increased rate of spontaneous abortions may be explained by older age if younger women with Sjögren's have delayed their first pregnancy. It is also important to consider antiphospholipid autoantibodies or immunologic pathways that might be involved.

Pregnancy in Sjögren's requires close cooperation between women and their healthcare providers. A multidisciplinary approach with rheumatologists, obstetricians, and pediatricians would be helpful for the optimal management of pregnancies complicated by Sjögren's. Vigilant surveillance by the multidisciplinary team throughout the perinatal period is warranted for these women and their infants.

Women should also be counseled before pregnancy about the risk of pregnancy loss, maternal morbidity, and neonatal morbidity and mortality. Patients should plan for pregnancy and discuss the pros and cons of various medications with their physicians prior to attempting to become pregnant. This may take several months of planning, as the effects and half-lives of some drugs are very prolonged. The other reason for planning for pregnancy is to ensure that the disease is inactive, as disease activity is known to affect pregnancy outcome. Many women with Sjögren's have successful pregnancies.

Summing Up

Sjögren's patients are at increased risk for a variety of gynecologic and urologic complications. Vaginal dryness and dyspareunia are among the most common manifestations of Sjögren's and can be successfully treated with topical products. The pathogenesis of gynecologic manifestations such as premature ovarian failure, endometriosis, amyloidosis, and IC in Sjögren's patients needs further research. The rare manifestation of lichen sclerosus needs to be addressed by the patient's gynecologist, as this condition can cause severe vulvovaginal atrophy and regression. Untreated lichen sclerosus can cause vulvar atypia and possibly vulvar carcinoma.

Pregnancy poses potential and unique problems. Autoantibodies such as Ro and La are associated with the risk for CHB in the infant, so if a woman with Sjögren's is positive for these autoantibodies, the fetus should be monitored for heart block. If a mother-to-be is positive for antiphospholipid autoantibodies, treatment reducing the chance of miscarriage should be initiated. A multidisciplinary approach with the rheumatologist, gynecologist, and pediatrician is key to the successful treatment and management of patients with Sjögren's.

For Further Reading

Bloch KJ, Buchanan WW, Wohl MJ, Bunnim JJ. Sjögren's syndrome: A clinical, pathological and serological study of sixty-two cases. *Medicine.* 1992;71(6):386–403.

Bui T, Duong H. Muscarinic Agonists. [Updated 2021 Jul 26]. In: StatPearls [Internet]. Treasure Island (FL): StatPearls Publishing; 2021 Jan-. Available from: https://www.ncbi.nlm.nih.gov/books/NBK553130/

Chen Jian S, Roberts Christine L. Pregnancy outcomes in women with rare autoimmune diseases. *Arthritis & Rheumatology.* 67;12 December 2015:3314–3323.

Cirpan T, Guliyeva A, Onder G, et al. Comparison of human papillomavirus testing and cervical cytology with colposcopic examination and biopsy in cervical cancer screening in a cohort of patients with Sjögren's syndrome. *Eur J Gynaecol Oncol.* 2007;28(4):302–306.

Dugué PA, Rebolj M, Hallas J, et al. Risk of cervical cancer in women with autoimmune diseases, in relation with their use of immunosuppressants and screening: Population-based cohort study. *Int J Cancer.* 2015;136(6):E711–E719.

Eutymiopoulou K. Aletras A, Ravazoula P, et al. Antiovarian antibodies in primary Sjögren's syndrome. *Rheumatol Int.* 2007;27:1149–1155.

Haga HJ, Gram Gjesdal C, Irgens LM, Ostensen M. Reprooduction and gynecological manifestations in women with primary Sjögren's syndrome: A case-control study. *Scand J Rheumatol.* 2005;34:45–48.

Haarala M, Alanen A. Lower urinary tract symptom in patients with SS SLE. *Int Urogneal J* 2000;1(1):84–86.

Hussein SZ, Jacobson LTH, Lindquist PG, Theander E. Pregnancy and fetal outcome in women with primary Sjögren's syndrome compared with women in the general population: A nested case-control study. *Rheumatology.* 2001;50:1612.

Kersemans P, Van Ongeval C, Van Steen A, Drijkoningen M. Amyloid deposition of the breast in primary Sjögren's syndrome. *JBR-BTR.* 2006;89(6):313–314.

Lee CK, Tsai CP, Liao TL, et al. Overactive bladder and bladder pain syndrome/interstitial cystitis in primary Sjögren's syndrome patients: A nationwide population-based study. *PLoS One.* 2019;14(11):e0225455.

Matorras R, Ocerin I, Unamuno M, et al. Prevalence of endometriosis in women with systemic lupus erythematosus and Sjögren's syndrome. *Lupus.* 2007;16:736–740.

Mulherin DM, Sheeran TP, Kumararatne DS, et al. Sjögren's syndrome in women presenting with dyspareunia. *Br J Obstet Gynaecol.* 1997;104(9):1019–1023.

Nielsen NM, Jørgensen KT, Pedersen BV, et al. The co-occurrence of endometriosis with multiple sclerosis, systemic lupus erythematosus and Sjögren's syndrome. *Hum Reprod.* 2011;26(6):1555-1559.

Pereira E, Silva R, Romão VC, et al. Overactive bladder symptom bother and health-related quality of life in patients with systemic lupus erythematosus and primary Sjögren's syndrome. *Lupus.* 2019;28(1):27-33.

Piccioni MG, Merlino L, Derma M, et al. The impact of primary Sjögren's syndrome on female sexual function. *Minerva Ginecol.* 2020;72(1):50-54.

Raposo A, Tani C, Costa J, Mosca M. Human papilloma virus infection and cervical lesions in rheumatic diseases: A systematic review. *Acta Reumatal Port.* 2016;41:184-190.

Rosen R, Brown C, Heiman J, et al. The Female Sexual Function Index (FSFI): A multidimensional self-report instrument for the assessment of female sexual function. *J Sex Marital Ther.* 2000;26(2):191-208.

Stephenson KR, Meston CM. The conditional importance of sex: Exploring the association between sexual wellbeing and life satisfaction. *J Sex Marital Ther.* 2015;41(1):25.

Tayal SC, Watson PG. Dyspareunia in undiagnosed Sjogren's syndrome. *Br J Clin Pract.* 1996 Jan-Feb;50(1):57-58.

Van de Merwe J, Kamerling R, Arendsen E, Mulder D, Hooijkaas H. Sjögren's syndrome in patients with interstitial cystitis. *J Rheumatol.* 1993 Jun;20(6):962-966.

Van Nimwegen JF, Arends S, van Zuiden GS, et al. The impact of primary Sjögren's syndrome on female sexual function. *Rheumatology.* 2015;54(7):1286-1293.

Walker J, Gordon T, Lester S, et al. Increased severity of lower urinary tract symptoms and daytime somnolence in primary Sjögren's syndrome. *Rheumatology.* 2003;30(11):2406-2412.

36

Management of Vasculitis in Sjögren's

Ghaith Noaiseh

Sjögren's is a chronic autoimmune disease (a disease in which the immune system recurrently or sporadically attacks the body over the long term). It is characterized by lymphocytic infiltration of exocrine glands (such as the salivary and lacrimal glands), leading to dryness and other symptoms.

It is useful to think of Sjögren's as a spectrum ranging from common symptoms affecting the majority of patients, such as dryness, fatigue, and joint pain, to less common and more serious complications, such as lung or kidney inflammation. The culmination of inflammatory processes can lead, in some patients, to the development of lymphoma. In general, the presence of vasculitis in Sjögren's patients denotes a more severe disease and requires careful monitoring to allow early identification and treatment of complications.

What is vasculitis? The word vasculitis is a combination of two roots: *vascul*, meaning "blood vessels," and *itis*, meaning inflammation. Thus, vasculitis means inflammation of the blood vessels. In general, vasculitis can affect large, medium, or small vessels. The narrowing and/or complete occlusion of blood vessels causes decreased blood flow, ischemia, and damage to the supplied tissue, which then leads to a wide variety of symptoms.

Vasculitis syndromes can be classified based on the size of blood vessel involved. For example, in Takayasu's arteritis, a large vessel vasculitis, major vessels such as the aorta and its main branches are involved; in antineutrophil cytoplasmic antibody (ANCA) vasculitis, the small vessels are involved. Takayasu's arteritis and ANCA vasculitis are distinct rheumatic entities and are considered primary vasculitis disorders, whereas vasculitis in Sjögren's is considered secondary to the disease. Similarly, vasculitis may occur in the context of other autoimmune rheumatic diseases such as rheumatoid arthritis and systemic lupus erythematosus. Vasculitis in Sjögren's is almost universally small vessel vasculitis involving different organs, concurrently or sequentially. Medium-sized vessel involvement is rare but has been reported.

Ghaith Noaiseh, *Management of Vasculitis in Sjögren's* In: *The Sjögren's Book*. Edited by: Daniel J. Wallace, Oxford University Press. © Sjögren's Foundation 2022. DOI: 10.1093/oso/9780197502112.003.0036

Clinical Spectrum

The most commonly involved organs are the skin and peripheral nerves. The severity of symptoms can vary widely from mild to severe to life-threatening.

Skin Involvement

Cutaneous vasculitis has been reported in 9% to 32% of patients with Sjögren's (Ramos-Casals et al., 2004, 2008). While about half of patients with cutaneous vasculitis only have one episode in their lifetime (Ramos-Casals et al., 2004), the presence of cutaneous vasculitis in a Sjögren's patient suggests a higher likelihood of developing more severe disease, including other extraglandular manifestations and development of lymphoma.

Patients usually present with slightly raised red lesions on the lower extremities, typically on the shins, called purpura. The lesions may be painful and associated with a burning sensation or pruritus, or they can be asymptomatic. An increase in pigmentation in the area usually persists after the lesion resolves.

Cutaneous vasculitis should be distinguished from hypergammaglobulinemic purpura, a benign phenomenon that looks similar but is not associated with an increased risk of severe extraglandular manifestations or lymphoma. A skin biopsy is required to distinguish the two entities.

Peripheral Nervous System Involvement

The disease of peripheral nerves is referred to as neuropathy. In Sjögren's, several types of neuropathies can occur, a few caused by a vasculitic process. Nerve damage leads to sensory symptoms (numbness and tingling in the distal part of the upper and lower extremities), motor symptoms (muscle weakness), or combined sensorimotor symptoms.

Multiple mononeuropathies (mononeuritis multiplex) is a type of neuropathy almost exclusively caused by vasculitis. It is usually suspected when a patient presents with sensory and motor symptoms that correspond to different nerves in an asymmetrical fashion—for example, new-onset left foot numbness occurring simultaneously with right foot weakness. The nerve conduction study can be very useful, and the diagnosis is usually confirmed by obtaining a nerve biopsy (usually the sural nerve, a small sensory nerve that innervates the lateral aspect of the calf).

When suspected, an expedited work-up and prompt initiation of therapy are essential to prevent irreversible neurologic damage.

Other potential body organ involvement includes the following:

1. Central nervous system involvement (brain and spinal cord): The diagnosis of vasculitis usually requires obtaining a tissue biopsy, which is not an easy procedure to do on brain tissue. For this reason, it can be challenging to determine that an inflammatory process in the brain or spinal cord is vasculitic. There are few reports of biopsy-proven vasculitis of the central nervous system in patients with Sjögren's (Alexander et al., 1986). The central nervous system manifestations in Sjögren's are discussed in more detail in Chapters 13, 30, and 31.
2. Muscle involvement may lead to muscle pain and occasionally muscle weakness.
3. Kidney involvement may lead to the presence of protein in the urine (proteinuria), blood in the urine (hematuria), hypertension, and renal failure that can be severe enough to require replacement therapy (dialysis).
4. Gastrointestinal manifestations with vasculitic features are uncommon, but patients with such features can present with abdominal pain due to ischemia of the bowel wall. In severe cases, bowel perforation can occur, which is a surgical emergency.
5. Vasculitis and Sjögren's may rarely affect the pancreas and the gallbladder (Ramos-Casals et al., 2004; Tsokos et al., 1987).

Diagnosis of Vasculitis in Sjögren's

Clinicians rely on suggestive clinical features; for example, lower extremity purpura in a patient with Sjögren's may suggest cutaneous vasculitis. Specific neurologic presentations such as inability to move the ankle upward (foot drop) should prompt consideration of mononeuritis multiplex.

Laboratory testing can be very useful. Elevation of inflammatory markers, such as erythrocyte sedimentation rate (ESR) and/or C-reactive protein (CRP), is common. Certain laboratory abnormalities tend to accompany vasculitic features; for example, low levels of complement C3 and C4; abnormal immunoglobin protein, or a paraprotein, in the blood or urine (monoclonal gammopathy); low white blood cell count (leukopenia); and the presence of abnormal proteins in the blood, called cryoglobulins, that precipitate under cold conditions.

Imaging studies, such as computed tomography (CT) and magnetic resonance imaging (MRI), can be helpful in assessing brain and spinal cord lesions. Nerve conduction studies are essential when evaluating for suspected neuropathies. Tissue sampling (biopsy) remains the most important diagnostic test, when feasible.

Treatment

Treatment is tailored to the specific clinical syndrome caused by vasculitis. Vasculitic rashes frequently respond to oral corticosteroids such as prednisone and methylprednisolone (Medrol) and/or other immunomodulatory therapies such as hydroxychloroquine (Plaquenil), azathioprine (Imuran), and methotrexate. Associated pain can be managed with nonsteroidal anti-inflammatory drugs (NSAIDs) such as ibuprofen or naproxen. Topical corticosteroids and second-generation antihistamines such as fexofenadine (Allegra) and loratadine (Claritin) can be helpful in managing pruritus without worsening sicca symptoms. For difficult-to-manage vasculitic rashes, topical tacrolimus is also an option. More serious complications such as mononeuritis multiplex typically require high-dose corticosteroids and potent immunosuppressive therapy such as cyclophosphamide (Cytoxan) and rituximab (Rituxan).

Prognosis

Cutaneous vasculitis usually responds well to therapy but may recur. Other body organ involvement can be severe and potentially life-threatening. Sjögren's patients who exhibit vasculitic features have an increased risk of developing other severe extraglandular manifestations and exhibit a higher risk for lymphoma development. Such patients should be carefully monitored.

Summing Up

Vasculitis is characterized by inflammation of the blood vessels and can occur in small, medium, or large vessels. When it occurs in Sjögren's, vasculitis commonly affects the small blood vessels; the most commonly involved organs are the skin and peripheral nerves. When vasculitis occurs, treatment is tailored to the specific cause and may include oral corticosteroids or immunomodulatory therapies. Vasculitis severity can range from mild to severe, and the presence of vasculitis in Sjögren's usually represents a more serious disease course.

Acknowledgment

The author would like to thank Sandra Burkett for her valuable comments on the contents of this chapter.

For Further Reading

Alexander EL, Lijewski JE, Jerdan MS, Alexander GE. Evidence of an immunopathogenic basis for central nervous system disease in primary Sjögren's syndrome. *Arthritis Rheum.* 1986 Oct;29(10):1223–1231.

Carsons SE, Vivino FB, Parke A, et al. Treatment guidelines for rheumatologic manifestations of Sjögren's syndrome: Use of biologic agents, management of fatigue, and inflammatory musculoskeletal pain. *Arthritis Care Res.* 2017;69(4):517–527. doi:10.1002/acr.22968

Ramos-Casals M, Anaya JM, García-Carrasco M, et al. Cutaneous vasculitis in primary Sjögren syndrome: Classification and clinical significance of 52 patients. *Medicine (Baltimore).* 2004 Mar;83(2):96–106.

Ramos-Casals M, Solans R, Rosas J, et al. Primary Sjögren syndrome in Spain: Clinical and immunologic expression in 1010 patients. *Medicine.* 2008;87(4):210–219.

Scofield RH. Vasculitis in Sjögren's syndrome. *Curr Rheumatol Rep.* 2011;13:482.

Tsokos M, Lazarou SA, Moutsopoulos HM. Vasculitis in primary Sjögren's syndrome. Histologic classification and clinical presentation. *Am J Clin Pathol.* 1987 Jul;88(1):26–31.

37

Management of Lymphoma and Other Cancers in Sjögren's

Kieron Dunleavy and Katherine M. Hammitt

One of the most serious potential complications of Sjögren's is the development of lymphoma or other blood and non-blood cancers. The risk in Sjögren's is highest for B-cell non-Hodgkin's lymphoma (NHL), which is reported to have an incidence of 5% to 10%. Most lymphomas in Sjögren's have an indolent course, meaning that they progress very slowly and as such typically call for close monitoring (a "watch and wait" approach without aggressive treatment). It is important, however, for patients and their healthcare professionals to be aware of the possibility of malignancy in Sjögren's, so that patients can be monitored and managed appropriately. It is also important to recognize that our knowledge about lymphoma and other cancers in people with Sjögren's is constantly expanding, and investigators across the globe are working hard to find potentially new and better treatments.

Why Do Lymphoma and Other Cancers Occur in Sjögren's?

Development of cancer in Sjögren's is complex and most likely involves the interplay of multiple factors. While we do not fully understand why malignancy sometimes arises in Sjögren's, chronic inflammation and prolonged stimulation of the immune system likely contribute to its development. The risk of lymphoma is increased with most autoimmune and rheumatic diseases; a positive rheumatoid factor (RF) and the presence of certain autoantibodies are viewed as risk factors for lymphoma development.

A higher incidence of lymphoma occurs in Sjögren's than in any other autoimmune rheumatic disease. One Scandinavian study examining data from about 30,000 patients with autoimmune disease and NHL found that NHL occurred in Sjögren's at a 6.6-fold higher rate than that of the normal

Kieron Dunleavy and Katherine M. Hammitt, *Management of Lymphoma and Other Cancers in Sjögren's*
In: *The Sjögren's Book*. Edited by: Daniel J. Wallace, Oxford University Press. © Sjögren's Foundation 2022.
DOI: 10.1093/oso/9780197502112.003.0037

population. Corresponding rates were a 2.7-fold increase in patients with systemic lupus erythematosus (SLE) and a 1.0-fold increase for rheumatoid arthritis (RA) patients. Other studies have found up to a 44-fold increase in lymphoma in association with Sjögren's compared to a seven-fold increase in SLE and a four-fold increase in RA.

Lymphoproliferation that occurs in the moisture-producing glands and mucosa in Sjögren's—including the salivary glands, oral cavity, stomach, gastrointestinal tract, and lungs—can transform from a benign process to a malignant one. The most frequent cancer in Sjögren's is B-cell lymphoma of the mucosa-associated lymphoid tissue (MALT), which can occur in any mucosal tissue but most often occurs in the salivary glands. Ninety percent of lymphoma cases in Sjögren's are made up of MALT lymphomas (58%), diffuse large B-cell lymphomas (20%), and non-MALT marginal zone lymphomas (MZLs; 12%). Additionally, thyroid, breast, colorectal, and stomach cancer as well as other blood cancers (hematologic cancers) such as myeloid neoplasia/leukemia and multiple myeloma also have been identified at a higher rate in Sjögren's than in the normal population.

Who Is Most at Risk?

We know more about lymphoma than other cancers in Sjögren's, as this link was established as far back as 1978 and more studies have been done in this area than in any other. Those who develop lymphoma are more likely to have certain clinical signs and lab findings (Table 37.1).

In addition, high disease activity as measured by the European Alliance of Associations for Rheumatology (EULAR) Sjögren's Syndrome Disease Activity Index (ESSDAI) is equated with a higher risk of B-cell MALT lymphoma and non–B-cell cancers. Other risk factors for malignancy overall in Sjögren's include being male, being older, and having a longer duration of disease. The latter might be related to the longer time of chronic inflammation and stimulation of the immune system. Malignancy, however, can occur prior to diagnosis with Sjögren's or earlier in the disease course and at any age. The median time from diagnosis of Sjögren's to development of any type of cancer is about 5 years.

Risk also might be attributed to environmental and genetic factors. Environmental triggers, including viruses and bacteria, can contribute to development of malignancy. The best-known example is the bacterium *Helicobacter pylori* (*H. pylori*), which is associated with stomach cancer. Hepatitis C (HCV) is linked with both autoimmune disease development and lymphoma. Other bacteria and viruses are associated specifically with MALT

Table 37.1 Clinical and Lab Risk Factors for Lymphoma Development

Clinical Findings	Lab Findings
Major salivary gland swelling	Low complement factor 3 (C3)
Lymph node swelling (lymphadenopathy)	Low complement factor 4 (C4)
Skin vasculitis (including palpable purpura)	Monoclonal components in serum or urine
Enlarged spleen (splenomegaly)	Cryoglobulinemia
Peripheral neuropathy	High levels of anti-SSB/La
Glomerulonephritis (inflammation of filters in the kidney)	Anemia
Low-grade fever	Leukopenia
Germinal centers in minor salivary gland biopsy	Lymphopenia
	Neutropenia
	Hypogammaglobulinemia
	Elevated serum beta2 microglobulin
	Anti-SSA/Ro positivity
	Elevated B-cell activating factor (BAFF)
	Rheumatoid factor positivity

lymphoma or other cancers. These, too, can further stimulate the immune system and contribute to a higher risk of lymphoma development. Genes can affect the way the immune system responds to environmental triggers and can play a role in cell death and elimination (apoptosis) that occurs with the lymphoproliferation in Sjögren's and contributes independently to development of malignancy.

Prognosis and Management

Prognosis varies depending on the type of cancer. Most lymphomas that occur in Sjögren's are very slow-growing; the types of lymphoma include MALT lymphoma, follicular lymphoma, chronic lymphocytic leukemia/small lymphocytic lymphoma, and splenic MZL. These often call for a "watch and wait" approach over many years. More aggressive lymphomas that can occur include diffuse large B-cell lymphoma, Burkitt lymphoma, lymphoblastic leukemia/lymphoma, and some T-cell lymphomas. These more commonly have acute onset with fever, night sweats, and weight loss and always call for an aggressive treatment approach.

Interestingly, many of the therapies used to treat systemic symptoms of Sjögren's were first approved for use in cancer. For example, methotrexate was used for certain types of cancer and is now a first-level therapy used separately or in conjunction with hydroxychloroquine to manage Sjögren's. The biologic rituximab was first approved by the U.S. Food and Drug Administration (FDA) for use in NHL and may be prescribed to treat more severe cases of Sjögren's. Since these drugs modulate the immune system, they have been used successfully in some autoimmune diseases, including Sjögren's, although this is an off-label use.

Preventing severe complications in Sjögren's can be a better approach than treating them after the fact. As such, treating the underlying disease of Sjögren's when symptoms are severe, disease activity is high, and the patient has many of the known risk factors for lymphoma development is important to reduce the incidence of cancer. Reducing inflammation and impeding disease progress can play an important role in preventing further complications, as can identifying and eradicating viral and bacterial infections associated with malignancy.

That said, all therapies have potential side effects, and these must be weighed carefully and risks and benefits discussed by patients and healthcare professionals as part of determining the patient's healthcare plan. Once a cancer develops, traditional cancer treatments such as radiation and chemotherapy can be combined with some of the newer biologics and other drugs such as rituximab for better outcomes. Newer monoclonal therapies with very specific targets and other therapies are in development and will lead to better outcomes and a brighter future for those with Sjögren's who do develop cancer as part of their autoimmune disease.

Can Sjögren's Treatments Increase the Chance of Developing Malignancy?

Treating Sjögren's can be an intricate balance. Suppressing the immune system in any way, such as with the use of corticosteroids, might contribute to the development of malignancy. At the same time, reducing an overactive immune system that occurs in Sjögren's and other autoimmune diseases can decrease the inflammation and chronic immune stimulation that can lead to increased susceptibility. Some medications used to treat Sjögren's and related diseases have been potentially linked with development of lymphoma; however, the connection is not clear and is controversial. Tumor necrosis factor

(TNF) inhibitors (including infliximab [Remicade], etanercept [Enbrel], and adalimumab [Humira]), which are commonly used to treat RA, have been linked with potential increased susceptibility to NHL. This, too, most likely involves an intricate balance, as normal levels of TNF can be protective in preventing B-cell proliferation and are important to normal apoptosis, but too little TNF has been shown to contribute to the development of autoimmune disease and B-cell lymphoma.

Summing Up

Lymphoma, especially B-cell MALT lymphoma, is the most common malignancy associated with Sjögren's, and physicians and patients should be alert to this potential development and the risk factors that increase susceptibility. Other hematologic and solid cancers can occur in the setting of Sjögren's, so awareness of and monitoring for these is also an important part of a patient's care. Prognosis and management and treatment differ according to the type of cancer. Most lymphomas that occur in Sjögren's are slow-growing and do not need aggressive treatment.

For Further Reading

Brito-Zerón P, Kostov B, Fraile G, et al. Characterization and risk estimate of cancer in patients with primary Sjögren's syndrome. *J Hematol Oncol.* 2017;10(1):90.

Flores-Chávez A, Kostov B, Solans R, et al. Severe, life-threatening phenotype of primary Sjögren's syndrome: Clinical characterization and outcomes in 1580 patients (GEAS-SS Registry). *Clin Exp Rheumatol.* 2018;36 Suppl 112(3):121–129.

Jonsson MV, Theander E, Jonsson R. Predictors for the development of non-Hodgkin lymphoma in primary Sjögren's syndrome. *Presse Med.* 2012;41(9 Pt 2):e511–e516.

Nocturne G, Mariette X. Sjögren syndrome-associated lymphomas: An update on pathogenesis and management. *Br J Haematol.* 2015;168(3):317–327.

Retamozo S, Brito-Zeron P, Ramos-Casals M. Prognostic markers of lymphoma development in primary Sjögren syndrome. *Lupus.* 2019;28(8):923–936.

Tomi AL, Belkhir R, Nocturne G, et al. Brief report: Monoclonal gammopathy and risk of lymphoma and multiple myeloma in patients with primary Sjögren's syndrome. *Arthritis Rheumatol.* 2016;68(5):1245–1250.

Weng MY, Huang YT, Liu MF, Lu TH. Incidence of cancer in a nationwide population cohort of 7852 patients with primary Sjögren's syndrome in Taiwan. *Ann Rheum Dis.* 2012;71:524–527.

38

Management of Hepatic and Pancreatic Involvement in Sjögren's

Chadwick R. Johr

Hepatic Involvement

The liver is a large organ in the right upper portion of the abdomen abutting the diaphragm. Just below it lies the gallbladder and pancreas. Together, these organs produce and store fluids such as bile that aid in digestion. The liver helps maintain proper blood glucose levels and is an essential manufacturer of important proteins and lipids. Furthermore, it is largely responsible for processing medications, toxins, and waste products in preparation for excretion from the body.

When a liver cell (hepatocyte) is sufficiently injured, it releases its contents into the bloodstream. Some of the released compounds, such as asparagine aminotransferase (AST) and alanine aminotransferase (ALT), are found in greater concentrations in hepatocytes than in other cell types and are thus frequently referred to as "liver enzymes." When enough hepatocytes become damaged, there is a detectable increase in blood levels of liver enzymes. The degree of liver enzyme elevation is typically proportional to the extent of hepatocyte damage.

Abnormal levels of liver-related blood tests have been noted in 10% to 40% of Sjögren's patients. They are often mild and not of any significant consequence; however, their detection should prompt consideration of further evaluation.

Non-autoimmune Causes

The most common liver problems in Sjögren's patients are not autoimmune in nature. Some medications used to treat various aspects of Sjögren's occasionally cause liver inflammation (hepatitis). Generally, the inflammation is mild and resolves with adjustments in medication dosage or discontinuation.

Chadwick R. Johr, *Management of Hepatic and Pancreatic Involvement in Sjögren's* In: *The Sjögren's Book*. Edited by: Daniel J. Wallace, Oxford University Press. © Sjögren's Foundation 2022. DOI: 10.1093/oso/9780197502112.003.0038

The hepatitis C virus (HCV) is a common cause of hepatitis in many populations. The virus can cause a clinical syndrome that mimics Sjögren's, and some studies note an increased prevalence of HCV in Sjögren's patients. The diagnosis of HCV infection can be made with blood testing. Testing for HCV should be strongly considered in Sjögren's patients with evidence of liver disease.

Non-alcoholic fatty liver disease (NAFLD) is a common cause of liver inflammation in the general population, affecting up to 5% of American adults and up to 20% of those who are obese. Because of its high prevalence, evaluation for NAFLD should be considered in Sjögren's patients with persistently elevated liver enzymes. Imaging such as ultrasound or computed tomography (CT) can help make the diagnosis. Occasionally, liver biopsy is needed for confirmation.

Autoimmune Hepatitis

The most common autoimmune liver manifestations in Sjögren's are autoimmune hepatitis (AIH) and primary biliary cholangitis (PBC) (Table 38.1).

In AIH, the immune system attacks hepatocytes, leading to chronic liver inflammation. It has been noted in 1% to 4% of Sjögren's patients and can occur alongside other autoimmune conditions or all by itself. It affects women more often than men. Typically, the onset is insidious and manifests prior to 45 years of age. Symptoms of AIH may include fatigue, diminished appetite, and a yellow hue to the skin (jaundice). The diagnosis of AIH should be suspected in those with abnormal results of liver-related blood tests, especially when levels are persistently elevated. In such patients, the diagnosis may be established with blood tests demonstrating the presence of anti-smooth

Table 38.1 Autoimmune Liver Manifestations in Sjögren's

Autoimmune Manifestation	Prevalence in Sjögren's	Typical Symptoms	Recommended testing	Treatment	Prognosis
Primary biliary cholangitis	2–5%	Fatigue, itchy skin	Anti-mitochondrial antibody levels	Ursodeoxycholic acid (ursodiol)	Good
Autoimmune hepatitis	1–4%	Fatigue, decreased appetite, jaundice	Anti-smooth muscle antibody and anti-nuclear antibody levels	Prednisone or prednisolone +/− azathioprine	Good

muscle antibodies or other related autoantibodies. Occasionally, a liver biopsy may be necessary to confirm the diagnosis. The liver inflammation in AIH is chronic and may eventually lead to scarring and irreversible liver dysfunction (cirrhosis); however, most AIH patients do not develop cirrhosis, and the 10-year survival rate is greater than 90%. The treatment of AIH typically consists of glucocorticoids such as prednisone. Occasionally other immunosuppressant medications such as azathioprine are used.

Primary Biliary Cholangitis

Instead of attacking hepatocytes, the immune system sometimes attacks the ducts that collect bile produced by the liver. This autoimmune condition is known as PBC. PBC has been reported in 2% to 5% of Sjögren's patients. The age of onset is typically between 40 and 60 years, and it affects women far more often than men. The biliary duct damage and inflammation in PBC leads to obstruction of biliary flow and elevated serum levels of bilirubin, gamma-glutamyl transferase (GGT), and alkaline phosphatase.

Typical symptoms of PBC include fatigue and itchiness of the skin (pruritus), though about half of patients are asymptomatic at the time of diagnosis. The diagnosis is suspected in those with elevated serum levels of GGT or alkaline phosphatase and confirmed with elevated serum levels of anti-mitochondrial antibodies. As with AIH, a liver biopsy may be necessary to establish the diagnosis.

PBC is ordinarily treated with ursodeoxycholic acid (ursodiol), a medication that protects the bile duct cells from damage. The prognosis is good in those undergoing treatment. Only a minority develop cirrhosis, and most live a normal lifespan.

Pancreatic Involvement

The pancreas is the chief organ responsible for regulating blood sugar levels. It also secretes enzymes like amylase and lipase that help digest carbohydrates, fats, and proteins. Pancreatic inflammation (pancreatitis) is rare in Sjögren's but not uncommon in a disease known to mimic Sjögren's, IgG4-related disease. As with hepatitis, some of the medications used in Sjögren's management are known to cause pancreatitis. Whenever pancreatitis is suspected in a patient with Sjögren's, IgG4-related disease should be considered and the medication list evaluated for offending agents.

Summing Up

Basic lab tests that evaluate liver health and function should be checked at least yearly in Sjögren's patients. It's not unusual to find liver-associated blood test abnormalities in Sjögren's patients. When noted, common causes should be considered, such as side effects from medications, HCV infection, and NAFLD. AIH and PBC, though infrequent, are the most common autoimmune liver manifestations in Sjögren's. When these are suspected, testing for anti-mitochondrial antibodies and anti-smooth muscle antibodies can help make the diagnosis. Occasionally, imaging and/or biopsy is required to confirm the diagnosis. Pancreatic involvement in Sjögren's is rare. In patients with symptoms of Sjögren's, the development of chronic pancreatitis suggests an underlying diagnosis of IgG4-related disease.

For Further Reading

Brito Zeron P, Retamozo S, Bove A, et al. Diagnosis of liver involvement in primary Sjogren syndrome. *J Clin Transl Hepatol.* 2013;1:94–102.

Ebert EC. Gastrointestinal and hepatic manifestations of Sjogren syndrome. *J Clin Gastroenterol.* 2012;46(1):25–30.

Selmi C, Generali E, Gershwin ME. Rheumatic manifestations in autoimmune liver disease. *Rheum Dis Clin North Am.* 2018;44:65–87.

39

Management of Kidney-Associated Involvement in Sjögren's

Daniel J. Wallace

The kidneys remove waste products from the blood and form urine. The prevalence of renal involvement in Sjögren's ranges from 5% to 15%, but with sophisticated studies that detect mild abnormalities it averages 27%. Box 39.1 lists the renal manifestations of Sjögren's. Patients present with hypertension, protein or blood in the urine, or abnormal renal blood tests. It is usually discovered at onset or in the first 10 years of disease.

Interstitial Nephritis

The most common kidney problem in patients with Sjögren's is inflammation of the tissue around the kidney filters (interstitial nephritis). Interstitial nephritis is found early in the disease and has a benign course. It generally causes mild deterioration in kidney function, manifested as a mild elevation in the plasma creatinine concentration. This usually requires no treatment, and progression to end-stage renal disease is rare.

When there is progressive deterioration of kidney function in a patient with Sjögren's, a kidney biopsy is often done. This involves taking a small piece of kidney tissue with a needle while the patient is awake but under local anesthesia. The tissue is examined under the microscope, and if the diagnosis of interstitial nephritis is made, a course of corticosteroids is given as treatment. Kidney function usually improves within a few weeks unless irreversible scarring in the kidneys has already occurred.

Interstitial nephritis can cause abnormalities in the kidney tubules, which are part of the kidney's filtering mechanism. One such abnormality is renal tubular acidosis (RTA), in which the kidney tubules cannot excrete acid in the urine. This can occur in up to 25% of patients with Sjögren's. As a result, the urine becomes more alkaline (high urine pH) and the blood becomes

Daniel J. Wallace, *Management of Kidney-Associated Involvement in Sjögren's* In: *The Sjögren's Book*. Edited by: Daniel J. Wallace, Oxford University Press. © Sjögren's Foundation 2022. DOI: 10.1093/oso/9780197502112.003.0039

Box 39.1 Renal Manifestations of Sjögren's

Tubulointerstitial nephritis
- Can be also due to infection, drugs, sarcoidosis, lymphoma, toxins

Renal tubular acidosis
- Distal RTA with hypokalemia and hypercalciuria is the most common
- Proximal RTA
- Rule out myeloma, monoclonal gammopathy, drugs, toxins, sarcoid, congenital metabolic diseases, sickle cell anemia, diabetes, obstructive nephropathy

Glomerulonephritis
- With or without cryoglobulinemia
- Consider lupus, vasculitis, IgG4 in overlap patients
- Rule out viral, bacterial, lymphoma

---

more acidic (low blood pH). This can lead to low levels of potassium in the blood and can give rise to kidney stones. Patients with RTA usually have no symptoms. Rarely, when the blood potassium level is very low, muscle weakness or even paralysis can occur. Also, recurrent pain in the loin area from kidney stones can sometimes be the presenting symptom. The treatment of RTA depends on its severity. If the potassium level is very low, then the patient is given potassium supplements. Alkaline agents (sodium bicarbonate) are given to correct the acidity of the blood to prevent the formation of renal stones.

Nephrogenic Diabetes Insipidus

Another rare abnormality of the renal tubules in Sjögren's is nephrogenic diabetes insipidus. In this condition the renal tubules become insensitive to the effects of anti-diuretic hormone and as a result cannot concentrate the urine. Patients with nephrogenic diabetes insipidus complain of thirst and of passing large amounts of urine frequently. The diagnosis is suspected if the urine remains dilute when the patient is deprived of water (when a normal person becomes dehydrated, the kidneys try to save water by concentrating the urine). Nephrogenic diabetes insipidus can be treated by a number of means, including the use of diuretics, nonsteroidal anti-inflammatory drugs (NSAIDs), and a low-salt, low-protein diet.

Glomerulonephritis

The glomeruli, which also form part of the kidney's filtering mechanism, are rarely affected in Sjögren's. Antibodies produced by the immune system sometimes become deposited on the glomeruli and cause inflammation (glomerulonephritis). As a result, the function of the kidneys deteriorates. This can be picked up on routine testing of a urine sample and by looking at the blood tests and observing a deterioration of kidney function. Symptoms include high blood pressure and leg swelling due to water retention (edema). Glomerulonephritis is rare in patients with Sjögren's and occurs mainly in patients who also have other overlapping conditions such as systemic lupus erythematosus, cryoglobulinemia (a condition whereby protein complexes circulating in the blood become deposited during cold weather), and vasculitis (inflammation of blood vessels). If left untreated, glomerulonephritis may lead to severe kidney failure. Therefore, in a patient with suspected glomerulonephritis, a kidney biopsy should be performed to confirm the diagnosis and assess the severity of the kidney disease. Treatment involves corticosteroids as well as other immunosuppressive drugs such as cyclophosphamide, mycophenolate mofetil, or rituximab.

Differential Diagnosis

When working up a patient, IgG4-associated diseases, sarcoidosis, amyloid, lymphoma, or overlap syndromes with features of scleroderma, vasculitis, or lupus also should be considered in the differential. Inflammation of the bladder (interstitial cystitis) can occur in patients with Sjögren's. The symptoms are frequent urination and pain in the lower abdomen over the bladder area.

Summing Up

Kidney involvement is clinically evident in about 10% of Sjögren's patients. Usually manifested as mild interstitial nephritis, some patients develop RTA and kidney stones. Fewer individuals have inflammation of the glomerulus and many have features that overlap with other autoimmune disorders. These patients warrant more aggressive management. All Sjögren's patients should have their renal function assessed with a urinalysis.

For Further Reading

Bossini N, Savoldi S, Franceschini F, et al. Clinical and morphological features of kidney involvement in primary Sjögren's syndrome. *Nephrol Dial Transplant.* 2001;16(12):2328–2336. doi:10.1093/ndt/16.12.2328

Francois H, Mariette X. Renal involvement in primary Sjogren syndrome. *Nature Rheumatol.* 2016;12:82–93.

Ren H, Wang WM, Chen XN, et al. Renal involvement and follow-up of 130 patients with primary Sjögren's syndrome. *J Rheumatol.* 2008;35(2):278–284.

40

Complementary, Alternative, and Integrative Approaches to Health in Sjögren's

Matthew Makara

Complementary and alternative approaches to health vary widely and may include lifestyle changes related to nutrition and physical or psychological activities—alone or in combination. While traditional medicine can often help treat, manage, or cure a disease, that is not always the case (as those with Sjögren's well know), and these approaches provide additional ways in which those living with Sjögren's, or any disease, can try to improve their quality of life. It is important to note up front that randomized controlled trials in Sjögren's have not been conducted in many of the approaches mentioned in this chapter, though current knowledge supports that these are generally safe to pursue. Additionally, not everyone who has a given disease (especially those with Sjögren's, who may experience a wide range of symptoms and limitations) will have the same ability to participate in or use the approaches discussed in this chapter. As has been suggested many places throughout this book, it is always important to inform and consult with your healthcare provider(s).

Defining the Terms

What are the differences between the terms *complementary*, *alternative*, and *integrative*? While similar, these terms should not be used interchangeably. To help shed light on the differences, we look to the National Center for Complementary and Integrative Health, a part of the U.S. National Institutes of Health. In brief:

- A *complementary* approach to health is a non-mainstream approach used together with conventional medicine.

Matthew Makara, *Complementary, Alternative, and Integrative Approaches to Health in Sjögren's* In: *The Sjögren's Book*. Edited by: Daniel J. Wallace, Oxford University Press. © Sjögren's Foundation 2022. DOI: 10.1093/oso/9780197502112.003.0040

- An *alternative* approach to health is a non-mainstream approach used in place of a conventional medical approach.
- An *integrative* approach to health incorporates both conventional and complementary approaches to health in a coordinated way. This approach emphasizes multimodal interventions and emphasizes treating the whole person.

Thus, it is not the approaches being referenced that differentiate these terms but rather how these approaches are used (or not used) in conjunction with more traditional medicine.

For the purpose of this chapter, and unless stated otherwise, the term *complementary* will be used to describe these approaches. When reading the literature on these topics, readers may also see the acronym CAM (complementary and alternative medicine).

Types of Complementary Therapies

The type of complementary therapies a person may use can generally fall into one of five categories (Table 40.1): alternative medical systems, nutrition, dietary supplements, movement and exercise, and mind–body medicine.

Alternative Medical Systems

A variety of alternative medical systems exist that readers may want to be familiar with. In the United States, there is a distinct branch of medicine known as osteopathic medicine, which emphasizes the interrelatedness of all body systems.

Naturopathic medicine is also a common practice in the United States and involves a variety of treatment approaches, including dietary and lifestyle

Table 40.1 Types of Complementary Therapies and Examples

Alternative medical systems	Chinese medicine, ayurvedic medicine
Mind–body interventions	Meditation
Biologically based treatments	Diets, herbs
Manipulative and body-based methods	Chiropractic, massage
Energy therapies	Reiki, therapeutic touch

changes, stress management, exercise therapy, and psychotherapy, among other things.

Chinese medicine, which consists of psychological, physical, and herbal approaches, has been studied in various disease groups with varying results. One meta-analysis of Chinese versus traditional Western medicine claimed superiority of Chinese medicine when looking at the effectiveness of treating Sjögren's. However, bias has been noted in many of these studies, so the claims being made should be taken with that in mind.

Ayurvedic medicine, which originated in India, relies on natural and ho-listic approaches to physical and mental health. This approach combines the use of plant products, and to a lesser degree animal, metal, and mineral products, with diet, exercise, and lifestyle changes. Little information exists on the safety and effectiveness of this system in the published literature as it relates to immune disease and Sjögren's, but we mention it here because it is a familiar result for those who may be searching for alternative medical systems.

Nutritional Approaches

Much of the food consumed in the Western world today is pro-inflammatory. Many common foods include or consist of refined sugars and carbohydrates and processed grains, all of which have pro-inflammatory qualities. Other foods with pro-inflammatory properties include red meats, dairy products, and eggs. (Of course, this is not an exhaustive list but rather some examples of things that many individuals consume on a regular basis.)

Taking this in the context of inflammatory diseases, including Sjögren's, we can see the potential benefits of our nutritional choices in disease management. While there is no Sjögren's-specific diet to date, and nutritional management in Sjögren's is not well studied, an anti-inflammatory approach to nutrition is often recommended.

So, what foods are suggested in an anti-inflammatory diet and why are they anti-inflammatory? Typically, components of an anti-inflammatory diet include an abundance of colorful vegetables and moderate amounts of fruits, minimally processed fats, olive oil, fatty fish, moderate intake of whole grains, and moderate meat consumption (Table 40.2). These types of food are considered anti-inflammatory for a variety of reasons, including:

- Foods in their natural state tend to have a carbohydrate, fat, and protein ratio that moderates fluctuations in blood sugar and minimizes pro-inflammatory insulin surges.

Table 40.2 Components of an Anti-Inflammatory Diet and Examples

Plant-based	Fruits and vegetables
Minimally processed whole foods	Fruits and vegetables
High in anti-inflammatory fats	Avocado; olive and coconut oils
Moderate free-range/organic meat	Poultry, bison
Moderate in whole grains	Whole wheat bread, oatmeal
Low in food additives	Artificial sweeteners, high-fructose corn syrup
Low in common food allergens	Eggs, wheat
Low in refined oils	Vegetable oil, margarine

- Minimally processed foods naturally have fewer additives that can pose an antigenic load on the immune system.
- Focusing on these foods eliminates many common pro-inflammatory allergens.
- There is a higher nutrient content of vitamins, minerals, and phytonutrients.
- There are more essential fats, which are naturally anti-inflammatory.

Products containing alcohol and caffeine can also exacerbate symptoms of oral dryness, so limiting their use may be helpful in that regard.

The Mediterranean diet, which includes many anti-inflammatory foods (e.g., avocado, salmon, olive oil), was recently found to be associated with a lower likelihood of having Sjögren's. The 2020 study by Machowicz et al. noted that fish intake had the highest correlation with reduced inflammation.

Dietary Supplements

Supplements can provide nutrients that are deficient in an individual's normal diet. While few studies exist, a variety of nutrients have been found to be deficient in patients with Sjögren's; supplementation may be beneficial for these nutrients.

Vitamin D helps to regulate calcium and phosphate within our bodies, and deficiencies have been associated with an increased risk of developing autoimmune diseases. Up to 30% of Sjögren's patients are believed to be deficient in vitamin D, and this deficiency is associated with extraglandular manifestations of Sjögren's, including lymphoma. Chapter 41 of this book is dedicated solely to the topic of vitamin D, including the recommended consumption.

Omega-3 fatty acids are highly beneficial to health and have been studied in relation to joint pain and dry eye. One recent study that readers may be familiar with in connection to dry eye from the Dry Eye Assessment and Management (DREAM) group compared omega-3s to a placebo (olive oil) to gauge the effectiveness in reducing the signs and symptoms of dry eye. While this study showed that the impact of omega-3s was comparable to that of the placebo, it is important to note that this did not mean omega-3s were not effective; rather, the investigators found that both were effective and a majority of patients did see improvement, so their continued use should still be considered. Omega-3s have been used as a longstanding supplement for those suffering from dry eye and are available in fish oil capsules.

Other nutrients that have been found to be deficient in patients with Sjögren's, and that should be considered for supplementation, include:

- Vitamin A: an important nutrient for vision, immune system health, and reproductive and organ health
- Vitamin B$_{12}$: an important nutrient for blood and nervous system health; contributes to DNA synthesis
- Folic acid: a B vitamin important to the formation of new cells
- Iron: a mineral that aids in growth and development

To address a variety of deficiencies, multivitamins are often recommended and used as a broad-spectrum approach. Particularly for those living with autoimmune disease, it is important to be aware of any additives, fillers, binders, or colorings that may be added to these (or any other) supplements.

While further study is needed as it relates to nutrition, supplementation, and Sjögren's, the recent work into these areas is encouraging, and coupled with our increasing knowledge on the microbiome (see Chapter 9), it is not a far-fetched thought that we could soon have a Sjögren's-specific diet.

Movement and Exercise

Regular exercise is known to be one of the best ways to prevent and manage many different health conditions and is generally considered beneficial for a multitude of reasons (Table 40.3). Of course, those who are suffering from a

Table 40.3 Effects of Moderate Exercise

Improvements in:	Aerobic capacity
	Joint mobility
	Balance
	Muscle mass
Reductions in:	Fatigue
	Depression
	Anxiety
	Blood pressure
	Cholesterol
	Body fat

given health condition may be hindered in their ability to participate in physical activity. This is, of course, true in many of those with Sjögren's.

People with Sjögren's have diminished cardiovascular conditioning (aerobic capacity), stamina, and joint mobility. They also are impaired significantly by fatigue, anxiety, and depression. In 2007, Strömbeck et al. studied over 50 people with Sjögren's compared to age-matched control subjects and measured their baseline aerobic conditioning by stress testing; their mobility, balance, and stamina by standardized tests; and fatigue, anxiety, and depression by self-administered questionnaires. Compared to control subjects, aerobic capacity was reduced by 11% in Sjögren's, the equivalent of adding 10 years onto a person's age. There was also a significant increase in fatigue, depression, and anxiety. The researchers estimated that nearly 50% of the fatigue experienced by Sjögren's patients was due to a combination of poor aerobic capacity, reduced functional abilities, and depression.

Since fatigue is a dominant problem in Sjögren's, exercise to improve aerobic capacity would be expected to improve fatigue. This has been confirmed through a variety of studies, including one that evaluated the safety and effectiveness of a supervised walking program in patients with Sjögren's; improvements were found in aerobic fitness, tolerance for exercise, fatigue, and the patient's perception of improvement. An earlier study noted significant differences in aerobic capacity, fatigue, and other factors between those who participated in a walking program versus those who did not.

Anaerobic exercise is also recommended. Commonly, resistance training falls into this category as the exercises, though more intense at times, are performed for a shorter duration, do not require oxygen, and break down glucose for energy. A study investigating the effectiveness of a supervised resistance-training exercise program in functional fitness in patients with Sjögren's saw an increase in functional capacity and overall quality of life.

Exercise is strongly recommended in the Sjögren's Foundation treatment guidelines (Carsons et al., 2017). Developing an exercise plan with a qualified health professional is recommended. A combination of aerobic, anaerobic, and balance exercises can be beneficial to both Sjögren's-related and general health.

Mind–Body Interventions

Mind–body interventions are based in the belief that our mental and emotional state impacts our physical health. Examples include acupuncture, massage, mindfulness, meditation, and yoga, among others. As with most other topics noted in this chapter, little formal research has been done in the context of Sjögren's, but the concepts will be introduced for the reader's consideration.

Mindfulness is the concept of being fully present and aware of an experience in a given moment. Conversely, meditation is the practice of being aware of and finding peace within. These concepts have been studied in autoimmune disease populations, including Sjögren's, with positive results. See Chapter 43 for detailed coverage of this and other topics, including guidance for incorporating the practice.

Acupuncture, which is often associated with Chinese medicine, involves inserting thin metallic needles into the skin, which are then activated through movement or electrical stimulation. Acupuncture is widely used and has been found to be beneficial in a variety of conditions, including nausea, headache, fibromyalgia, osteoarthritis, and lower back pain.

Yoga and tai chi are two other practices that incorporate both physical and mental aspects and from which Sjögren's patients may benefit. These gentle forms of exercise can help with relaxation, fatigue, and joint pain and can be scaled to the user's ability to perform the movements. No equipment is needed and an individual can participate in a group or on their own, in nearly any setting.

Choosing a Complementary or Alternative Care Provider

When choosing to use complementary medicine, many patients feel they are faced with an "either/or" choice of working with their conventional medical doctor or choosing an alternative practitioner. This is unfortunate, since complementary medicine should not limit the care available but rather provide additional options for patients. Ideally, patients should be actively involved in their care and seek out conventional and alternative practitioners who are open to working with each other.

Finding an alternative medical provider can be challenging since their training, experience, and certification and their familiarity with the therapies may vary considerably. Here are some basic questions that can help your selection. Recommendations from your current physician can also provide additional guidance.

Questions to ask of an alternative medical physician or provider:

1. Do they have a current license recognized by the ruling state/national agency or jurisdiction?
2. Have they graduated with a degree from a recognized institution?
3. Do they carry malpractice insurance? This typically provides an additional level of verification of professional credentials.
4. Are they a member in good standing of their professional organization? Does their organization have a process of self-regulation and ethical codes that would warrant a practitioner's removal if not adhered to?
5. Is their practice facility and manner professional?
6. Do they provide diagnoses, treatment plans, and reasonable expectation of results and side effects?
7. Do they keep accurate records and are they willing to share them with other providers?
8. Are they willing to suggest second opinions to assess their care and judgment of your health condition?

It is not easy to choose a new healthcare provider, traditional or alternative. Therefore, a careful medical consumer should obtain advice from multiple trusted sources, such as current medical providers, family, friends, and certifying organizations, in order to make the best possible decisions.

Summing Up

For a more holistic approach to health, people often incorporate non-mainstream or nontraditional approaches in hopes of achieving a better quality of life. These approaches can complement traditional medical treatment (complementary health), replace traditional treatment (alternative health), or be used in a coordinated fashion (integrated health) toward achieving these goals.

Examples of these nontraditional approaches include nutritional changes (including supplementation), mind–body techniques, and exercise and body-based methods. In Sjögren's and other autoimmune disease populations, a relatively limited body of research is available, but as our understanding of the disease continues to increase, there is reason to be optimistic that a more precise approach and guidance will be available to manage the many complications of Sjögren's.

For Further Reading

Asbell PA, Maguire MG, Peskin E, et al. Dry Eye Assessment and Management (DREAM©) study: Study design and baseline characteristics. *Contemp Clin Trials*. 2018;71:70–79.

Carsons SE, Vivino FB, Parke A, et al. Treatment guidelines for rheumatologic manifestations of Sjögren's: Use of biologic agents, management of fatigue, and inflammatory musculoskeletal pain. *Arthritis Care Res*. 2017;69(4):517–527.

Geneen LJ, Moore RA, Clarke C, et al. Physical activity and exercise for chronic pain in adults: An overview of Cochrane reviews. *Cochrane Database Syst Rev* 2017;1(1):CD011279.

Machowicz A, Hall I, de Pablo P, et al. Mediterranean diet and risk of Sjögren's syndrome. *Clin Exp Rheumatol*. 2020;38 Suppl 126(4):216–221.

Minali PA, Pimentel C, de Mello MT, et al. Effectiveness of resistance exercise in functional fitness in women with primary Sjögren's syndrome: Randomized clinical trial. *Scand J Rheumatol*. 2020;49(1):47–56. doi:10.1080/03009742.2019.1602880

National Center for Complementary and Integrative Health. Complementary, alternative, or integrative health: What's in a name? https://www.nccih.nih.gov/health/complementary-alternative-or-integrative-health-whats-in-a-name

Sjögren's Foundation. Conquering Sjögren's Blog. Nutrition to Improve Symptoms of Sjögren's. https://www.sjogrens.org/blog/2021/nutrition-to-improve-symptoms-of-sjogrens

Strömbeck BE, Theander E, Jacobsson LTH. Effects of exercise on aerobic capacity and fatigue in women with primary Sjögren's syndrome. *Rheumatology*. 2007;46(5):868–871.

Wouters EJ, van Leeuwen N, Bossema ER, et al. Physical activity and physical activity cognitions are potential factors maintaining fatigue in patients with primary Sjögren's syndrome. *Ann Rheum Dis*. 2012 May;71(5):668–673.

41

Vitamin D and Sjögren's

Jeffrey W. Wilson

In the past, vitamin D deficiency was associated primarily with metabolic bone disease. Deficiency caused rickets in children and softening of bone (osteomalacia) in adults. These patients presented with diffuse severe skeletal pain and often muscle weakness. Osteoporosis has received greater attention with the development of tests to assess bone strength and medicines to treat the disorder. Bone mass normally begins to decrease from peak levels after 30 years of age. This is an asymptomatic process unless osteoporotic (fragility) fractures occur. Bone density studies and the Fracture Risk Assessment Tool (FRAX) allow physicians to predict osteoporotic fracture risk and intervene with calcium, vitamin D, and medicines such as bisphosphonates, denosumab, teriparatide, and, more recently, romosozumab.

Until 2007 the normal range for 25-hydroxyvitamin D was considered to be 8 to 50 ng/mL. This prior standard accounted for an underestimation of vitamin D deficiency and insufficiency. The accepted normal range now is 32 to 100 ng/mL. While less than 32 ng/mL indicates deficiency, the wide disparity between the past and present normal ranges for vitamin D makes it difficult to define which vitamin D level represents insufficiency or optimal replacement.

For the Sjögren's patient, as with our general patient population, vitamin D is increasingly important. In addition to its role in treating osteoporosis with special consideration for Sjögren's patients taking corticosteroids or with associated autoimmune liver disease (primary biliary cirrhosis), vitamin D is also mentioned as a possible treatment for the arthralgias and fatigue seen so commonly in Sjögren's patients.

A 2003 article by Plotnikoff and Quigley related low vitamin D levels to persistent, nonspecific musculoskeletal pain and prompted us to check vitamin D levels in all our patients. The findings were in line with subsequent review articles by Holick in 2006 and 2007. Vitamin D deficiency is common, affecting over 70% of our general patient population, including our Sjögren's patients.

The reviews and subsequent investigations involve a wide array of diseases possibly associated with vitamin D deficiency, including many forms of

Jeffrey W. Wilson, *Vitamin D and Sjögren's* In: *The Sjögren's Book.* Edited by: Daniel J. Wallace, Oxford University Press.
© Sjögren's Foundation 2022. DOI: 10.1093/oso/9780197502112.003.0041

cancer, cardiovascular disease, multiple sclerosis, type 1 diabetes, psoriasis, and autoimmune disorders such as lupus and rheumatoid arthritis. How could vitamin D be related to so many varied illnesses? Some researchers feel it should be considered a hormone rather than a vitamin. "Vitamin" is derived from "vital amine" and implies something from exogenous sources; it is not manufactured by our bodies. This is clearly different for vitamin D, which is produced by the skin in response to sun exposure. The discovery that most cells and tissues have vitamin D receptors and respond to the active form of vitamin D (1,25-dihydroxyvitamin D) suggests that the biological functions of vitamin D extend far beyond those of calcium homeostasis and bone health.

Diagnosis

The diagnosis is made by a blood test checking the 25-hydroxyvitamin D level (*not* the 1,25-dihydroxyvitamin D level, which is of limited usefulness). While levels less than 32 ng/mL define vitamin D deficiency, it is less clear what constitutes insufficiency. What is a target goal of therapy? It should be no surprise after 50 years of considering deficiency to be less than 8 ng/mL that the optimal level is not clearly defined. A level of 50 to 60 ng/mL is the goal of our treatment. How do we achieve that?

Treatment

The treatment regimen includes a prescription for 50,000 IU of vitamin D_2 (ergocalciferol) weekly, with 2,000 IU of over-the-counter vitamin D_3 (cholecalciferol) daily (including the day that the 50,000 IU of D_2 is taken) for 8 to 12 weeks. A follow-up 25-hydroxyvitamin D level is checked at that time and adjustments are made in the regimen. The most common maintenance regimen is 50,000 IU of D_2 every other week (we have our patients take it on the first and fifteenth day of the month to facilitate compliance) and 2,000 IU of D_3 daily. Vitamin D levels are then checked every 6 months.

Maintenance regimens, however, vary greatly. Most of our lupus patients have very low initial levels—often less than 7 ng/mL (with little difference according to race). Some of them require 50,000 IU of D_2 every Monday and every Thursday, with 5,000 IU D_3 daily. On the other hand, an older patient with osteoarthritis may need only 50,000 IU of D_2 monthly or 2,000 IU of D_3 daily. The only way to determine the proper regimen is with follow-up testing.

Frequently family members present with similar initial vitamin D levels and end up requiring similar subsequent maintenance regimens. This suggests a role of pharmacogenetics in some cases (Wang et al., 2010).

Toxicity

With such widely varying treatment regimens, there is concern about possible vitamin D toxicity. However, this is extremely rare and relates to the effect of the vitamin D supplementation on the patient's serum calcium level. A 2015 article by Holick suggests that daily vitamin D_2 doses of 50,000 IU for 3 or more months would be required to produce toxic levels. For example, a 93-year-old nursing home patient who was taking that exact regimen (50,000 IU D_2 daily for 3 months) due to an error on the admission orders was evaluated at our office. Her 25-hydroxyvitamin D level was 144 ng/mL (the highest I had seen), but her calcium level was normal and she had no signs or symptoms of hypercalcemia. In our practice, hypercalcemia is most often related to a developing cancer (usually breast or lung cancer) or hyperparathyroidism.

Other Features of Vitamin D Treatment

Patients on vitamin D supplementation often notice that their hair, fingernails, and toenails grow faster. There is frequently a subjective increase in strength and energy. Several patients report fewer seasonal allergy symptoms and less frequent cold and flu episodes. Long-term studies in the future will be required to determine if the hoped-for decreases in the incidence of associated cancers or cardiovascular events are realized.

Sjögren's Lessons

Are there special considerations regarding vitamin D supplementation and the Sjögren's patient? The following case history is instructive.

My 56-year-old White female patient had been followed since 1994 with a history of Sjögren's. Her 25-hydroxyvitamin D levels were normal in 2003 (43 ng/mL) and 2004 (37 ng/mL), but the level in November 2005 was less than 4 ng/mL. For more than 25 years the patient had been diagnosed with irritable bowel syndrome. Subsequent testing included a tissue transglutaminase IgA level of more than 250 U (normal 0–30 U), and a small bowel biopsy confirmed the diagnosis of celiac disease. Her clinical symptoms of "irritable bowel syndrome" resolved with the usual dietary modifications for celiac disease.

Her story reminds us that our patients are dynamic and more prone to other autoimmune diseases, and their vitamin D level should be followed at least yearly. It also suggests that, especially in our Sjögren's patients, we need to remain vigilant for the development of other autoimmune diseases, such as hypothyroidism, B_{12} deficiency, and celiac disease.

The antimalarial drug hydroxychloroquine (Plaquenil) is a frequent part of the treatment regimen for lupus and Sjögren's patients. In our experience, vitamin D supplementation often allows the usual dose of Plaquenil to be reduced from 200 mg twice per day to 200 mg once per day without worsening in sicca or other Sjögren's-related symptoms, such as arthralgias. This not only can save money but also decreases the potential for ocular toxicity.

The Future

A 2007 article by Bizarro et al. raises some hopeful considerations for the future. The authors write:

> The capability of prediction will be valuable only if preventive measures can be adopted. Knowledge is accumulating to recommend an avoidance of exposure to ultraviolet light, specific diet, avoidance of specific chemicals (silica, mercury, toxic oil and the like), use of specific contraceptives or vaccines, and, based on animal studies, administration of vitamin D.

For the patient with Sjögren's, beyond the general benefits of vitamin D, will supplementation prevent the development of other autoimmune manifestations such as B_{12} deficiency, Addison's disease, celiac disease, or hypothyroidism? With an appreciation of the familial tendency for these illnesses, perhaps there is a more intriguing question for the future: If other family members are deficient in vitamin D, will vitamin D supplementation help prevent Sjögren's or other autoimmune diseases from developing? I encourage my vitamin D–deficient patients to be the champion in their family and arrange vitamin D testing for children and relatives.

Summing Up

While there have been no well-designed studies specifically looking at the role of vitamin D in Sjögren's, a large number of patients with rheumatoid arthritis, lupus, and scleroderma have vitamin D deficiency. Up to 30% of them have Sjögren's as well. Sjögren's patients should have 25-hydroxyvitamin D levels checked yearly, with vitamin D supplementation when levels are low. Vitamin D insufficiency may be associated with musculoskeletal pain and increased disease activity.

For Further Reading

Bizarro N, Tazzoli, R, Shoenfeld Y. Are we at a stage to predict autoimmune rheumatic diseases? *Arthritis Rheumatol.* 2007;56:1736–1744.

Holick MF. High prevalence of vitamin D inadequacy and implications for health. *Mayo Clin Proc.* 2006;81:353–373.

Holick MF. Vitamin D deficiency. *N Engl J Med.* 2007;357:266–281.

Holick MF. Vitamin D is not as toxic as was once thought: A historical and an up-to-date perspective. *Mayo Clin Proc.* 2015;90:561–563.

Plotnikoff GA, Quigley JM. Prevalence of severe hypovitaminosis D in patients with persistent, nonspecific musculoskeletal pain. *Mayo Clin Proc.* 2003;78:1463–1470.

Wang TJ, Zhang F, Richards JB, et al. Common genetic determinants of vitamin D insufficiency: A genome-wide association study. *Lancet.* 2010;376:180–188.

PART VI
TAKING CHARGE OF YOUR SJÖGREN'S

42

Sjögren's

The Self and Others

Teri P. Rumpf and Lynn C. Epstein

> *Chronic*: Of an illness lasting for a long time. Persisting or constantly
> recurring, as opposed to acute.
>
> **Oxford English Dictionary, 2018, online edition**

Chronic Versus Acute Illness

Until you have one, living with a chronic disease is difficult to imagine.
Sjögren's means having an illness that may relapse and remit but is chronic.
Healthy people are occasionally sick, generally well.

We tend to think of most episodes of illness as acute or, if it recurs, as intermittent. We get sick, the episode ends, we get better. The constant and recurrent nature of a chronic illness is completely different. It gets better and worse
but is always there; sometimes foreground, sometimes background, permanently present.

An understanding of what chronicity means comes slowly, with the passage
of time, and this awareness is different for each person. Signs and symptoms
of Sjögren's may initially be regarded independently—that is, dry eyes unrelated to dry mouth and further unrelated to frequent infections, joint pain, or
fatigue. Multiple medical specialists treat the problems of Sjögren's, and it is
often not until months or years have gone by that someone thinks about putting them together as a unified disease entity. Since the diagnosis of Sjögren's
takes time, an individual is left wondering, "What's wrong with me?" Even
before Sjögren's is diagnosed, this increase in uncertainty generates an intensified level of stress. Unlike an acute illness with obvious manifestations,
Sjögren's is both invisible and unpredictable, which creates stressful obstacles
for those who have it.

Once the diagnosis is made, more questions follow. Is the diagnosis definitive? What do these symptoms mean for me? Is this it? Will things ever get

Teri P. Rumpf and Lynn C. Epstein, *Sjögren's* In: *The Sjögren's Book*. Edited by: Daniel J. Wallace, Oxford University Press.
© Sjögren's Foundation 2022. DOI: 10.1093/oso/9780197502112.003.0042

better again, or will they get worse? When symptoms are minimal, the illness seems to recede. Life goes on almost as before—but perhaps not quite. When there is a flare or something acute occurs, Sjögren's takes over, perhaps to the point where life occurs around it. Emotions fluctuate, with more emotional discomfort when the disease flares and less when it diminishes.

A diagnosis may be received with a mixture of both relief and anxiety. There is relief that someone knows what is wrong and also dismay that this seemingly disparate compendium of symptoms is an actual disease with a name. Individuals simultaneously experience relief that the disease is not all in their head and alarm that Sjögren's is real and that they must live with it. A sense of chronicity and the diagnosis of a disease are different, but with diagnosis, a shift in comprehension begins. Recognition of chronicity occurs at whatever point a person realizes that their medical problems represent an illness, and the illness is not going to go away. Changes in awareness can then begin to emerge: "If I do too much one day, I will pay for it the next. Stress makes things worse. I am tired. I cannot do what I used to do. I have to pace myself differently." For some, the perception is quick, almost immediate; for others, it takes years to fully comprehend.

Individuals and their families ask additional questions: What will happen to me? How will I be able to cope? How can I continue to work, be a parent, multitask, take care of myself and perhaps others? How can I live my life as I have been living it? What if I cannot? What if we as a family cannot continue because of this illness? Does Sjögren's change the way I see myself or the way others see me? Can I be the vital, effective person I was before Sjögren's? What does the future hold? One person, interviewed by one of the authors, remembers asking herself constantly: "What do I do now? What am I supposed to do now? How can I get through this?" for a number of years after she was diagnosed. The question faded with the passage of time, but only after years of living with the illness had passed and many adjustments and adaptations had been made.

The time of life at which diagnosis occurs makes a difference in terms of life tasks, stressors, and relationships. Traditionally, Sjögren's has been described as a disease of middle age, but increased awareness and better diagnostic methods have led to the disease being increasingly identified in younger people. In her 2018 book *Invisible*, Hirsch describes issues particular to young people with significant health issues that set them apart from their peers. With youth, she says, there is the expectation of unlimited energy and a body that functions perfectly. With a chronic disease, there is often the absence of both. There are issues of separation and independence. Life choices, distance from family, and where to live, work, or go to school may all have to be modified because of the disease.

Stress and Sjögren's

Ever since the work of Hans Selye in the 1930s, we have understood that there are different kinds of stress and that stress in the body affects the mind and vice versa. Many years of research have documented this strong connection between the mind and body. Hafen et al. (1996), offer an excellent description of the stress response. They describe three distinct kinds of stress: physical, psychological, and psychosocial:

- Physical stressors may be in the environment or the body, such as noise, physical discomfort, injury, inflammation, or illness.
- Psychological stressors include both reactions to real events and events perceived as real and that usually carry some level of threat.
- Psychosocial stress involves relationships with family, friends, employers, and spouses or partners. Psychosocial stress may result from interactions with others, but it may also be the result of isolation from others.

Van Houtem et al. (2015) note that "being chronically ill is a continuous process of balancing the demands of the illness and the demands of everyday life." They find that stress arises from basic life problems, including finances, housing, work and social problems, such as relationships with children, friends and a partner, sex and leisure pursuits. To these, we would add a separate category of stress: being immersed in the medical system, which includes everything from long waits for appointments; having to schedule a doctor's visit at an inconvenient time; waiting for lab or test results that may be indicative of further disease or inconclusive; or having an interview with an unsympathetic physician. The medical system all too frequently lacks the ability to deal with the "human side" of illness and fails to recognize the physical and emotional toll that an illness takes on both the patient and the family.

The stresses and uncertainty of a chronic illness evoke a variety of emotions: sadness, anxiety, loss, demoralization, confusion, and the frustration of not being able to do things as before. The losses are real, and it is natural to react to them. The line between being able to cope and not cope is often quite thin. A single experience may be all that's needed to push a patient too far—for example, a physician who doesn't believe a person's set of symptoms or experiences, or a family member who instead of being supportive is judgmental or indifferent. How people react to stress and their illness is a function of their life histories and personal circumstances, of who they are and what is going on in their lives.

What do Sjögren's patients have to say about living with their illness? In a 2016 survey conducted by the Harris Poll on behalf of the Sjögren's Foundation, in addition to dry eyes and dry mouth, the majority of patients surveyed experienced fatigue, joint pain, trouble sleeping, difficulty thinking, forgetfulness, and brain fog. Interestingly, those newly diagnosed (0–4 years) felt that their overall mood had been negatively affected to a greater extent than those who had been diagnosed 5 to 9 years previously. One hypothesis for this is that the initial stages of the disease present more challenges and require the most adaptation. However, we emphasize that adaptation is required throughout the course of living with Sjögren's. Chapter 4 provides more specific information from this survey and the many ways in which patients are impacted.

Emotions occur on a continuum from manageable to overwhelming, from grief and loss to clinical depression. States of clinical anxiety and depression may be part of a biological response to a stressful reality or may be part of the disease itself. They may be fluctuating, transitory, or enduring. When necessary, medication can be helpful. Antidepressants may do double duty since they are often used in the treatment of chronic pain. People cope, but not always consistently: "Chronically ill people struggle to cope day-by-day, as do their families and health practitioners. We cope well on Tuesday, badly on Wednesday morning, better Wednesday afternoon" (Kleinman, 1988, p. 144). Resilience and the ability to cope mean being able to develop new strategies and learn new ways of being in the world.

Illness and the Self

What does living with a chronic illness do to an individual's sense of self? While the answer to this question depends on many variables (e.g., age, personality, family structure, illness severity, energy level, finances, coping style, resiliency, support system), it is certain that it will affect at least some if not all of these aspects of living.

Among the extensive and eloquent literature on illness and the self, Frank's 1991 book *At the Will of the Body* stands out. Having had experiences at an early age with both a heart attack and cancer, he notes that "Being ill is just another way of living, but by the time we have lived through illness we are living differently" (p. 3). Disease is what the doctor sees, what the laboratory measures. "Illness is the experience of living through disease. If disease talk measures the body, illness talk measures the fear and frustration of living inside a body that is breaking down" (Frank, 1991, p. 13).

Charmaz (1991) describes people who define their illness in terms of a series of temporary crises. This implies full recovery and may present an alternative way of viewing and coping with having a chronic disease. Without chronicity, individuals can assume that except for these "illness episodes," they can continue to think of themselves as healthy and able-bodied, or at least relatively so. Charmaz, whose book is entitled *Good Days, Bad Days*, says that a good day is one with "minimal intrusiveness of illness, maximal control over mind, body and actions, and a greater choice of activities. . . . A bad day means intensified intrusiveness of illness . . . and limited choices about activities. Illness and regimen take center stage" (pp. 50–51). Bad days mean changes of plans, revisions of activities and expectations. With repeated or frequent bad days, an individual's sense of what they can expect of themselves begins to change.

Years ago, one respondent told one of the authors:

The two major emotions that come to mind when I'm asked about what it's like to live with Sjögren's are frustration and a sense of loss, which tend to intertwine. There's the reality of continually needing to reinvent myself as I decline physically, but at the same time trying desperately to hold on to my former self. It seems like a constant struggle, and there are times when the urge to abandon those activities that I love but lack the energy for creeps into my brain. For now, it comes in spurts of moments or days, but the need to hold on to as much as I can eventually wins out over those urges. I feel like I'm living on the edge of a precipice, wondering what will be the next symptom to put me out of action.

There have been many losses both large and small: the loss of a career, the inability to be physically active . . . the lack of energy to do things spontaneously, little everyday things that used to be taken for granted . . . Thankfully, I am a resilient person and that is what keeps me going, keeps me trying to be active in the things that matter most to me. Each day is a compromise of what I'd like to do and what I can do. I have never been a quitter, always someone managing to rethink my goals, adapt my lifestyle around the barriers that Sjögren's creates . . . I impatiently wait for better treatments and perhaps, eventually, a cure. (personal communications with T. Rumpf, 2011)

Eight years later (2018), she has had to make further adjustments but continues to do well. It is important to note the indications of resilience in this individual. She feels the limitations of her illness but struggles to hold on to what she considers important in her life. She considers herself resilient. There are threats from the illness, but she can meet them. She acknowledges the compromises she is forced to make, but she prioritizes, adapts, and gets by. She looks to the future. It is worth noting that this respondent was of middle age, with a stable family situation and adequate finances. When life circumstances are challenging, individuals have more difficulty meeting the stresses presented by the disease.

Hirsch (2018) uses the expression "off time" to describe the feeling of having a body that is out of sync with her young, healthy peers. Her peers are not concerned about making and attending multiple doctors' appointments and pacing their life. They can do something spontaneously with friends without having to pay a serious price for it the next day. Hirsch details how she walks a tightrope between fitting in and taking care of herself. That kind of daily adaptation is both exhausting and "off time." Her book paints a vivid picture of the lengths people will go to in order to fit in, and how fearful they are of being negatively judged by physical limitations they cannot control.

At any age, a chronic illness creates multiple stresses related to identity, but this is especially true for young people, who are in the process of forming adult identities. Plans need to be changed or deferred and must be adapted to the illness. While sometimes these adaptions are fortuitous, it is problematic to be in a situation where your peers can work 60 hours a week and still go out on the weekends when you cannot. A process of grieving for the loss of the healthy self may occur, although it is not always perceived as such or given that name.

The issue of authenticity is not limited to any particular age group. Frank notes that society praises people who are ill with words like "courageous, optimistic and cheerful" (1991, p. 64). But what about when none of those feelings are present? Authenticity is tied to disclosure: How much should I pretend? How much should I reveal? How disturbing is it to be different from my peers, and what are the consequences of making those differences known? Many who have Sjögren's look better than they feel. Therefore, it is possible to pretend to be well, even to the extent, as Hirsch describes, of harming oneself in the process. Pretending is stressful. For a limited time, it may be less stressful than disclosing the truth about one's illness and disability, but not always. Sometimes these consequences of disclosure can be severe, such as when the person finds their job "eliminated" or transferred to someone else.

Illness and Relationships

Biological changes affect relationships. Family and friends may not understand why a patient no longer functions as they used to. A person who suffers from severe fatigue may not feel like participating in an event, since it takes all of their energy just to arrive at the activity and they become exhausted even before they begin to participate. It can also be difficult for friends and relatives to appreciate the disparity between the way a person looks and feels. Unlike better-known diseases or acute medical crises, with Sjögren's, assistance and support may not be forthcoming. Patients are often reluctant to request help until circumstances become extreme and they are forced to ask. Their need for help may pass unnoticed. Asking for help takes the disease from the private into the public realm and represents an admission that "I am not able to handle this on my own." Not asking for help may make personal suffering seem invisible.

The revelation of illness carries the risk of being judged, stigmatized, or, even worse, abandoned. Having an illness that is largely invisible creates a choice. People can choose not to disclose, but at a certain point they are forced to confront and explain their limitations. As long as disclosure is a choice, individuals may feel that they are able to control the way the illness interacts with their life and with the way they interact with the world (Charmaz, 1991). Once the illness shifts from the private to the public domain, there is the risk that the illness becomes a prevailing factor in the way they are perceived by others. As Charmaz points out, "Most men and women want to be known for attributes other than illness" (1991, p. 113). Indeed they do, and the more extensive and pervasive the illness, the more it impinges on their identity and requires increased efforts to adapt to its demands.

Wall writes about living with fibromyalgia:

> Passing as a well person can be an act of self-preservation, allowing dignity, control and a chance to maintain a pre-illness identity, often vital to one's sense of self. . . . And, depending on how ill you are, it can be folly, exacting a cruel price. (2005, p. 13)

Once an illness is made known, the fact that it exists cannot be withdrawn.

Other people's reactions can either help or hinder an individual's ability to cope, so much so that the extent of the disease may not matter as much as the level of support. In unpublished research with breast cancer patients, one of the authors found that patients who have at least one friend or family member with whom they could communicate unreservedly were less depressed than those who lacked such a relationship (Rumpf, 1980). When friends and family don't know what to say, they often do or say nothing, even if their intentions are kind. Alternatively, they can be critical or judgmental, assuming that the disease is the result of not taking care of oneself or engaging in some form of harmful living (Sontag, 1977).

Criticism in the guise of being helpful is neither supportive nor useful for the person with the disease. Johnson and Webster (2002) note that people with chronic or debilitating illnesses are forced to live with their illness and their hopes and fears on a daily basis. In the best of all possible worlds, there are people willing to support them, and this support in turn improves and helps maintain their quality of life. However, they note that sometimes little or no support exists. Social isolation is one of the very real consequences of an illness such as Sjögren's. The indifference of others can be painfully demoralizing. By isolating themselves, individuals retain a certain amount of control, but at the cost of being separated from others.

In a marriage or partnership, the limitations of chronic illness can destabilize longstanding relationship patterns. For those who are not part of a couple, finding a partner willing to accept these limitations may be even more difficult. Some people offer emotional support but cannot help with tasks of daily living, while the reverse is true for others—say, they can bring in the groceries but are no help during an emotionally laden crisis. Most people need emotional as well as instrumental support at various times. Even those who basically have both may not always have support available. Caretakers need support and in the course of a long marriage or relationship, it is possible that circumstances change and roles switch and it is the caretaker who needs to be cared for.

The internet has facilitated communication among a wide variety of patient groups. People with Sjögren's now have access to information and each other in ways formerly unimaginable, even if they are separated by geography and age. Support groups are available both in person and online and help diminish isolation. Being able to compare notes with others about symptoms and treatments offers the sense that there are other people dealing with similar issues and provides information about what to ask about with regards to medical problems. When looking around the room in a Sjögren's support group meeting, these authors saw a collection of remarkably normal-looking people, so much so that it was impossible to differentiate those who had the disease from those who were accompanying spouses or friends.

The Role of Doctors, the Medical System, and Finding a New Normal

A relationship with a medical professional is like any other: Sometimes the personalities involved work well together and sometimes they don't. The doctor–patient relationship is extremely powerful in its ability to help or hurt. Without any other intervention, a relationship with a physician may heal because it allows the patient to share the burden of the illness, and it offers hope. In contrast, a physician who is cold or unkind has great power to hurt. Physicians can validate the changes in patients' lives and encourage them to take steps that maximize a sense of well-being. Alternatively, for patients who feel overly immersed in the medical system and who have limited energy, it can feel as if living is what takes place in between doctors' appointments.

Physician styles vary: They can be collaborative, authoritarian, interrogative, formal, informal, and paternalistic—or some combination of these. The physician's own personality influences his or her style and communication with patients. It is important that there be a match between patient and physician. A physician who makes a patient uncomfortable is not likely to heal. Choice of physicians is sometimes limited by geography or by insurance plans. Patients should be encouraged to find a physician they can work with, but if this is not possible they should prepare for their appointments and be as specific as they can with regard to what they need.

The use of the word "heal" in the previous paragraph is deliberate. Sjögren's is a disease that cannot be cured, but patients can be healed to the extent that they can go on with life despite the intrusions and accommodations demanded by the disease. As Garrett (2001) notes:

> In the absence of a cure, there may still be healing. This is what we recognize when we see people living full lives in spite of their illness . . . healing is not achieved at a single time, once and forever. It is a process the person actively constructs from day to day with a growing understanding of its meaning.

Healing or adapting means finding a new normal. With time and experience, patients learn that there are choices to be made about how to live and learn to look for opportunities to make them. It means making adjustments, recognizing the need to pace oneself and changing what can be changed. Sjögren's is the proverbial uninvited guest. Adaptation, like coping, is continuous, difficult, and rife with frustration. Changes are best made one at a time or in baby steps to the extent possible. Finding a new normal requires making modifications again and again. It is a struggle:

Illness is the night side of life, a more onerous citizenship. Everyone who is born holds dual citizenship, in the kingdom of the well and in the kingdom of the sick. Although we all prefer to use only the good passport, sooner or later each of us is obliged, at least for a spell, to identify ourselves as citizens of that other place. (Sontag, 1977, p. 3)

Summing Up

- Having Sjögren's is stressful on a variety of levels: physiologic, psychological, and interpersonal. It is an invisible, chronic disease with no cure— but people with Sjögren's can still lead meaningful, productive lives.
- Sjögren's may vary in its intensity and effects but it never goes away.
- Patients with Sjögren's often look better than they feel, so other people may not believe they are "really" sick.
- A chronic illness generates stress and uncertainty. Patients do not know what will happen next and can't predict how they will feel. Anxiety, confusion, frustration, and depression are all common emotions. They may be mild, moderate, or severe.
- Challenges brought on by the disease can lead to changes in relationships with family and friends.
- Coping is not static. People may cope well at times, not well at others. Adaptation can be difficult.
- Physicians can help validate the changes in patients' lives and encourage them to maximize a sense of well-being.
- Eventually, a new normal develops for most people. However, even after it does, the parameters shift with the disease.
- The bottom line: Sjögren's is more of a marathon than a sprint. It is also an uninvited guest that must be accommodated.

For Further Reading

Charmaz K. *Good Days, Bad Days: The Self in Chronic Illness and Time.* Rutgers University Press; 1991.

Charmaz K, Paterniti D, eds. *Health, Illness and Healing: Society, Social Context and Self.* Roxbury Publishing Company; 1999.

Cobb S. Social support as a moderator of life stress. *Psychosom Med.* 1976;38:5.

Cousins N. *Anatomy of an Illness.* Basic Books; 1979.

Cousins N. *Head First: The Biology of Hope.* E.P. Dutton; 1989.

Frank A. *At the Will of the Body: Reflections on Illness* (first Mariner Books ed.). Houghton Mifflin; 2002.

Fremes R, Carteron N. *A Body Out of Balance*. Avery; 2003.

Garrett C. Sources of hope in chronic illness. *Health Sociol Rev*. 2001;10(2):99–107.

Gawande A. *Being Mortal*. Henry Holt and Company; 2014.

Groopman J. *The Anatomy of Hope: How People Prevail in the Face of Illness*. Random House; 2004.

Hafen B, Karren K, Frandsen K, Smith NL. *Mind/Body Health*. Allyn and Bacon; 1996.

Halpern S. *The Etiquette of Illness: What to Say When You Can't Find the Words*. Bloomsbury; 2004.

Hirsch M. *Invisible: How Young Women with Serious Health Issues Navigate Work, Relationships and the Pressure to Seem Just Fine*. Beacon Press; 2018.

Johnson C, Webster D. *Recrafting a Life: Solutions for Chronic Pain and Illness*. Routledge; 2002.

Kleinman A. *The Illness Narratives*. Basic Books; 1988.

Lown B. *The Lost Art of Healing*. Houghton Mifflin; 1996.

Ornstein R, Sobel D. *Healthy Pleasures*. Perseus Books; 1989.

Piburn G. *Beyond Chaos: One Man's Journey Alongside His Chronically Ill Wife*. Arthritis Foundation, 1999.

Rumpf T. Breast Cancer Patients: Depression and Satisfaction with Support Systems. Unpublished Master of Science thesis, University of Massachusetts, 1980.

Rumpf T, Epstein L. Lifestyle issues, emotional. In Wallace D, ed. *The Sjögren's Book*. Oxford University Press; 2012:293–300.

Rumpf T, Hammitt K. *The Sjögren's Syndrome Survival Guide*. New Harbinger Publications; 2003.

Sontag S. *Illness as Metaphor*. Farrar, Strauss and Giroux; 1977.

Sternberg EM. *The Balance Within: The Science Connecting Health and Human Emotions*. WH Freeman and Company; 2001.

Telford K, Kralik D, Koch T. Acceptance and denial: Implications for people adapting to chronic illness: Literature review. *J Adv Nurs*. 2006;55(4):457–464.

Van Houtem L, Rijken M, Groenewegen P. Do everyday problems of people with chronic illness interfere with their disease management? *BMC Public Health*. 2015;15:1000.

Wall D. *Encounters with the Invisible*. Southern Methodist University Press; 2005.

Wells SM. *A Delicate Balance: Living Successfully with Chronic Illness*. Perseus Books; 2000.

43

Enhancing Resilience Through Mind–Body Interactions

Margaret Baim

It is easy to see why living with a chronic and unpredictable condition such as Sjögren's can be a stressful experience. The disease adds to the stress of daily life that is unavoidable for everyone, healthy or not. Any perception of threat—either real or imagined—is a trigger for stress, and Sjögren's patients can face both. Stress can come from many sources for Sjögren's patients, whether from the biological inflammation that accompanies the disease, or from the multiple symptoms and their repercussions (including dryness, pain, fatigue, and sexual dysfunction), or from the fear of potential complications, such as developing cancer or having a baby with heart block. Stress is also exacerbated by the need to make lifestyle changes brought on by Sjögren's and the not always helpful expectations and reactions from family, friends, and colleagues.

Although stress leads to negative feelings such as worry, fear, sadness, and frustration, it can also prompt us to heal and develop greater resilience. In this chapter we explore how stress works within the body and review findings from the new science of mind–body medicine. You will learn how certain attitudes and behaviors can offset stress and create a greater sense of well-being.

The Stress System

Resilience is defined as the body's ability to meet a demand, mount an appropriate response, and turn that response off when it is no longer needed. The body's vast communication network designed to perform these functions is the stress system. For example, when your body needs energy, the brain releases signals leading to hunger and food-seeking behaviors. Once this need is satisfied, those signals are replaced by other signals that lead to feelings of satisfaction. Another example is the release of signals and responses when you need to run and catch a bus. Blood flow is diverted from your stomach to your

Margaret Baim, *Enhancing Resilience Through Mind–Body Interactions* In: *The Sjögren's Book*. Edited by: Daniel J. Wallace, Oxford University Press. © Sjögren's Foundation 2022. DOI: 10.1093/oso/9780197502112.003.0043 arms and legs and your heart rate and breathing rate increase. After you either catch the bus or determine that it's a lost cause, further signals return the body to its baseline state.

The control center of the stress system is the brain. Weighing in at a mere three pounds, the brain requires one-third of our total daily caloric requirements to perform its extensive functions. Just think: During waking hours the brain is a constant surveyor of the world around us. Every movement and sound must be interpreted as threat or non-threat. Internally, every thought, memory, exertion, and emotion alters its activity. Repeated activity has been shown to alter its structure over time, a property termed *neural plasticity*. One notable influence on the brain's activity and subsequent neural plasticity is psychological stress. For those coping with the daily challenges and unpredictable nature of Sjögren's, periods of stress are to be expected. However, recent findings show that long periods of psychological stress can lead to changes within the brain's neural pathways that can lead to self-perpetuating activation of the stress system. Just as a road surface wears down where car tires hit it, thinking the same thoughts and experiencing the same moods day after day can create a well-worn pattern in our brains. Living in a stressful state of mind caused by fear, anxiety, worry, and sadness can lead to deeply rooted neural pathways.

However, mood is just one way stress steals our sense of well-being. Psychological stressors activate the stress system, beginning from brain responses and terminating in certain cells within our immune system. Stress induces these cells to work harder, and this overexertion leads to a series of toxic byproducts. Collectively, these byproducts impose a new type of stress on the body known as *oxidative stress*. Too much oxidative stress is damaging, because it overtaxes the mechanisms in place for our body to cope with these toxic byproducts. Among the consequences of unchecked oxidative stress is the production of pro-inflammatory proteins. These proteins, in turn, interfere with the production of hormones needed to stabilize mood and support feelings of well-being. The more the stress system is activated through psychological pathways, the more demand is placed on cells and the more wear and tear our bodies suffer. Ultimately, too much wear and tear leads to imbalances that we experience as mood disturbances, physical symptoms, and exacerbation of preexisting conditions and disease states.

So what is the good news? You have the power to cope with stress, thereby reducing the burden on your stress system and offsetting the effects of oxidative stress. Just as it is physiologically supportive to eat a balanced, antioxidant-rich diet, to engage in routine physical activity, and to obtain recuperative sleep—all of which offset oxidative stress and work to restore balance within the stress system—our attitude and state of mind also work to restore mind–body balance and support resilience.

Perception and Cognitive Reappraisal

> The mind is its own place and in itself, can make a Heaven of Hell, a Hell of Heaven.
>
> **John Milton**

The way we think matters. Years of study have demonstrated how our brains and bodies change between stressed and non-stressed states of mind. We all understand what it feels like to be stressed, but this awareness is only the tip of the iceberg—beneath it rests a host of physiologic processes that also play a part in the stress response. Under the influence of stress, the lower regions of our brain are most active; this is referred to as *bottom-up control*. In non-stressed states, in contrast, the upper regions of the brain associated with higher processing are most active; this is termed *top-down control*. Figure 43.1 shows the differences in activity between stressed and non-stressed brains. Greater activity in the upper, prefrontal regions is associated with enhanced executive function, regulation of emotions, and positive, adaptive perspectives (Arnsten, 2009).

As neurobiologist Robert Sapolsky outlines in his book *Why Zebras Don't Get Ulcers*, humans, unlike other animals, remember threats. This memory can be recalled to reactivate the stress system even when the threat is no longer present. Having this ability to remember is part of our advanced development, but it becomes a curse rather than a blessing if not used wisely. The perception of threats is a call to *adapt*; without adaptive coping, threats remain in memory to activate and sustain activation of the stress system long after the fact. Research on coping suggests that adaptive attitudes lead to a greater sense of well-being and longevity. Specifically, the deployment of problem-solving strategies, the acceptance of stressors beyond our control, and a general attitude of positivity correlate to feelings of well-being and longevity. Most recently, the role of these adaptive perspectives is understood to offset activation of the stress system as they lead to top-down control of the brain.

In cognitive theory, emotions correspond with a particular perception. For example, anger is felt in response to the perception of injustice, and sadness is felt in response to the perception of loss. Since these perceptions cause suffering and the wearing- and tearing-down effects of oxidative stress, it is wise to see them as challenges for adaptation rather than succumb to their grip. When a particular negative emotion is felt, we must learn to reflect on the

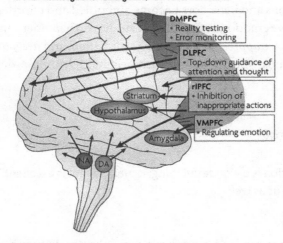

a Prefrontal regulation during alert, non-stress conditions

DMPFC
• Reality testing
• Error monitoring

DLPFC
• Top-down guidance of attention and thought

rlPFC
• Inhibition of inappropriate actions

VMPFC
• Regulating emotion

Striatum

Hypothalamus

Amygdala

NA DA

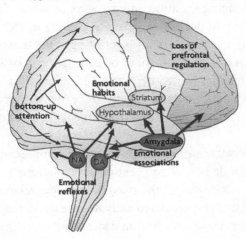

b Amygdala control during stress conditions

Loss of prefrontal regulation

Emotional habits

Striatum

Bottom-up attention

Hypothalamus

Amygdala

Emotional associations

NA DA

Emotional reflexes

Figure 43.1 Differences in activity between stressed and non-stressed brains.
Arnsten AF. Stress signalling pathways that impair prefrontal cortex structure and function. *Nat Rev Neurosci.* 2009;10:410–422.

underlying perception at work. Negative emotions focus on what we do not want, whereas adaptation works with what is. Choosing to adapt can provide an opportunity to redirect our perceptions toward those of greater service to us. Adaptive perspectives lead to positive emotions and behaviors such as compassion, wisdom, change, process, humor, gentleness, kindness, strength, patience, persistence, and influence. Positive and adaptive qualities turn off the stress system and restore top-down control of the brain. Hundreds of positive emotions and adaptive behaviors are available to counteract psychological and emotional suffering. As we apply these perspectives and behaviors to a stressful experience, the more adaptive and resilient we becomes. Over time, these perceptions and behaviors become embodied and effortless.

Three positive emotions often cited in studies on happiness and coping with chronic illness are *appreciation*, *positive expectation*, and *acceptance*. Each can be applied to most situations, and each originates from top-down control of the brain.

Appreciation

> Appreciation is a wonderful thing: It makes what is excellent in others belong to us as well.
>
> **Voltaire**

Two perspectives can lead to appreciation: valuing what we have and understanding that a challenging situation could always be worse. Living in a state of appreciation can help buffer against stress. A useful practice is to begin and close each day with *appreciations*, or an accounting of the things we appreciate in our life. To deepen this practice, focus on any memory of an appreciation until you relive the feeling. Generally, it takes less than 30 seconds to relive an emotion evoked by a particular memory. Once the memory is recalled, its neural effect becomes strengthened and over time it becomes more accessible and easily felt.

Appreciations typically fall into three categories: appreciation of ourself, the world, and others. It is wise to practice appreciations of each type. As appreciation for ourself develops, the need to feel appreciation from others lessens. Since feeling underappreciated activates the stress response, building self-appreciation can provide an additional stress buffer. Although the world has its troubles, it also can bring countless appreciations to mind, such as its abundant resources, ever-changing beauty, or endless opportunity for creative endeavors. Finally, feeling and expressing appreciation of others enhances resilience for not only the giver but also the receiver. In a culture where much of our communication is negative, this attitude is a welcome influence.

Positive Expectation

The placebo response is activated through positive expectation and is well known to buffer against pain and depression. It originates from upper brain regions associated with top-down control, motivation, and reward. Positive expectation can lead to the development of desirable qualities and abilities. Ellen Langer, professor of psychology at Harvard University, has studied the influence of positive expectations and has shown that expecting to lose weight can actually influence weight loss; the expectation is, in a sense, a self-fulfilling prophecy (Crum & Langer, 2007). Through recent brain-mapping studies, this phenomenon is understood through two mechanisms: release of dopamine and activation of the brain's reward and motivation circuitry. A general attitude of positive expectation not only allows the brain to release mood-stabilizing chemicals but also provides the motivation necessary to accomplish what is desired. Unlike negative expectations that bring on feelings of anxiety and stress, positive expectation feels good, buffers stress, and contributes to achieving what is positively expected.

Acceptance

Resisting "what is" leads to stress. As outlined in theologian Reinhold Niebuhr's "Serenity Prayer," wisdom is knowing when to accept what is beyond our control. Surrendering to what is beyond our control stops resistance and allows the mind to begin the process of acceptance. Acceptance empowers us to find whatever is good in the midst of a challenging situation. Patience, perseverance, strength, giving and receiving support, compassion, kindness, gentleness, and learning are only a few of the many potential qualities developed and expressed through this acceptance. When Sjögren's patients explore problem-solving strategies and define what can be changed, acceptance of what remains limits stress and enhances overall resilience. Given the role stress plays in promoting inflammation and in compromising the body's natural ability to heal, accepting what is unavoidable makes good therapeutic sense.

According to neuroscientist Joseph LeDoux, we are who we remember ourselves to be. This valuable understanding of how the brain works and how malleable the brain appears to be explains the influence that our self-perceptions have on our coping. Long-held views or self-identifications can be either empowering or self-defeating. Viewing yourself as weak, victimized, or anxious activates stress and limits the development of adaptive, positive perceptions such as learning, strength, and acceptance.

Meditation

Meditation makes it easier to cultivate adaptive perspectives and to heal stressful memories. Scientific investigation into meditation's influence on mind–body interactions is based on neural imaging, cognitive science, and the stress systems' regulation of neuroimmune, endocrine, and metabolic activity. Modern science helps us understand the healing influence of meditation on both mind and body, which helps us understand why all the world's wisdom traditions recommend its use. One essential benefit of meditation is increased awareness developed through non-thinking, feeling states of mind, known as interoceptive awareness. We will discuss three functions derived from this form of awareness (Conklin et al., 2018). Each function has been shown to enhance positive emotions, facilitate effective coping through adaptive perspectives, and inhibit stress, thus improving mood and physical symptoms:

1. *Attentional processes develop*: The brain regulates attention through the ability to sustain focus and experience. Negative habits of thinking begin to lose their grip as information processing becomes more top-down. This shift is called meta-awareness, where we gain control over our thoughts rather than being at their mercy.

2. *Threatening and maladaptive perspectives fade away*: As our non-thinking, meditative awareness develops, insight into maladaptive perceptions emerges and negative self-talk reflective of our emotional suffering begins to fade away. We begin to recognize thoughts, feelings, and perceptions as temporary and flexible rather than fixed and perpetually impactful. It seems as if the brain is naturally aligned to the reality of life's challenges, by giving us our own guidance system that rewards us with equanimity and other positive feelings when we choose to adapt appropriately. Inherent perspectives tucked in the deep recesses of our top-down selves (the very regions of the brain that keep evolving through human existence) move us from the suffering ramifications of life's threats to positive and rebalancing ramifications of a life well lived.

3. *Positive feelings and adaptive perspectives emerge*: By regaining the ability to sustain experiential focus, we are naturally drawn to see ourselves, others, and life through the lens of these inherent adaptive perspectives. Over time, rehearsal of these perspectives through meditation makes them more readily accessible. As our top-down brain develops, we evolve and benefit from the felt experience of mind–body balance, free from the "stuck-ness" of stress. In a nutshell, we become stronger, wiser, and more compassionate.

Accidental Stress

In addition to the top-down brain changes that guide you toward positive emotions and adaptive perspectives, several other brain changes develop through meditation that protect you from a pernicious and entirely unnecessary activation of stress. By sustaining moment-to-moment experiential awareness, the mind is protected from two common causes of chronic stress: mind wandering and splintered attention. It's estimated that our mind wanders into the future and into the past about 50% of our wakeful day, often triggering negative memories and expectations that then activate a low-grade noxious stress response (Killingsworth & Gilbert, 2010). This unintentional mind wandering results in more oxidative stress, systemic inflammation, and neuro-inflammation, wearing down the body's limited resources, increasing vulnerability to illness, or exacerbating current symptomatology.

Another mental habit cultivated through today's fast-paced, multi-sensory environment is splintered attention. Our brains are often pummeled by sounds and images coming at us from a variety of sources, such as television and computer monitors, smartphones, and highway traffic. As a result, we're becoming more easily distracted, losing the ability to simply be and deeply experience our top-down, positive and adaptive brain processes. Given the choice, would you prefer to think about sinking your teeth into a delicious sandwich or have the experience? With a distracted, wandering mind, the depth of our awareness and positive experiences becomes limited and diluted at best. However, if our thinking emanates from the stress-signaling, bottom-up brain, then negative or challenging aspects of an experience can easily become magnified or distorted while our inherent, natural ability to cope and experience stress-buffering feelings and emotions becomes compromised.

Reflect: How many times today have you been fully immersed in an experience? Did you experience the fragrances, sights, and feelings that came to you during breakfast? Did you give a friend or relative your full attention when they spoke to you today? How many times today has your attention split from what you were doing? For example, did you drive to the store while your mind was having a stressful conversation with a coworker? Was your mind busy filling up your to-do list while you were eating dinner?

Neural Processing

Meditation begins with the practice of sustaining focus and once this focus is held, the thinking regions of the brain quiet down. Although this sounds simple enough in theory, the mind wanders , and it can take many moments, even minutes, to realize that we've lost the intended focus . The process of reorienting is necessary before our attention returns fully to the intended focus. Appreciating how the brain builds the skill of sustaining focus against its habit of wandering may help you have patience with your own practice. With practice and time, the ability to sustain focus develops, along with all its adaptive and positive benefits.

In recent studies on brain function, alterations in both brain structure and activity can be measured after only 8 weeks of a daily meditation practice. These changes are consistent with greater top-down control of the brain, less stress activation, and improvement of mood and physical symptoms.

Before you begin a meditation practice, it's helpful to appreciate that it is a natural state of mind elicited through a focused and receptive mode of awareness. For example, drinking to quench thirst or enjoying a delicious piece of fruit can bring the mind into a meditative state. The drink or fruit is focused on, and the accompanying enjoyment leads to a receptive and positive attitude. Much as a perception of a threat activates the stress response and leads to bottom-up control of the brain, a focused and receptive awareness elicits the body's relaxation response and leads to top-down control of the brain. In a meditative state, negative emotions triggered from remembered threats are made less prominent by activating the regions of the brain responsible for storing positive memories, positive expectations, and other adaptive perspectives. Recent studies on meditation not only demonstrate neural changes consistent with reduced stress, greater top-down control, and more positive and adaptive perspectives but also show changes in gene expressions throughout the body that alter cellular functioning. Rather than overproducing oxidant toxins as cells do in response to stress, certain types of cells are known to reduce or even reverse their oxidative stress in response to meditation. Thus, building a meditation practice is well worth the time and effort.

Building a Meditation Practice

It may come as a surprise to you, but you actually already meditate. Every time you look at something or someone with a focused and receptive state of mind, you are in a meditative state. Viewing someone or something pleasing, new, and interesting naturally focuses the mind and activates top-down control of the brain. However, the ability to sustain and retain this state of mind and return to it at will when stressed requires practice. The first step toward controlling your own awareness is to build an ability to concentrate and sustain a particular focus.

The following strategies represent a few meditation methods to support your practice (Box 43.1). Just as there are many ways to activate stress,

---

Box 43.1 How to Begin Meditating

- **Frequency**
  Practice daily! Regular and frequent practice improves neural plasticity in a cumulative fashion.
- **Duration**
  After 10 minutes of practice, physiologic change is measurable. Begin with 10 to 20 minutes and slowly increase to 20 to 30 minutes.
- **Lifestyle**
  Meditating at the same time each day and in the same place helps integrate this new behavior into your normal routine. Placing a sacred or healing symbol in this environment serves as a positive reminder of this new state of mind.

  Developing and maintaining a meditative state of mind throughout the day is challenging. Try meditating first thing in the morning and again at bedtime. While meditating in the morning sets the right tone for the day, meditating at bedtime reduces stress hormones and other chemicals that interfere with your ability to obtain deep, recuperative sleep.
- **Redirecting the Wandering Mind**
  Each time the mind wanders from your intended focus (commonly every few seconds), gently return to it without recrimination. Simply noticing how often the mind wanders while sustaining an attitude of interest builds focus and receptive awareness. Your mind will wander less as you develop the ability to sustain your focus. Over time, lapses in this ability may indicate the influence of greater stress or of needing more recuperative sleep.

---

there are many ways to activate a non-stressed, meditative state of mind. Any mental activity that engages the mind toward a sustained focus of receptive interest will lead to desired change. Body-based practices such as hatha yoga, qigong, and tai chi are well-known meditation methods but are beyond the scope of this chapter. However, once you develop any meditation practice, expanding it through the use of other methods can bring added benefit.

Single-Pointed Focus

Concentrating on a soothing or empowering word, phrase, or image is one method for building concentration. Aligning your single-pointed focus to a natural rhythm such as the breath often helps sustain focus.

Imagine a Desirable Self

The mind's influence on behavior is well known. Olympic athletes have learned to imagine themselves performing their skill perfectly. Studies on rehabilitation after a stroke show greater recovery associated with imagining the use of pre-stroke abilities. If you are anxious, imagining yourself calm, balanced, powerful, and accepting is corrective. If you are inclined to feelings of sadness and depression, imagining yourself as appreciative and filled with positive expectancy brings about a more adaptive persona.

Safe Place

Rest your mind on the memory or creation of a safe, nurturing place. As with any mental focus, it is important to keep the perspective positive and supportive: A pleasing memory of an old friend can conjure up the loss of that friendship, or a wished-for experience can begin to feel remote or hopeless. Any stress-activating shift in perception can be instructive and useful if met with a receptive awareness. Understanding the nature of your stress is an expression of self-compassion. From the perspective of a safe place, you can ask yourself what you need to heal. Moving your mind away from stress-activating thoughts to those that heal is an integral aspect of developing a meditative state of mind.

Mindfulness

If the mind is in the present moment, and the present moment does not pose a threat, then the brain is functioning in non-stressed, top-down control. However, holding mental focus in a moment-to-moment awareness is challenging. To begin, pick a discrete and pleasant activity like eating an apple or drinking a cup of tea. To maintain that present awareness, bring your mind to the experience of seeing, tasting, smelling, touching, and hearing. Noticing how you feel or think in any given moment is also part of mindfulness when accomplished with an open, receptive attitude of interest. Negative judgments or memories of stress may come into your mind, but if you meet them in mindfulness, a deeper, more adaptive awareness is likely to follow from maintaining top-down control. In this non-judgmental state of self-awareness, clarity and wisdom are more accessible.

Time Travel

Reliving pleasant memories or focusing on a desirable outcome also frees the mind from the control of stress-activating regions. Holding awareness on the positive aspects of a memory or on a desirable expectation free of worry or negativity arouses the senses to relive the memory or begin enjoyment of a future expectation. Expectations influence language and behavior, and these in turn become influences themselves. Therefore, be careful to create expectations for your own good and for the good of others.

Insight

We frequently carry on a conversation with ourselves. We often ask ourselves questions such as "Should I buy this?" or "What time do I need to get up?" If we are stressed, answers to these questions are likely to come from bottom-up brain processes where the brain stores memories of threats. Perceiving through these pathways can activate stress and become a habitual way of sustaining stress and blocking positive or adaptive perceptions. Posing questions with an open, receptive attitude—as in a meditative state of mind—often brings new and more serviceable insights. To help sustain a positive and focused awareness, especially when asking a question whose answer can elicit stress, it is useful to first imagine a safe place. Once you are fully secure in this place, ask the question to an imagined wise person or a loving presence. If you prefer a particular answer, the stress response takes over and insight may be blocked.

Through the years I have taught thousands to meditate and have had the privilege of watching many heal from the stress of traumatic memories and stress imposed by chronic illness. Those with Sjögren's can use the tools described in this chapter to promote healing and cope positively with the added stress that is an inevitable part of this disease. The mind is an expression of free will; through both cognitive reappraisal and meditation, this free will can be used more wisely in support of adaptive and healing perspectives. Using psychological stress as a signal to heal enhances resilience. Although physical limitations may continue, a growing sense of well-being can be achieved.

Summing Up

Increasing awareness of mind–body connections and taking advantage of ways to reduce stress can help Sjögren's patients cope better with the emotional and physical challenges of their disease. Meditation and cognitive strategies to ease anxieties and stress and focus on more positive feelings and perspectives can be valuable tools in the struggle to develop a sense of well-being and more positive life experiences.

For Further Reading

Arnsten AF. Stress signalling pathways that impair prefrontal cortex structure and function. *Nat Rev Neurosci.* 2009;10:410–422.

Benson H, Proctor W. *Relaxation Revolution: Enhancing Your Personal Health Through the Science and Genetics of Mind Body Healing.* Scribner; 2010.

Conklin QA, Crosswell AD, Saron CD, Epel ES. Meditation, stress processes, and telomere biology. *Curr Opin Psychol.* 2018;28:92–101.

Crum AJ, Langer EJ. Mind-set matters: Exercise and the placebo effect. *Psychol Sci.* 2007;18:165–171.

Fontana D. *The Meditation Handbook: The Practical Guide to Eastern and Western Meditation Techniques.* Watkins; 2010.

Fredrickson B. *Positivity: Groundbreaking Research Reveals How to Embrace the Hidden Strength of Positive Emotions, Overcome Negativity, and Thrive.* Crown; 2009.

Kabat-Zinn J. *Wherever You Go There You Are: Mindfulness Meditation in Everyday Life.* Hyperion; 2005.

Killingsworth MA, Gilbert DT. A wandering mind is an unhappy mind. *Science.* 2010;330(6006):932.

Parallax Press. http://www.parallax.org/ [resources from Buddhist monk Thich Nhat Hanh, the most prolific writer on mindfulness]

Ricard M, Lutz A, Davidson RJ. Mind of the meditator. *Sci Am.* 2014;311(5):38–45.

Sapolsky R. *Why Zebras Don't Get Ulcers* (3rd ed.). Holt Paperbacks; 2004.

Sounds True. http://www.soundstrue.com/guide/meditation/ [online guidance, books, and audio from a variety of wisdom traditions]

44

Sleep Disorders

H. Kenneth Fisher and Daniel J. Wallace

Problems with sleep are seen in more than 70% of U.S. adults with rheumatic disorders. The main sleep complaint reported by Sjögren's patients is that their sleep is nonrestorative: about two-thirds report they are fatigued, both physically and mentally. Depression is not the principal cause, though it is often present as well. The characteristics of disabling fatigue in Sjögren's are indistinguishable from those of patients with rheumatoid arthritis (RA) or systemic lupus erythematosus. Sleep disturbances are rated moderate or severe in the majority of patients with Sjögren's, more than is found in RA alone, RA with sicca symptoms, or osteoarthritis. Among patients with Sjögren's, those who also have fibromyalgia symptoms have especially severe sleep complaints.

Prevalence of Sleep Disturbances

The Sjögren's research group at Newcastle University in the United Kingdom performed a systemic review of the literature (Hackett et al., 2017) and found nine studies that were acceptable for analysis. Perceived sleep disturbance, time spent in bed, total sleep time, sleep onset latency, sleep efficiency, number of night awakenings, arousal index, ventilator measurements, sleep apnea, and daytime somnolence were reviewed. Most patients underwent polysomnography. The major factors associated with Sjögren's and sleep disturbances were dry eye, sleep apnea, and nocturnal pain. Many patients had no sleep disturbances, and it is becoming increasingly appreciated that autonomic symptoms (palpitations, dizziness, and sweats) may play a role in sleep disorders in Sjögren's.

What Sleep Characteristics Do Sjögren's Patients Experience?

The somatic fatigue of Sjögren's patients is different from sleepiness and is commonly progressive during the day. Mental fatigue is also progressive

H. Kenneth Fisher and Daniel J. Wallace, *Sleep Disorders* In: *The Sjögren's Book*. Edited by: Daniel J. Wallace, Oxford University Press. © Sjögren's Foundation 2022. DOI: 10.1093/oso/9780197502112.003.0044

during the day, and both symptoms are associated with poor nocturnal sleep and physical discomfort during the night. Nocturnal awakenings due to musculoskeletal pain, anxiety, and other sleep-disturbing symptoms are all associated with daytime fatigue.

Besides daily progressive daytime fatigue, daytime sleepiness self-measured by the Epworth Sleepiness Scale is also common in Sjögren's patients. Bladder irritability and urinary urgency are seen more often in Sjögren's patients than in osteoarthritis patients and may play a role in poor sleep quality.

What Causes Poor Sleep in Sjögren's?

It seems unlikely that inflammation by itself explains the disturbed sleep of Sjögren's patients. When compared with both healthy controls and RA patients, Sjögren's patients differ in several ways that might result in worse sleep quality. They have more muscle tension at bedtime, more symptoms of restless legs syndrome, and more pains during the night. Not surprisingly, they have a larger sleep deficit. More frequently than those in the comparison groups, Sjögren's patients do not feel rested after sleep and complain of daytime fatigue and sleepiness.

Although sleep architecture is generally normal, time awake after sleep onset is considerably greater among Sjögren's subjects and reduces sleep efficiency from 94% in healthy controls to 70% among Sjögren's subjects. Half the Sjögren's subjects demonstrate alpha brain wave activity intruding into delta (deep) sleep, an anomaly seen commonly in fibromyalgia patients who also suffer from prominent daytime fatigue. The exact links between disturbed nocturnal sleep and daytime fatigue are not yet known, but one hint that the autonomic nervous system may be involved comes from the observation that those Sjögren's and fibromyalgia patients with the greatest levels of daytime fatigue are also the ones with the lowest diastolic blood pressures. Knowledge that the surface tension of airway-lining fluids in Sjögren's patients is abnormally high led to speculation that some of the daytime fatigue and sleepiness might be caused by increased risk of obstructive sleep apnea due to airway collapse. However, recent studies have found no increased airway collapsibility in patients with Sjögren's.

Can Commonly Coexisting Conditions and Medications Affect Sleep?

Dryness, musculoskeletal and chronic pain, neuropathies, and sensitivity to cold and heat are all commonly seen in Sjögren's and can interfere with sleep. Keeping inflammation, pain, and the patient's disease under control will improve sleep. If depression is part of the patient's medical picture, this condition can add to sleep problems. In addition, coexisting fibromyalgia and autoimmune thyroid disorders can complicate the clinical picture. Up to 25% of Sjögren's patients have autoimmune thyroid disease, which can occur as hypothyroidism (Hashimoto's thyroiditis) or hyperthyroidism (Graves disease). While these conditions would seem to have opposite impacts on sleep, both can interfere with the quality of sleep. Hashimoto's can add to the joint and muscle pain and stiffness already experienced by many Sjögren's patients, and the anxiety and restlessness that occur in Graves disease can diminish sleep quality. Thyroid disease often is underdiagnosed, and thyroid function should be checked in Sjögren's patients.

Medication lists should be checked for side effects that include interference with sleep. Prednisone, especially when taken in the evening, can cause some patients to become nervous and have difficulty sleeping. Before trying medications for troubled sleep, basic rules of sleep hygiene should be followed. Regular exercise can increase a sense of well-being, can help with depression if it exists, and can improve sleep; however, patients should avoid exercise in the few hours before bedtime. Finally, relaxation techniques can help before bedtime and if a patient awakens in the middle of the night.

What Can Be Done for Sjögren's Patients with Poor Sleep?

Now that we understand more about the nature of the disabling fatigue in Sjögren's patients, what can we do about it? Only very tentative answers are available so far. Exercise has been shown to improve both aerobic capacity (as expected) and fatigue levels.

Most Sjögren's patients do not require sleep medication, and if they do, their choice is limited because of the drying properties of commonly used agents such as tricyclic antidepressants and antihistamines. Patients who are sleep-deprived may benefit from counseling on "sleep hygiene" (Box 44.1). In Sjögren's, nocturnal dryness of the eyes and mouth may also disturb sleep. A room air humidifier can be helpful. Patients are encouraged to use ocular lubricants (e.g., Refresh PM) or gels (e.g., GenTeal gel) instead of artificial tears before bed for longer-lasting relief. Bedtime doses of oral secretagogues (e.g., pilocarpine [Salagen] or cevimeline [Evoxac]) are also very useful. The mouth and inner cheeks can also be coated with over-the-counter moisturizing gels (Oral Balance, Orajel) or vitamin E oil to alleviate night symptoms.

Box 44.1 Tips To Achieve Restful Sleep

---

1. Keep a regular sleep schedule for going to bed and getting up.
2. Avoid taking daytime naps.
3. Try to get at least 8-1/2 hours of sleep per night, or longer if you wake up a lot.
4. Do not use caffeine or alcohol within 6 hours of bedtime.
5. Try to exercise regularly for at least 20 minutes a day, but don't exercise right before bed.
6. Create a dark, cool, quiet, and secure environment for sleep.
7. Do not go to bed hungry.
8. Do not work or watch TV in the bedroom.
9. Try a warm bath before bedtime to relax aching muscles and relieve stress.
10. Don't sleep with pets, children or bed partners who snore

---

Summing Up

Sleep problems are common in Sjögren's patients, with the most frequent complaint being nonrestorative sleep. Sleep efficiency and time spent in deep sleep appear reduced in many Sjögren's patients. Those with both Sjögren's and fibromyalgia have the severest complaints. The causes of sleep problems in Sjögren's are unknown, but autonomic nervous system involvement is suspected of playing a role. While few studies have been done, medications under investigation for use in Sjögren's and other autoimmune disorders or on the market for sleep problems in fibromyalgia patients might prove useful.

For Further Reading

Abad VC, Sarinas PS, Guilleminault C. Sleep and rheumatologic disorders. *Sleep Med Rev.* 2008;12:211–228.

Au NH, Mather R, To A, Malvankar-Mehta MS. Sleep outcomes associated with dry eye disease: A systematic review and meta-analysis. *Can J Ophthalmol.* 2019;54(2):180–189.

Chung SW, Hur J, Ha YJ, et al. Impact of sleep quality on clinical features of primary Sjogren's syndrome. *Korean J Intern Med.* 2019;34(5):1154–1164.

d'Elia HF, Rehnberg E, Kvist G, et al. Fatigue and blood pressure in primary Sjögren's syndrome. *Scand J Rheumatol.* 2008;37:284–292.

Goodchild CE, Treharne GJ, Booth DA, Bowman SJ. Daytime patterning of fatigue and its associations with the previous night's discomfort and poor sleep among women with primary Sjögren's syndrome or rheumatoid arthritis. *Musculoskel Care.* 2010;8(2):107–117.

Gudbjornsson B, Broman JE, Hetta J, Hallgren R. Sleep disturbances in patients with primary Sjögren's syndrome. *Br J Rheumatol.* 1993;32:1072–1076.

Hackett KL, Gotts ZM, Ellis J, et al. An investigation into the prevalence of sleep disturbances in primary Sjogren's syndrome: A systematic review of the literature. *Rheumatology.* 2017;56:570–580.

Hilditch CJ, McEvoy RD, George KE, et al. Upper airway surface tension but not upper airway collapsibility is elevated in primary Sjögren's syndrome. *Sleep.* 2008;31:367–374.

Strombeck BE, Theander E, Jacobsson LT. Effects of exercise on aerobic capacity and fatigue in women with primary Sjögren's syndrome. *Rheumatology.* 2007;46(5):868–871.

Theander L, Strombeck B, Mandl T, Theander E. Can we detect treatable causes of tiredness in primary Sjögren's syndrome? *Rheumatology.* 2010;49(6):1177–1183.

Tishler M, Barak Y, Paran D, Yaron M. Sleep disturbances, fibromyalgia and primary Sjögren's syndrome. *Clin Exp Rheumatol.* 1997;15:71–74.

45

Sex and Sjögren's

Anne E. Burke

Sjögren's can affect women's sexual function. Physical symptoms that can occur with Sjögren's include vaginal dryness and pelvic pain. The age at which people are diagnosed with Sjögren's may also coincide with perimenopause or menopause, with accompanying hormonal changes. Other factors, such as mood, fatigue, and general challenges of living with a chronic illness, can in turn affect sexual function and sexual satisfaction for women with Sjögren's.

Sjögren's affects more women than men. This may be because hormones such as estrogen play a role in its cause. Nonetheless, previous studies suggested that fewer than half of women with Sjögren's ever had a doctor ask them about vaginal or sexual symptoms. There is now growing recognition of these connections.

Vaginal Dryness

Women with Sjögren's often experience vaginal dryness, along with dry mouth and dry eyes (see Chapter 26). Vaginal dryness is common in women who have Sjögren's, with the proportion affected possibly as high as 75%. Vaginal dryness may be caused by inflammation of the glands that would usually lubricate the vagina. In addition, just as the function of other moisture-producing glands such as the salivary and lacrimal glands is affected by the lymphocytic infiltration that occurs in Sjögren's, a perivascular lymphocytic infiltrate has been seen on vaginal biopsy in Sjögren's patients (Skopouli et al., 1994). Recent research suggests that it may also be due to Sjögren's-linked dysfunction of the blood vessels. The physical stress of chronic illness can also contribute to vaginal dryness.

Diagnosis of Sjögren's often coincides with the start of the hormonal changes that lead into menopause. This perimenopausal stage is characterized by less regular menstrual periods and some symptoms of menopause, such as hot flashes. Hormone levels may follow unpredictable patterns. Perimenopause

Anne E. Burke, *Sex and Sjögren's* In: *The Sjögren's Book*. Edited by: Daniel J. Wallace, Oxford University Press.
© Sjögren's Foundation 2022. DOI: 10.1093/oso/9780197502112.003.0045

can last for several years, and as a woman transitions into menopause, her estrogen levels decrease. However, while the lower estrogen levels associated with menopausal status can contribute to vaginal dryness, younger women with Sjögren's may also experience this symptom.

Vaginal dryness can affect sexual function. Without enough lubrication, vaginal intercourse may be painful. The friction caused by having sex without enough moisture can cause abrasions or small cuts in the vagina, which can increase pain levels. This can also contribute to low sex drive, as our normal instinct is to avoid things that cause pain.

There are several treatment options for vaginal dryness. It is often reasonable to start with vaginal moisturizers. These over-the-counter products generally do not contain hormones. They are used two or three times a week, not during intercourse, and increase vaginal moisture through a variety of mechanisms. Several products are available in pharmacies or online. Water-based lubricants (as distinct from moisturizers) may help to increase lubrication for intercourse. Other products may contain botanical or oil-based natural ingredients, such as aloe vera or vitamin E. Some products may damage condoms, so it is important to read labels carefully. Vaginal moisturizers are effective for many individuals with dryness.

Vaginal estrogen treatments also help with dryness, and in some cases may be more effective than moisturizers for those in menopause. Several forms of estrogen can be used in the vagina, such as creams, pills, and rings. For women whose dryness is caused at least in part by low estrogen levels (such as women who have gone through menopause), these medications can improve the health of the vaginal cells and increase moisture over time. These usually require a prescription. Some women may use hormone pills or patches for a limited time, primarily if they have other symptoms of menopause such as hot flashes. "Natural" hormone treatments, such as soy supplements or black cohosh, have not been well studied.

Sometimes a more creative approach is necessary to achieve sufficient relief or improvement if treatments are not effective. Alternatives to vaginal intercourse include oral sex or masturbation. It may also help to talk with a partner about new ways to approach vaginal sex. Sometimes more foreplay is helpful. Women may also opt to limit vaginal intercourse to shorter periods of time to decrease painful friction. Some women with Sjögren's have also found that it helps to plan sex around times of the menstrual cycle when natural lubrication is greatest. Women with Sjögren's should not be afraid to discuss this with their doctors or healthcare providers, who will often be able to address concerns or refer them to appropriate specialists.

Dry Mouth

Dry mouth is a common symptom of Sjögren's. Women with Sjögren's may find that even kissing can be uncomfortable. Just as dry mouth can affect chewing and swallowing, it can also affect activities like deep kissing or giving oral sex to one's partner.

Treatments that improve dry mouth may also make things like deep kissing more comfortable. These can range from simple things like chewing gum (to stimulate saliva) to prescription medications used to manage symptoms of Sjögren's. Women can discuss these options with their healthcare provider. Some options are discussed in Chapter 24.

Pelvic Pain and Painful Sex (Dyspareunia)

Many women with Sjögren's suffer from neuropathic pain in different parts of the body. This can include pelvic pain and feelings of bladder or urinary irritation. Often these types of pain can be difficult to treat, which can be frustrating. Any of these symptoms can make sexual intercourse painful, a condition referred to as dyspareunia. How common is this? The research varies. One study reported that over 60% of women with Sjögren's complained of dyspareunia. However, others have found that if there are no other medical problems, women with Sjögren's may not have dyspareunia any more frequently than other women.

Dyspareunia can either be deep (felt with deep vaginal penetration) or superficial (felt with initial vaginal penetration). Many causes of dyspareunia and/or pelvic pain are not related to Sjögren's. Causes of deep dyspareunia can include ovarian cysts, endometriosis, infection, or scarring from any previous surgeries. Vaginal dryness or vulvar pain can cause superficial dyspareunia. Dyspareunia can result in avoidance of sex due to pain. Persistent dyspareunia can also cause involuntary tension to develop in the pelvic muscles, which may increase pain. Individuals with dyspareunia should have an evaluation to assess for other causes that can be treated.

Some treatment strategies can help. Some sexual positions may be more comfortable than others. Treating vaginal dryness may also help. Women with chronic pain or pelvic pain may benefit from pelvic physical therapy (PT). This involves spending several sessions with a physical therapist trained in pelvic rehabilitation. Some pelvic PT techniques include biofeedback, electrical stimulation, physiotherapy, and vaginal dilator therapy. With a prescription or referral, insurance will often cover several pelvic PT sessions. Therapists often also discuss techniques that women can use at home. Some women may benefit from cognitive therapy that focuses on improving sexual function, especially if such therapy is part of a larger treatment approach. Dealing with any psychological effects of the pain through counseling and learned coping skills can be helpful as well.

Other Symptoms

The quality of one's sex life is affected by numerous factors. A condition like Sjögren's can play a role in sexual function, as it shares characteristics with other common chronic illnesses. Systemic inflammation can itself lead to diminished libido. Further, fatigue or depressed mood can affect sexual function. Fatigue may be due to the illness itself or to medication side effects.

Many women with Sjögren's struggle with depression, often due in part to the stress of dealing with illness. In some cases, too, women had symptoms of Sjögren's for years before it was actually diagnosed. Years of dealing with frustrating or debilitating symptoms with no diagnosis can contribute over time to depressed mood. Decreased self-esteem and depression can also result when Sjögren's-related disability causes significant life changes. When depression is properly treated, its effects on sexual function may lessen.

Some treatments for depression may affect sexual function. A commonly used type of antidepressant is a selective serotonin reuptake inhibitor (SSRI). Examples include fluoxetine (Prozac), sertraline (Zoloft), and paroxetine (Paxil); these can be associated with a higher incidence of sexual problems than some other medications. If one of these medications affects a woman's sexual function, options include trying a different medication or lowering the dose to the lowest that is effective.

Issues such as physical disability, stiffness, chronic pain, emotional stress, and altered self-image can have a negative impact on overall quality of life and, in turn, on sexual function. Problems like fatigue or depression may have similar effects. Some women with Sjögren's have found that it helps if they plan when they are going to have sex. This can include scheduling times with a partner and allowing more time for foreplay. For women who suffer from fatigue, it may help to target times of the day or days in the week when fatigue is less severe. Pain or stiffness may require different techniques to minimize discomfort. Women who take medications should consider asking their healthcare providers if a change may lessen any sexual side effects. Seeing a healthcare provider or counselor with specific expertise in sexual health may also be beneficial.

Partnerships

A woman's relationship with her partner is an important contributor to sexual function and satisfaction. This can be especially true for women with chronic conditions like Sjögren's, when the condition affects aspects of the relationship. It is important to acknowledge such feelings. It may also be helpful to remind oneself, and one's partner, that Sjögren's can physically affect sexual function. Counseling can be helpful for many couples who are having resultant difficulties in their partnerships.

Sexual Well-Being

Sexual well-being is a measure of satisfaction with one's sexuality. Women with Sjögren's may experience changes in sexual function, due to the reasons we have just described or perhaps to other reasons as well. Women with Sjögren's may have physical or psychological reasons to have sex differently or less frequently. However, many other women with Sjögren's continue to enjoy sexual activity and satisfaction. Even with the limitations of Sjögren's, women and their partners can maintain a state of sexual well-being. This may require more patience, effort, and creativity as well as altered expectations if symptoms progress over time.

Summing Up

People living with Sjögren's may have symptoms that affect their sexual health. These can include vaginal dryness, pain (pelvic, muscle, joint, and neuropathic pain), fatigue, dry mouth, and depression. Perimenopause, menopause, and/or medications can exacerbate dryness or low libido. In addition to treating Sjögren's itself, moisturizing products and lubricants, prescription hormones, specialized physical therapy, and counseling, when needed, can alleviate symptoms that interfere with sexual health.

For Further Reading

Basson R. Sexual function of women with chronic illness and cancer. *Womens Health.* 2010;6(3):407–429.

Schoofs N. Caring for women living with Sjögren's syndrome. *J Obstet Gynecol Neonatal Nurs.* 2003;32(5):589–593.

Sjögren's Foundation. Patient Education Sheet: Sex & Sjögren's. https://www.sjogrens.org/sites/default/files/inline-files/Sex%20and%20Sjogren%27s%20Patient%20Education%20Sheet.pdf

Sjögren's Syndrome News. Tips for Dealing with Vaginal Dryness in Sjögren's Syndrome. 2011. https://sjogrenssyndromenews.com/2020/02/06/tips-for-dealing-with-vaginal-dryness-in-sjogrens-syndrome/

Skopouli FN, Papanikolaou S, Malamou-Mitsi V, et al. Obstetric and gynaecological profile in patients with primary Sjogren's syndrome. *Ann Rheum Dis.* 1994;53(9):569–573.

Tristano AG. The impact of rheumatic diseases on sexual function. *Rheumatol Int.* 2009;29(8):853–860.

van Nimwegen JF, van der Tuuk K, Liefers SC, et al. Vaginal dryness in primary Sjögren's syndrome: A histopathological case-control study. *Rheumatology.* 2020;59(10):2806–2815.

Verschuren JE, Enzlin P, Dijkstra PU, Geertzen JH, Dekker R. Chronic disease and sexuality: A generic conceptual framework. *J Sex Res.* 2010;47(2):153–170.

46

Vaccinations in Sjögren's

Richard D. Brasington Jr.

One of the most important aspects of preventive health care is receiving the appropriate vaccinations. This is particularly important for patients with autoimmune disease with compromised immune function, especially when immunosuppressive medications are used. We can think of vaccinations in three broad categories: (1) those everyone should receive; (2) those that are particularly appropriate for patients with autoimmune diseases; and (3) those that may be dangerous for such patients and therefore should be avoided. Updating vaccinations is particularly important before taking some immunosuppressive medications, because these can seriously blunt a person's response to appropriate vaccination.

Nowadays, the "standard" vaccinations are administered during the preschool and elementary school years and include mumps, measles, rubella, tetanus, diphtheria, and so forth. For purposes of this discussion, we will assume that all patients who are ultimately diagnosed with Sjögren's have received all of the appropriate childhood immunizations.

At least every 10 years, all adults should receive a tetanus and diphtheria (Td) booster. In reality, this booster is often administered when a question arises as to whether tetanus immunity is current; if there is no documentation of a Td booster in the previous 10 years, it is given at that point.

The varicella vaccine is a live virus vaccine and should not be given to immunosuppressed persons. Sjögren's patients generally are not considered to be immunosuppressed unless they are taking medications that suppress the immune system (examples are listed in the next paragraph). Note that hydroxychloroquine (Plaquenil) does not suppress the immune system.

However, patients with autoimmune disorders such as Sjögren's are generally considered to have some compromise of the immune system and increased susceptibility to infection. A simple way to think of this is to consider that if the immune system is "misdirected" toward self, it probably is not doing an ideal job of protecting against infectious agents. Obviously, someone with mild Sjögren's who does not have pronounced systemic disease will not

Richard D. Brasington Jr., *Vaccinations in Sjögren's* In: *The Sjögren's Book*. Edited by: Daniel J. Wallace, Oxford University Press.
© Sjögren's Foundation 2022. DOI: 10.1093/oso/9780197502112.003.0046

be as susceptible to infection as a patient with systemic disease requiring immunosuppressive agents such as prednisone, azathioprine, methotrexate, mycophenolate mofetil, rituximab, or cyclophosphamide. Nonetheless, I recommend that all patients with Sjögren's undergo vaccination for influenza, pneumococcal pneumonia, and shingles.

While some patients fear that vaccines can activate the immune system and cause systemic flares, no scientific evidence exists to indicate that this is the case. In fact, studies in systemic lupus erythematosus do not suggest disease activation with Pneumovax. Vaccines need to be avoided only when a previous reaction has occurred, and a reaction to one vaccination does not mean that all future vaccinations should be avoided.

The flu shot each fall is familiar to everyone. This vaccine is different each year and must be given every year. The vaccine for a given flu season is developed based on scientists' best predictions of which strains of influenza virus will be dominant that particular year. Hence, immunity in one year does not necessarily carry over until the next year. Even when vaccination does not prevent the occurrence of influenza in those vaccinated, it is likely that the illness will not be as severe in those who have been vaccinated.

The pneumonia shot (Pneumovax, or pneumococcal polysaccharide vaccine) specifically protects against one kind of bacterial pneumonia, pneumococcal pneumonia, and covers 23 serotypes. Those who are elderly or chronically ill are particularly at risk of developing severe, even fatal, pneumococcal infections. For some persons, a second dose is recommended.

There has been an important advance in vaccination against pneumococcal pneumonia with the advent of Prevnar, or pneumococcal 13-valent conjugate vaccine. Prevnar provides additional protection and should also be given. The order in which one receives Pneumovax and Prevnar depends upon a number of issues, so you should consult with your physician about this. Everyone with Sjögren's should receive these vaccines, unless there are specific medical reasons to the contrary.

The third category of vaccines to consider is the "live virus" vaccines. The vaccines we have just discussed are made of killed viruses or bacteria and pose no risk of infection. However, vaccination with a live virus does pose some risk of infection, and in someone with an autoimmune disease who is taking immunosuppressive medication, this may be quite dangerous. One such live attenuated vaccine is FluMist, which is administered as a nasal spray. FluMist should not be given to immunosuppressed patients. The definition of immunosuppressed is open to interpretation but clearly includes patients taking immunosuppressive agents such as prednisone, azathioprine, methotrexate, cyclophosphamide, rituximab, or mycophenolate mofetil.

There has been a major new development in the shingles vaccine. Zostavax is an attenuated live virus vaccine that cannot safely be administered to patients who are significantly immunosuppressed. The new vaccine, Shingrix (recombinant zoster vaccine), is a "killed virus" vaccine and therefore is not as risky to immunosuppressed persons. Furthermore, it appears that it is much more effective than Zostavax in preventing shingles. The Centers for Disease Control and Prevention recommends Shingrix over Zostavax and recommends two doses separated by 2 to 6 months in "immunocompetent persons" 50 years of age and older, including patients on "low dose immunosuppression." This latter term is open to interpretation, so ask your doctor which vaccination is right for you.

Human papillomavirus quadrivalent (Gardasil) protects against human papillomavirus infection and the complication of cervical cancer. Experience with this vaccine in young women with Sjögren's is limited. Talk to your physician about whether you are in a high-risk group and should consider receiving this immunization. For patients taking chronic steroids, doses of prednisone higher than 30 mg/day may alter antibody production. Ideally, vaccines should be administered at the lowest possible steroid dose. For patients taking Rituxan, vaccines should be given at least 3 weeks before the infusion in order to optimize antibody production. Similarly, vaccines should be given prior to a course of Cytoxan, which can also suppress B-lymphocyte function. Intravenous immunoglobulin (IVIg) should not pose a problem and, in fact, may provide what is known as passive immunity to many microbes.

Lastly, the pandemic caused by COVID-19 is something our global society has had to endure, and vaccines against this virus have recently become available. With input from a team of medical and scientific advisors, the Sjögren's Foundation is recommending that Sjögren's patients receive a COVID-19 vaccine. To date, no adverse reactions specific to Sjögren's have been reported in the peer-reviewed literature. We will learn more about COVID-19 as well as the available vaccines as time goes on, and Sjögren's patients are encouraged to speak with their care providers and reference the Sjögren's Foundation for up-to-date information as it becomes available.

Table 46.1 summarizes the recommendations made within this chapter.

Summing Up

I recommend that all patients with Sjögren's should have the pneumococcal pneumonia vaccine, yearly influenza vaccine, and a Td booster at least every

Table 46.1 Vaccinations and Sjögren's Patients

Killed or Other Vaccines (Recommended if indicated)	Live Vaccines (Not advised except in special circumstances)
Pneumococcus (Prevnar; Pneumovax)	Polio (Sabin)
Influenza	Influenza (FluMist)
Meningitis	Herpes zoster/shingles (Zostavax)
Shingles (Shingrix)	Varicella
COVID-19	
Human papillomavirus quadrivalent (Gardasil)	

10 years. Vaccination against shingles is now less complicated and should be strongly considered. Live virus vaccines such as FluMist and Zostavax should be avoided except in special circumstances to be determined by the physician. Sjögren's patients should receive a COVID-19 vaccine.

For Further Reading

Abdelahad M, Ta E, Kesselman MM, Demory Beckler M. A review of the efficacy of influenza vaccination in autoimmune disease patients. *Cureus.* 2021;13(5):e15016.

Centers for Disease Control and Prevention. CDC's Advisory Committee on Immunization Practices (ACIP) recommends universal annual influenza vaccination. February 4, 2010. http://www.cdc.gov/media/pressrel/2010/r100224.htm

Centers for Disease Control and Prevention. Healthy People 2030: Objectives and Data. https://health.gov/healthypeople/objectives-and-data/browse-objectives

Fiore AE, Shay DK, Broder K, et al. Prevention and control of seasonal influenza with vaccines: Recommendations of the Advisory Committee on Immunization Practices (ACIP), 2009. *MMWR Recomm Rep.* 2009;58:1.

Gardner P, Eickhoff T, Poland GA, et al. Adult immunizations. *Ann Intern Med.* 1996;124:35.

Hornberger J, Robertus K. Cost-effectiveness of a vaccine to prevent herpes zoster and postherpetic neuralgia in older adults. *Ann Intern Med.* 2006;145:317.

Kroger AT, Atkinson WL, Marcuse EK, Pickering LK. General recommendations on immunization: Recommendations of the Advisory Committee on Immunization Practices (ACIP). *MMWR Recomm Rep.* 2006;55:1.

Markowitz LE, Dunne EF, Saraiya M, et al. Quadrivalent human papillomavirus vaccine: Recommendations of the Advisory Committee on Immunization Practices (ACIP). *MMWR Recomm Rep.* 2007;56:1.

Oxman MN, Levin MJ, Johnson GR, et al. A vaccine to prevent herpes zoster and postherpetic neuralgia in older adults. *N Engl J Med.* 2005;352:2271.

Sjögren's Foundation. Sjögren's and COVID-19 Vaccination Statement. January 8, 2021. https://www.sjogrens.org/news/2021/sjogrens-and-covid-19-vaccination-statement

47
Disability

Thomas D. Sutton and Katherine M. Hammitt

The manifestations of Sjögren's can be disabling and impact a patient's ability not only to handle routine day-to-day activities but also to engage in paid work. This chapter will provide an overview of the ways Sjögren's can be disabling, tips for staying employed, and how to weigh the decision about whether to apply for disability. We offer advice on how to apply for disability and what to expect, with a focus on obtaining disability through the U.S. Social Security Administration (SSA).

Work and Sjögren's

The Sjögren's Foundation 2016 "Living with Sjögren's" national patient survey illustrates the profound and disabling effect that Sjögren's can have on a patient's ability to work. Even when patients can maintain a job, they often need special accommodations in the workplace, including flexible schedules and time off from work for medical appointments and major flares. As a recent German study on disability poignantly points out, even when Sjögren's patients work, they can face extreme job vulnerability when it comes to maintaining their job.

The inability to pursue a career or work in the kind of job for which a patient has been educated and trained also can add greatly to the already high financial burden of the disease. This survey found that 54% of Sjögren's patients had to make changes related to their work status, including 28% who had to stop working altogether, another 28% who had to reduce the number of working hours, and 30% who had to take days off from work (Figure 47.1).

The survey also found that 66% of Sjögren's patients say that living with Sjögren's adds a significant financial burden overall. Chapter 5 provides details on the high price tag that comes with having Sjögren's and cites several recent international studies showing that Sjögren's causes significant increases in disability. A 2017 study by Mandl et al. in Sweden found that disability rose significantly in the 2-year period following diagnosis with

Thomas D. Sutton and Katherine M. Hammitt, *Disability* In: *The Sjögren's Book*. Edited by: Daniel J. Wallace, Oxford University Press. © Sjögren's Foundation 2022. DOI: 10.1093/oso/9780197502112.003.0047

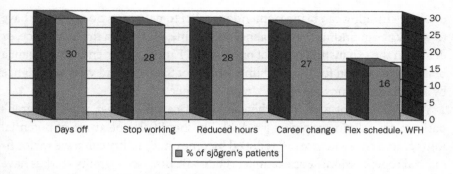

Figure 47.1 Changes at work due to Sjögren's.

Sjögren's. At diagnosis, 26% of patients were work-disabled; at 12 months, this figure rose to 37%, and at 24 months it rose to 41%. A 2018 Canadian study of patients with Sjögren's, lupus, and scleroderma found significant increases in lost productivity costs for those employed and a high incidence of complete lack of employment among all three groups, with 30% of Sjögren's patients not employed at all. This figure is similar to the 28% found by the Sjögren's Foundation survey.

Many Sjögren's patients are able to hold full- or part-time jobs, but for some who want to work, the symptoms and complications of the disease prevent them from doing so. Any one of the many symptoms included in this book and/ or listed under the SSA's "Listing of Impairments for Sjögren's Syndrome" can interfere with regular activities and result in disability. For example, fatigue, joint and muscle pain, numbness and nerve pain, gastrointestinal problems, vasculitis, cognitive issues ("brain fog"), or sleep problems can interfere with one's ability to work. Symptoms that wax and wane can prevent a patient from committing to a set schedule. Dry mouth can lead to difficulty speaking and swallowing and can cause loss of teeth and oral pain and infection, problems that might interfere with some jobs. Dry eyes can hinder the ability to read and use a computer and may be made worse by working under bright lights. One study from the Schepens Eye Research Institute found that 37.5% of employed Sjögren's patients reported that their dry eye symptoms interfered with their ability to work. The work environment also can aggravate symptoms and impairment through low humidity, fluorescent lights, drafts, and fumes.

Weighing the Decision to Apply for Disability

Whether to apply for disability can be a major decision, and all potential benefits and risks should be considered. On the positive side, access to disability funding can bring tremendous relief to patients who no longer have to worry about finding ways to generate income, manage in the workplace, or deal with the exhaustion brought on by work. Family and friends might gain a better appreciation for the disabling aspects of Sjögren's and view acceptance by a disability agency as legitimizing these aspects.

While often not a choice when a patient can no longer work, Sjögren's patients considering applying for disability should also be aware of potential unintended consequences. A reduced income on disability can have major financial repercussions. For example, rheumatic disease disability studies have documented that some recipients have been unable to manage major bills, such as car and house payments, and face a decreased standard of living, disconnection with intimate partners, loss of hobbies, and reduced self-esteem, independence, and socialization with friends from the workplace. These issues should be anticipated at the time of a disability filing, and if another job is not appropriate in a patient's situation, mitigations should be strategized in advance to prevent unwanted emotional, physical, and financial repercussions. Remember that Sjögren's patients may be "differently abled" because of their disease; in other words, a patient might or might not be disabled, but the tasks a patient can handle may be different and vary with each individual. Box 47.1 offers suggestions for improving your ability to stay employed.

Disability Pensions Around the World

The process for applying for a disability stipend or pension varies with each country. For example, the Swedish Social Insurance Agency handles disability in Sweden, and the United Kingdom and Australia have a Department for Work and Pensions. Disability can be relatively difficult to obtain in Asia, where disability may be stigmatized more than in many other locations. The United Nations has tackled the issue of disability from all causes and throughout the world through its Department of Economic and Social Affairs. The UN Convention on the Rights of Persons with Disabilities and the UN Economic and Social Commission for Asia and the Pacific are examples of the many initiatives led by the UN to ensure that those who are disabled and cannot work obtain the proper care. Because systems vary widely around the world, for simplicity's sake, we will focus on the disability process in the United States. Remember that many of the tips you gather from learning about the U.S. process may carry over to other countries.

Box 47.1 What Can You Do to Improve Your Ability to Stay Employed?

- Take care of yourself and see your healthcare professionals regularly.
- Understand your skills and the value you can offer an employer.
- Be positive about your ability to contribute to an organization.
- Know your limitations. (If you are exhausted and make a serious mistake, your boss is more likely to remember this than a time when you "saved the day.")
- Be honest about what you can and cannot do.
- Recognize that your employer has specific goals to accomplish. Make sure you understand your employer's needs so you can suggest ways that you can help meet them.
- Talk with your employer to see if accommodations can be made that satisfy both your and your employer's requirements. For example, can tasks or schedules be modified and at the same time meet your employer's needs?
- Know your rights. Familiarize yourself with or talk to a lawyer specializing in the Americans with Disabilities Act.
- Consider investigating private disability insurance in case you reach a point at which you can no longer work.
- If your current or prospective job will not allow the flexibility or changes you need, search for other positions or career paths that will.

Private Disability in the United States

Some individuals in the United States are fortunate to have private disability insurance, either as a benefit provided by an employer or as the result of an individually purchased policy. Remember that the definitions of disability in such policies may differ somewhat from the standard of the public disability programs administered by Social Security and should be carefully consulted before a claim is made. In addition to providing financial compensation for job loss due to disability, policies may include vocational rehabilitation and training for another job if one is permanently disabled from performing one's current job. For most Americans, however, the disability insurance programs administered by the SSA are the only source of income available when medical problems result in an inability to work.

U.S. Social Security Disability

Because of advocacy efforts on the part of the Sjögren's Foundation, SSA regulations now include specific disability criteria for Sjögren's. These criteria were added in 2010 and mean that Sjögren's patients no longer have to meet criteria set for another, related disease, and the need to educate SSA officials on the symptoms of Sjögren's and how these can be disabling has been reduced. However, while the listing of impairments for Sjögren's is now in use, patients and the attorneys who represent them still must be prepared to offer thoroughly documented medical records and a detailed presentation regarding the many facets of the disease and its effects on the individual's ability to function in a workplace.

Two SSA disability programs exist, each of which uses the same statutory definition of disability: the inability to engage in substantial gainful activity (SGA) because of medically determinable impairment(s) that have lasted for 12 months or are expected to last for 12 months or to result in death (42 U.S.C. § 416(i)). Disabled individuals with substantial work histories in covered employment are eligible for disability insurance benefits (DIB) and, following a statutory waiting period, Medicare. In addition, the dependents of individuals found eligible for DIB may receive auxiliary benefits. Individuals without a substantial work history in covered employment may be eligible for Supplemental Security Income (SSI) if they meet not only the medical standard for disability but also income and resource limitations.

The Evaluation Process

When an individual applies for SSA disability benefits, a sequential evaluation process is followed in every case.

Step 1

At Step 1, the question is whether the claimant is performing substantial gainful activity (SGA), a term that is defined somewhat differently for employees and self-employed individuals. If the claimant is performing SGA, the claim is denied; if not, the process continues.

Step 2

At Step 2, the question is whether the claimant has a medically determinable impairment that is severe, a term SSA has defined to mean an impairment that is more than slight and has more than a minimal effect on the claimant's ability to perform physical and/or mental work-related activities. The severity test is intended only to screen out obviously unmeritorious claims of disability at an early stage and should not be an obstacle for most Sjögren's patients. There are numerous examples of functional limitations caused by Sjögren's—for instance, xerostomia can seriously interfere with the ability to communicate due to lack of saliva; sicca symptoms may cause significant impairment of vision; fatigue may be as severe as that caused by illnesses such as lupus or chronic fatigue syndrome. These and many other symptoms of Sjögren's may result in more-than-minimal functional limitations, so Sjögren's should rarely, if ever, be dismissed as a non-severe impairment at Step 2. If there is at least one severe impairment, the process continues.

Step 3

At Step 3, the claimant may be found disabled if his or her condition meets or is clinically equivalent to the criteria set forth in the SSA's listing of impairments, found at 20 C.F.R. Part 404, Subpart P, Appendix 1. In § 14.00, the preface to the immune system disorders listings, SSA states the following regarding Sjögren's:

   a. *General.* (i) Sjögren's syndrome is an immunomediated disorder of the exocrine glands. Involvement of the lacrimal and salivary glands is the hallmark feature, resulting in symptoms of dry eyes and dry mouth, and possible complications, such as corneal damage, blepharitis (eyelid inflammation), dysphagia (difficulty in swallowing), dental caries, and the inability to speak for extended periods of time. Involvement of the exocrine glands of the upper airways may result in persistent dry cough.
   (ii) Many other organ systems may be involved, including musculoskeletal (arthritis, myositis), respiratory (interstitial fibrosis), gastrointestinal (dysmotility, dysphagia, involuntary weight loss), genitourinary (interstitial cystitis, renal tubular acidosis), skin (purpura, vasculitis), neurologic (central nervous system disorders, cranial and peripheral neuropathies), mental (cognitive dysfunction, poor memory), and neoplastic (lymphoma). Severe fatigue and malaise are frequently reported. Sjögren's syndrome may be associated with other autoimmune disorders (for example, rheumatoid arthritis or SLE); usually the clinical features of the associated disorder predominate.

b. *Documentation of Sjögren's syndrome.* If you have Sjögren's syndrome, the medical evidence will generally, but not always, show that your disease satisfies the criteria in the current "Criteria for the Classification of Sjögren's Syndrome" by the American College of Rheumatology found in the most recent edition of the *Primer on the Rheumatic Diseases* published by the Arthritis Foundation.

The listing for Sjögren's is found at § 14.10 of the listing of impairments: 14.10 *Sjögren's syndrome.* As described in 14.00D7. With:

A. Involvement of two or more organs/body systems, with:
  1. One of the organs/body systems involved to at least a moderate level of severity; and
  2. At least two of the constitutional symptoms or signs (severe fatigue, fever, malaise, or involuntary weight loss).

OR

B. Repeated manifestations of Sjögren's syndrome, with at least two of the constitutional symptoms or signs (severe fatigue, fever, malaise, or involuntary weight loss) and one of the following at the marked level:
  1. Limitation of activities of daily living.
  2. Limitation in maintaining social functioning.
  3. Limitation in completing tasks in a timely manner due to deficiencies in concentration, persistence, or pace.

For purposes of the listing of impairments, constitutional symptoms or signs means

severe fatigue, fever, malaise, or involuntary weight loss. Severe fatigue means a frequent sense of exhaustion that results in significantly reduced physical activity or mental function. Malaise means frequent feelings of illness, bodily discomfort, or lack of well-being that result in significantly reduced physical activity or mental function. (§12.00(C))

In addition, § 12.00(I) of the listing defines the functional criteria for disability from immune system disorders as follows:

To satisfy the functional criterion in a listing, your immune system disorder must result in a "marked" level of limitation in one of three general areas of functioning: Activities of daily living, social functioning, or difficulties in completing tasks due to deficiencies in concentration, persistence, or pace. Functional limitation may result from the impact of the disease process itself on your mental functioning, physical functioning, or both your mental and physical functioning. This could result from persistent or intermittent symptoms, such as depression, severe fatigue, or pain, resulting in a limitation of your ability to do a task, to concentrate, to persevere at a task, or to perform the task at an acceptable rate of speed. You may also have limitations because of your treatment and its side effects (see 14.00G).

When "marked" is used as a standard for measuring the degree of functional limitation, it means more than moderate but less than extreme. We do not define "marked" by a specific number of different activities of daily living in which your functioning is impaired, different behaviors in which your social functioning is impaired, or tasks that you are able to complete, but by the nature and overall degree of interference with your functioning. You may have a marked limitation when several activities or functions are impaired, or even when only one is impaired. Also, you need not be totally precluded from performing an activity to have a marked limitation, as long as the degree of limitation seriously interferes with your ability to function independently, appropriately, and effectively. The term "marked" does not imply that you must be confined to bed, hospitalized, or in a nursing home.

Activities of daily living include, but are not limited to, such activities as doing household chores, grooming and hygiene, using a post office, taking public transportation, or paying bills. We will find that you have a "marked" limitation of activities of daily living if you have a serious limitation in your ability to maintain a household or take public transportation because of symptoms, such as pain, severe fatigue, anxiety, or difficulty concentrating, caused by your immune system disorder (including manifestations of the disorder) or its treatment, even if you are able to perform some self-care activities.

Social functioning includes the capacity to interact independently, appropriately, effectively, and on a sustained basis with others. It includes the ability to communicate effectively with others. We will find that you have a "marked" limitation in maintaining social functioning if you have a serious limitation in social interaction on a sustained basis because of symptoms, such as pain, severe fatigue, anxiety, or difficulty concentrating, or a pattern of exacerbation and remission, caused by your immune system disorder (including manifestations of the disorder) or its treatment, even if you are able to communicate with close friends or relatives.

Completing tasks in a timely manner involves the ability to sustain concentration, persistence, or pace to permit timely completion of tasks commonly found in work settings. We will find that you have a "marked" limitation in completing tasks if you have a serious limitation in your ability to sustain concentration or pace adequate to complete work-related tasks because of symptoms, such as pain, severe fatigue, anxiety, or difficulty concentrating, caused by your immune system disorder (including manifestations of the disorder) or its treatment, even if you are able to do some routine activities of daily living.

If the claimant meets or equals in clinical severity the criteria set forth under Section 14.10A or B, he or she will be found disabled at Step 3. If not, the sequential evaluation process continues.

Step 4

At Step 4, the question is whether the claimant is able to perform past relevant work, either as he or she performed it or as it is generally performed in the national economy. At this point in the evaluation, SSA evaluates the claimant's residual functional capacity (RFC) for work, which is what he or she can still do despite the effects of all medical impairments in combination. Under the regulations, work performed in the past 15 years that was SGA and lasted long enough to learn how to perform it is generally considered relevant. The claimant has the burden to show that his or her medically determinable impairment(s) preclude the performance of all past relevant work. If the claimant is found able to perform any of his or her past relevant work, the claim is denied; if not, the process continues.

Step 5

At Step 5, the question is whether the claimant is able to perform any other work in the national economy, taking into account age, education, work experience, and RFC. At this step, SSA has the burden of demonstrating that jobs within the parameters of the claimant's RFC exist in significant numbers. For claimants over the age of 50, a finding of disability may be directed by the regulations if exertional limitations reduce the RFC to sedentary or light work. However, for claimants under the age of 50, with few exceptions, a finding of disability will be made at Step 5 only if the individual proves that he or she is incapable of performing any kind of work on a regular and continuing (i.e., full-time) basis. If the claimant proves such inability, disability will be found; if not, the claim will be denied at this final step of the evaluation.

If the claimant meets the requirements in one step, she or he then moves on to the next step for consideration (Table 47.1).

Table 47.1 Steps of the Disability Evaluation Process

Step 1	Is the claimant performing SGA?
Step 2	Does the claimant have a medically determinable impairment that can be defined as severe?
Step 3	Does the claimant's condition meet or is clinically equivalent to the criteria set forth in the SSA's listing of impairments?
Step 4	Is the claimant able to perform past relevant work?
Step 5	Is the claimant able to perform any other work, taking into account age, education, work experience, and RFC?

The Role of the Treating Physician

As is obvious from the foregoing description, the SSA evaluation process is detailed and exacting. Sjögren's patients should review the 2010 listing criteria with their rheumatologists and should also review the criteria for other immune system disorders (e.g., lupus) if they, like many Sjögren's patients, also suffer from those disorders. Great care should be taken to document involvement in every relevant organ or body system, constitutional signs such as severe fatigue and weight loss, and functional impact on daily activities, social functioning, and task completion. The opinion of a treating physician (especially that of a rheumatologist) regarding the nature and severity of the Sjögren's, particularly if it is well supported by treatment notes, clinical findings, and laboratory tests, should be accorded great weight in the disability determination process. If it is not clear that the Sjögren's alone meets all of the criteria of the listing, all of the claimant's impairments in combination must be considered in determining whether he or she has the RFC to sustain employment. Sjögren's, along with other physical impairments that may be present (e.g., diabetes with neuropathy, arthritis, chronic heart failure), may cause such limitations in exertion (i.e., ability to walk, stand, sit, lift, carry, push, and pull) that the claimant is found disabled from a physical standpoint. In addition, all non-exertional limitations must be considered, including mental, vision, manipulative, speech and hearing, postural, and environmental limitations. For example, Sjögren's may cause central nervous system effects similar to those seen in cases of lupus cerebritis, and cognitive dysfunction may be so severe as a result of this (or from a comorbid condition such as depressive disorder) that the claimant is unable to perform the mental functional requirements of work (e.g., ability to concentrate, focus, deal with stress, accept criticism from supervisors). When all of the claimant's exertional and non-exertional limitations resulting from all of his or her impairments in combination are considered, disability may be found where the claimant cannot perform past relevant work or sustain alternative employment on a regular and continuing basis. Thus, a claimant's failure to meet or equal the criteria of the listing of impairments is by no means fatal to his or her disability claim.

Claimants' Rights and Promising U.S. Federal Court Decisions

Individuals whose applications are denied have the right to a hearing with an administrative law judge and to a review of adverse hearing decisions by the SSA's Appeals Council. Claimants who are administratively denied at every level of appeal may institute civil actions against SSA in the federal courts. Historically, U.S. federal courts have been receptive to Sjögren's claims, and the most recent decisions by these courts demonstrate an increasingly receptive response to disability claims of Sjögren's patients, particularly where the medical records document significant clinical findings and functional limitations caused by the disease.

Examples of significant U.S. federal court cases over the last few decades are *Mahoney v. Commissioner of Social Security*, 2018, WL 1684455 (E.D. Wash. 2018); *Flores v. Berryhill*, 2017, WL 3446291 (W.D. Okla. 2017); *Broussard v. Commissioner of Social Security*, 2015, WL 5025422 (W.D. La. 2015); *James v. Astrue*, 2013, WL 12109250 (S.D. Tex. 2013); *Steen v. Astrue*, 2008, WL 4449602 (N.D. Cal. 2008); *Phillips v. Barnhart*, 357 F.3d 1232 (11th Cir. 2004); *Swindle v. Sullivan*, 914 F.2d 222 (11th Cir. 1990); *Mack v. Secretary of HHS*, 747 F.Supp. 1208 (E.D. La. 1990); *Beusching v. Bowen*, 1988 U.S. Dist. LEXIS 15756 (C.D. Cal. 1988); and *Mansfield v. Barnhart*, 2005, WL 1476370 (S.D. Ind. 2005) (affirmed denial of benefits). Most cases reversed denial of benefits; two required SSA to obtain vocational expert testimony to justify their denial of disability; and one case (2005) affirmed denial of benefits. Four of the decisions to reverse denial of benefits came as recently as between 2013 and 2018. These decisions relied on the regulations governing the adjudication of Sjögren's claims that were published in 2010 as Section 14.10 of the listing of impairments (found at 20 C.F.R. Part 404, Subpart P, Appendix 1). Readers are encouraged to share these cases with attorneys assisting them with pursuing SSA disability claims.

Tips for Applicants

These cases illustrate the fact that it is not necessarily easy to succeed with a disability claim, even where a serious illness like Sjögren's is involved. Sjögren's patients are well advised not only to report all of their symptoms at each physician visit but also to keep a personal daily journal of problems from the onset of inability to work (Box 47.2). For example, if doing normal housework for one day results in being effectively bedridden for the next two to three days due to excessive fatigue or pain, the individual should document this in his or her journal. Of course, Sjögren's patients should have regular visits with a rheumatologist experienced in the treatment of this disease and should make certain that primary physicians receive copies of all treatment notes and test reports. Finally, patients who suffer from Sjögren's who have become unable to work should retain the services of an attorney experienced in SSA disability law early in the application process in order to facilitate communication with the physicians and proper presentation of the evidence of disability at every stage of the adjudication process. Attorneys who practice extensively in the disability arena can be quite helpful in obtaining favorable determinations at the early stages of the process, and where claims are denied their services are essential to improve the odds of prevailing on appeal, whether before a SSA administrative law judge or the federal courts. With the help of caring professionals in medicine and law, individuals disabled by Sjögren's should be able to obtain the disability benefits provided by the Social Security Act,

---

Box 47.2 Quick Tips for U.S. Claimants

- Visit your rheumatologist and other key healthcare professionals regularly.
- Report all symptoms at each physician visit.
- Make sure your physician documents involvement of every relevant organ or body system, constitutional signs, and impact on daily activities.
- Keep your own personal daily journal, noting symptoms and how they affect your ability to perform tasks.
- Make sure that primary physicians receive copies of all treatment notes and test reports.
- For more tips, visit the Sjögren's Foundation website at www.Sjögrens.org and download the fact sheet: Tips on Obtaining Disability Benefits from the Social Security Administration.

which are necessary to ensure at least partial replacement of lost work income and medical coverage to enable them to maintain as normal a life as possible while fighting this devastating illness.

Summing Up

Sjögren's can result in a high financial cost to patients and their families. With a potentially disabling disease, some Sjögren's patients are unable to work and face the loss of their income. At the same time, these patients face higher costs to manage and treat their disease and to hire help for household and other tasks that they can no longer do. For those outside the United States, we advise you to familiarize yourself with your country's disability processes. Many of the tips provided in this chapter may be useful to you. Sjögren's patients in the United States need to learn about the specific requirements and processes set by the SSA, consult with an experienced attorney, and follow the many tips available to present a better case. Now that Sjögren's is included in the SSA's listing of disabilities following recent efforts by the Sjögren's Foundation, the process for obtaining Social Security disability is more straightforward than in the past.

For Further Reading

Americans with Disabilities Act. http://www.ada.gov

Dumusc A, Bowman SJ. Sjögren syndrome and work disability. *J Rheumatol.* 2017;44(2):133–135.

Mandl T, Jørgensen TS, Skougaard M, et al. Work disability in newly diagnosed patients with primary Sjögren syndrome. *J Rheumatol.* 2017;44(2):209–215.

McCormick N, Marra CA, Sadatsafavi M, et al. Excess productivity costs of systemic lupus erythematosus, systemic sclerosis, and Sjögren's syndrome. *Arthritis Care Res.* 2019;71(1):142–154.Sjögren's Foundation. Fact Sheet, Tips on Obtaining Disability Benefits. https://www.Sjögrens.org/files/brochures/disability_benefits.pdf

Sjögren's Foundation. About Sjögren's. https://www.Sjögrens.org/home/about-Sjögrens

Social Security Administration. Social Security Disability Guidelines for Immune System Disorders in Adults. https://www.ssa.gov/disability/professionals/bluebook/14.00-Immune-Adult.htm#14_10

Social Security Administration. Social Security Disability Guidelines for Immune System Disorders in Children. https://www.ssa.gov/disability/professionals/bluebook/114.00-Immune-Childhood.htm

Sullivan RM, Cermak JM, Papas AS, et al. Economic and quality of life impact of dry eye symptoms in women with Sjögren's syndrome. *Adv Exp Med Biol.* 2002;506(Pt B):1183–1188.

Westhoff G, Dorner T, Zink A. Fatigue and depression predict physician visits and work disability in women with primary Sjögren's syndrome. *Rheumatology.* 2012;51:262–269.

PART VII
THE FUTURE

48

Recent and Promising Scientific Developments

Steven E. Carsons, Mabi Singh, Nancy McNamara,
and Katherine M. Hammitt

The number of clinical trials with potential therapies for Sjögren's symptoms such as fatigue, pain, neuropathies, pulmonary complications, and dryness has more than doubled over the last decade. This alone brings hope to patients and those who manage and treat them. In addition, key fields such as the immune system (see Chapter 6), the gut microbiome (see Chapter 9), and genetics (see Chapter 8), to name just a few, are experiencing an explosion in new information and are bringing more potential targets for treatment to the fore. Autoimmune symptoms experienced by those suffering the long-term effects of COVID-19 will bring promising knowledge to light and provide areas for new research. We currently are on the cusp of a new era in medicine with "precision medicine," in which therapies can be targeted to individual patients for greater success. The next decade is expected to bring discoveries that will enlighten us further about Sjögren's and offer the first-ever Sjögren's-specific therapies.

Immune System and Biological Therapies

Scientific discovery, particularly in the field of immunology has been proceeding at a rapid pace and promises to yield important discoveries and advances for the treatment of Sjögren's disease. Understanding the immunologic mechanisms involved in the interface between our environment and the immune system, those responsible for the activation and interplay of T and B lymphocytes, and those that explain how these cells damage the salivary and lacrimal glands should lead to effective therapies. In fact, therapeutic approaches, including B-cell–directed therapies, have already shown initial promising signals in clinical trials. We will explore four areas of significant

Steven E. Carsons, Mabi Singh, Nancy McNamara, and Katherine M. Hammitt, *Recent and Promising Scientific Developments* In: *The Sjögren's Book*. Edited by: Daniel J. Wallace, Oxford University Press. © Sjögren's Foundation 2022.
DOI: 10.1093/oso/9780197502112.003.0048

immunologic impact that have the potential to lead to specific therapeutic approaches for Sjögren's.

Host–Microbe Interactions in Sjögren's

We discussed in Chapter 6 how the first interface between our environment and the immune system occurs at the ocular mucosa, the oral mucosa, the respiratory tract, and the lining of our gut, and that these surfaces contain billions of microorganisms that largely live in harmony with us. These species of bacteria, viruses, and fungi are collectively referred to as the microbiome. Since the key targets of immune system dysfunction in Sjögren's disease involve these surfaces, particularly those of the eye and mouth, it is not surprising that there has been intense research into the microbiome in Sjögren's. In general, imbalances between pro-inflammatory T cells and regulatory T cells are associated with shifts in the types of bacteria that make up the microbiome. Several recent publications have documented such alterations in the microbiome (called dysbiosis) in the gut and mouth of Sjögren's patients. Products of the metabolism of these microorganisms (such as sugars and fatty acids) may affect the behavior of Sjögren's patients' T cells. Interestingly, one recent study found that a protein from a species of *Bacteroides* bacteria, which is overrepresented in the gut of Sjögren's patients, binds to the plasma of Ro (SS-A)-positive Sjögren's and lupus patients. Ro/SS-A is thought to be an important pathogenic factor in Sjögren's; approximately 70% of Sjögren's patients produce an antibody (Anti-Ro/SS-A). Dysbiosis may arise from a variety of micro-environmental changes, including diet, excessive treatment with antibiotics, and even the mode of delivery during one's birth (vaginal vs. cesarean section). Recently, a study from the United Kingdom compared a cohort of Sjögren's patients to nonspecific sicca controls and demonstrated that a Mediterranean diet lowered the risk of Sjögren's, suggesting that dietary manipulation of the microbiome may be a means to prevent or treat Sjögren's disease.

Innate Immunity and Interferons in Sjögren's

The immediate-response arm of our immune systems is referred to as the innate immune system and was reviewed in Chapter 6. Innate immunity provides prompt initial recognition of potential foreign invaders and marshals a brisk inflammatory response until the acquired or adaptive immune system can produce more specific and targeted immunity via antibodies and T cells. One of the first events during the initiation of innate immunity is recognition of a component of a microorganism, for instance a viral RNA fragment, by a specialized receptor (Toll receptor) on a type of dendritic cell (plasmacytoid DC). This interaction results in the production of a protein known as type I interferon. Type I interferon belongs to a class of small molecules (cytokines) that mediate a variety of downstream inflammatory responses by binding to cellular receptors, in this case a type I interferon receptor. Binding to the interferon receptor mediates activation of a series of genes known as interferon-stimulated genes (ISGs). Taken together, the expression of these genes is referred to as the type I interferon signature.

The type I interferon signature is a molecular profile that is very characteristic of lupus and Sjögren's and is felt to be important in maintaining the inflammatory state. Recently anifrolumab, a therapeutic antibody directed against the type I interferon receptor, has demonstrated positive results for the treatment of lupus. This suggests that this type of therapeutic approach could be applied in the future for the treatment of Sjögren's. Engagement of a type I interferon receptor is followed by activation of a protein signaling complex called JAK-STAT. JAK-STAT signaling leads to induction of ISGs, which can result in activation of other pro-inflammatory cytokines and immune cells, including natural killer (NK) cells. There are now three oral medications approved by the U.S. Food and Drug Administration (FDA) that function as inhibitors of JAK signaling and are in use for the treatment of rheumatoid arthritis (RA). Currently two of these JAK inhibitors are in early-phase trials for Sjögren's.

Immune Checkpoint Inhibition: Lessons from Cancer Therapy

It is not surprising that our immune system contains a series of checks and balances to prevent overactivity during times when it is not challenged by foreign invaders. Otherwise, we can assume that there would be a potential for the development of autoimmune reactions. These naturally occurring immune suppressive molecules, known as immune checkpoints, reside on T cells and serve as brakes to stop the immune response from going forward. Two such proteins are CTLA-4 and PD-1. To circumvent our immune system's ability to destroy cancer cells, the cancer cells can express CTLA-4 and PD-1, which can then inhibit the body's natural anti-tumor T-cell responses.

One of the most important recent breakthroughs in cancer treatment is the development of monoclonal antibodies to block the activity of CTLA-4 and PD-1. These are called immune checkpoint inhibitors (ICIs) and "remove the brakes" allowing T-cell activation, which in turn kills the tumor cells. Interestingly, cancer patients treated with ICIs can develop inflammatory reactions (side effects) related to enhancement of T-cell activity. One of these immune response adverse effects (ir-AEs) is eye and mouth dryness, which closely resembles Sjögren's.

Thus, we have learned that blocking molecules such as CTLA-4 and PD-1 can result in the infiltration of salivary and lacrimal glands with lymphocytes and resultant dryness. Furthermore, restoration of CTLA-4 and PD-1 function in autoimmune disease could theoretically inhibit the autoimmune process. This is exactly what occurs when the biological agent abatacept (Orencia) is administered for the treatment of RA. Abatacept is purified CTLA-4 linked to an immunoglobulin fragment for stability. Abatacept has been studied for the treatment of primary Sjögren's, and although a recent phase 3 trial did not meet its endpoint, some data does show efficacy of abatacept for certain Sjögren's parameters. Lessons learned from the use of ICIs for cancer therapy has led to additional potential targets for Sjögren's treatment.

Germinal Centers, Antibody Production, and Sjögren's Disease Severity

Not only do the innate and adaptive (acquired) arms of the immune system cooperate in initiating the immune response, but also T and B cells need to cooperate in order to optimize antibody production. This is essential for the normal immune protective function but may be detrimental in the face of autoimmunity. During an immune response, T and B cells interact in immune organs such as lymph nodes but in other tissues as well when these tissues are affected by autoimmune disease. When the immune response intensifies, structures called germinal centers (GCs) form in these tissues. GCs serve as factories for the production of normal or abnormal antibodies such as anti-Ro (SS-A) in the case of Sjögren's.

Molecules known as chemokines attract antibody-producing B lymphocytes to target tissues. A chemokine important in GC formation in CXCL13. GC formation is a significant event in Sjögren's since the number of GCs in salivary gland tissue correlates with the clinical severity of disease and the risk of lymphoma. One mechanism for T cells to help B cells produce enhanced levels of antibodies is through interaction of a molecule known as

CD154 on the surface of T cells with a molecule known as CD40 on the surface of B cells. A new therapeutic approach to Sjögren's involves treatment with an antibody to CD40. This monoclonal antibody, known as iscalimab, has shown promise in early-phase studies of Sjögren's; treatment has resulted in improvement in disease activity as measured by the European Sjögren's Syndrome Disease Activity Index (ESSDAI) and a decrease in CXCL13 levels.

Biomarkers

The identification of biomarkers in Sjögren's will open up a whole new world in terms of understanding the disease, diagnosing it, identifying risk factors for better clinical management, offering targets for treatment, and leading to better clinical trial design to test new therapies. Biomarkers could even lead to more precisely redefining Sjögren's and other autoimmune diseases. Currently, autoimmune diseases have been defined around symptoms, key features, and the very few biomarkers (such as anti-SSA/Ro) that we have.

With biomarkers, we are ushering in a new era that focuses on predictive, preventive, and personalized medicine. What if we could take a whole new look at Sjögren's by breaking the disease down into the most basic, cellular level? What if we could say that because you have biomarker "a" you might be more susceptible to lung or other specific complications, and patients who did not have that biomarker would not be susceptible? What if we could say one therapy will work for you while another will not because of the biomarkers you have or do not have? What a difference this could make in our knowledge and in managing an individual's Sjögren's!

The Sjögren's Foundation has prioritized the discovery of biomarkers through multiple venues. First, research grant applications looking for biomarkers in Sjögren's have been given top priority for those awarded by the Foundation in recent years. Second, the Foundation has taken on a leadership role in two major initiatives that will accelerate the discovery of biomarkers: the Foundation for the National Institutes of Health (FNIH) Biomarkers Consortium in Sjögren's and the National Institutes of Health (NIH) Accelerating Medicines Partnership*—Autoimmune and Immune-Mediated Disease (AMP*-AIM) program. Both efforts include the patient voice via the Sjögren's Foundation, Sjögren's medical leaders, industry, and NIH scientists and government regulators.

The FNIH Biomarkers Consortium aims to identify several key biomarkers that will enable stratification of patients into subgroups for better management and greater success in clinical trials and other research studies. Patients can then be grouped according to clinical features and symptoms. This $2 million to $3 million initiative started in 2019 and is estimated to take 5 to 6 years. The NIH AMP*-AIM program, coordinated by the FNIH, focuses on tissue analysis and crosstalk between cells. This massive $63 million to $77 million initiative will break Sjögren's down to its basic molecular level ("deconstruction") to index and map all cells and pathways, so that a fresh look can be taken at disease pathways ("reconstruction"). This initiative will also include lupus, RA, psoriasis, and psoriatic arthritis in addition to Sjögren's so that similarities and differences can be determined between Sjögren's and each of these. NIH announcements requesting applications for grants were posted in early 2021.

Advances in Oral Medicine

One of the hallmarks of Sjögren's disease is the loss of saliva from three major paired and hundreds of unpaired minor salivary glands. Multiple complications arise with the loss of "bulk fluid" (i.e., the saliva in the oral cavity), including a subjective sensation of dryness in the mouth and sialorrhea (excessive saliva) as homeostasis is decreased. The physical consistency of saliva is altered; it presents as thick, stringy, viscous, ropey, and tacky, which may at times result in a subjective feeling of too much saliva (subjective sialorrhea).

Most of the symptomatic treatments are directed toward reducing the subjective sensation of dryness (xerostomia) of the oral cavity by increasing qualitative and quantitative saliva levels. Personal choice plays a large role in which salivary products a patient prefers, but new ones are continually hitting the market, offering more choices. However, substantial developments to improve decreased salivary function due to permanent destruction by infiltration of lymphocytes into the salivary gland cells remain lacking.

Randomized clinical trials generally have not shown significant statistical differences in oral dryness or salivary function. Patients with some remaining salivary gland function (i.e., those who do not have advanced disease or high disease activity) can receive help in preserving the salivary gland function from sialogogues and perhaps agents that target B cells. However, once the salivary glands are permanently and irreversibly damaged, salivary production cannot be increased.

Promising therapeutic targets include those that affect serum and salivary B-cell activating factor (BAFF) of the tumor necrosis factor (TNF) family, which are elevated in Sjögren's. The anti-rheumatic drug hydroxychloroquine can reduce BAFF and has shown mixed results with improvement in salivary function by diminishing the protein complexes that stimulate CD4⁺ T cells. In addition, the depletion of B cells, including those in the salivary glands, can be achieved by administration of biologics, such as anti-CD20 monoclonal antibody. For example, the Sjögren's Foundation Clinical Practice Guidelines for Use of Biologics (published in 2017 in *Arthritis Care and Research*) provides this recommendation:

> Rituximab may be considered as a therapeutic option for xerostomia in patients with primary Sjögren's with some evidence of residual salivary production, significant evidence of oral damage as determined by the clinician, and for whom conventional therapies, including topical moisturizers and secretagogues, have proven insufficient.

This was rated as a weak recommendation because it was based on only two clinical trials, one of which used salivary flow as a secondary measure and the second being a much smaller, randomized placebo-controlled trial. Since the B cells repopulate in the salivary glands, frequent treatment with the monoclonal antibodies may be needed.

With so many more clinical trials for biologics and small-molecule therapies in progress, hope is increasing that a systemic therapeutic will prove helpful for xerostomia. Potential future targets could include pathways that enable immune dysregulation of the epithelium of the salivary glands and infiltration of B and T cells into glandular tissues. Genetic, genomic, and proteomic studies could lead to novel targeted therapies. Further investigation into microRNA regulation of genes or proteins and subsequent alteration of lymphocyte characterization with microRNA may reduce autoimmune complications and consequently decrease glandular damage and manifestations of salivary hypofunction.

Gene therapy is a tool on the horizon that is expected to increase saliva and has been under investigation by government and university researchers as well as industry. This process introduces genetic material into cells to make them function better. It uses a delivery system called viral vectors for the gene transfer and is coupled with ultrasound and gene-editing technologies to accomplish this.

Gene therapy might be used to increase aquaporin expression. Aquaporins are involved in opening and closing water channels and thus contribute to salivary flow. These transmembrane proteins are expressed in the salivary glands' acinar, ductal, and myoepithelial cells. They allow for the movement of fluid across the semipermeable membrane. In addition to gene therapy, pharmacological solutions might be used to alter aquaporin expression for xerostomia.

Further study is warranted on the impact of omega-3s and omega-6s, disease-modifying anti-rheumatic drugs (DMARDs), and interferon-alpha in xerostomia. Some studies have found low levels of omega-3 and omega-6 fatty acids in Sjögren's patients. Subjective improvement has been seen in the oral cavity following dietary supplementation of omega-3s, possibly due to the anti-inflammatory nature and potential decrease in the fat mass and salivary cortisol levels with omegas. The administration of DMARDs, such as hydroxychloroquine, has demonstrated significant improvement in objective (but not subjective) measures of unstimulated salivary flow rates. Oromucosal administration of low-dose (150 IU TID) or weekly intramuscular injection of interferon-alpha has been shown in studies to increase unstimulated and stimulated salivary flow.

Various pharmacological and non-pharmacological agents have been tried to improve salivary function on the parasympathetic nervous system, and cholinergic drugs are the choice for improving salivary flow. The resulting saliva production depends on the dose and the remaining functional volume of the salivary glands. Pilocarpine HCl and cevimeline HCl are the sialogogues that have been most often researched and most often used to treat the subjective sensation of dryness in the oral cavity. These parasympathomimetic drugs act on the muscarinic receptors; hence, side effects may include sweating, increased acid production, tearing, change in vision, chills, and so forth. No serious side effects have been encountered with the long-term use (20-plus years) of pilocarpine in our clinical experience and in patients for whom tolerability is not an issue. Future research might bring more options for this class of drugs.

Ocular Advancements

When we think of Sjögren's and what is occurring on the ocular surface, we recognize that chronic and persistent dryness, another hallmark component of Sjögren's, causes chronic stress, and that stress leads to a local inflammatory response. This response sets off a cycle of inflammation that stimulates the release of inflammatory mediators from cells lining the ocular surface and resident immune cells. With the activation of antigen-presenting cells and T cells their associated pathways are "turned on," and, together with a variety of extrinsic factors, damage to the ocular surface ensues. Ongoing ocular surface damage further exacerbates the chronic nature of dry eye disease, and many Sjögren's patients experience other stressors like meibomian gland dysfunction and irritation from contact lens wear and environmental conditions. Taken together, the ocular surface in Sjögren's is a hotbed for chronic inflammation, which must be carefully controlled to prevent disease progression.

During the 2017 Tear Film and Ocular Surface's international Dry Eye Workshop II (DEWS II), the research community came together to (1) update the definition and classification of dry eye disease (DED); (2) evaluate critically the epidemiology, pathophysiology, mechanism, and impact of this disorder; (3) develop recommendations for the diagnosis, management, and therapy of this disease; and (4) recommend the design of clinical trials to assess future interventions for DED treatment. One outcome from this process was the introduction of a novel subcategory of dry eye resulting from damage to peripheral nerve terminals of the highly innervated cornea. In Sjögren's, we are now learning that the combination of systemic and local immune responses can result in significant neuropathic disease throughout the body, including the sensitization, depression, and/or loss of sensory nerves innervating the cornea. It is projected that the disruption to corneal nerves resulting from chronic dryness is more extensive than that resulting from inflammation.

This is an exciting area as it relates to new potential therapies and interventions for Sjögren's patients who suffer from dry eye. At present, there are few FDA-approved medications on the market (cyclosporine A in multiple doses and lifitegrast). All target the inflammatory response and, specifically, the T-cell pathway. While these medications are helpful for some, there remain numerous patients who do not benefit from their use—and in that respect, we know that there is still more work to be done in deciphering the underlying disease mechanism to gain a better understanding of more effective therapeutic strategies. Addressing the neuropathic component mentioned earlier will be an important part of this effort. As a research community, we currently have a limited understanding of how neuropathic changes occur in the cornea, the impact of these changes on ocular surface health, and effective mechanisms to reverse these pathogenic processes. There is considerable potential for scientific discovery, and we are working hard to grow our knowledge in this area. A few examples of exciting areas of dry eye research are provided next.

Tivanisiran is a small interfering RNA (siRNA) currently in development for the treatment of the signs and symptoms of dry eye. siRNA is a relatively new approach to treating disease in general. Tivanisiran is an inhibitor of the transient receptor potential vanilloid-1 (TRPV1), which is an important receptor in terms of corneal sensation and one that is believed to be impacted in the presence of DED. TRPV1 is a nociceptor that functions to sense, transmit, and regulate pain, as well as acting as a mediator of an inflammatory response. Given that the major pathogenesis of DED is a chronic immune response, tivanisiran is an attractive treatment to pursue as it addresses both the neuropathic and inflammatory components of DED.

Lacripep is a bioactive 19-amino acid peptide of the naturally occurring tear glycoprotein lacritin. Lacritin has pro-secretory and mitogenic properties that make it an interesting candidate for the treatment of DED. Interestingly, lacritin has also been found to be deficient in the tears of Sjögren's patients, and this deficiency is correlated to changes in corneal innervation as well as other clinical signs of dry eye in animal studies. We have demonstrated Lacripep's exciting potential to restore ocular surface health in the setting of Sjögren's-associated DED. In phase 1/2 clinical trials, Lacripep has shown further promise as an effective dry eye therapy through reduced disruption of the ocular surface epithelium and improvement in symptoms of burning and stinging. While Lacripep's therapeutic potential is attractive for a variety of reasons, perhaps most compelling is that it is a naturally occurring tear protein that replaces a component of the tears that has been shown to be deficient in individuals with Sjögren's.

Probiotics, or microorganisms to address gut dysbiosis, represent another area that holds promise in the field of dry eye research. As mentioned in Chapter 9 on the microbiome, data on probiotic use has been encouraging, though we are still in the early stages of fully understanding this field. A few specific examples in this area currently under evaluation are (1) the use of IRT-5, a mixture of five probiotic strains, which has shown benefit in the clinical manifestations of autoimmune-related uveitis and dry eye and (2) fecal microbiota transplantation (FMT), a procedure that involves transferring healthy stool from one person to the colon of another in an effort to reintroduce or boost helpful organisms.

Future technologies, namely the use of stem cells, development of organoids, spatial transcriptomics, and use of single-cell/nuclear RNA sequencing, hold promise in facilitating important discoveries in the field of Sjögren's disease. Using these technologies together with high-level genetic association studies, we will continue to learn more about the underlying basis of disease processes that drive Sjögren's development and progression.

Of course, as science is always evolving, opportunities beyond those listed here will certainly be unveiled and pursued.

Clinical Trials

Advances in outcome measures for clinical trials in Sjögren's and other clinical trial design elements are under way and will lead to a greater number of trials and more successful ones. Patient recruitment and retention will improve as industry reaches out to patients to better understand their needs and takes advantage of trends to decentralize trials by increasing the use of telehealth and virtual platforms. See Chapters 49 and 50 for more information on clinical trials.

Summing Up

Great strides are under way that promise a brighter future for Sjögren's patients and the healthcare professionals who manage and treat them. We are learning more about the immune system and how immune function might go awry, including the role of the microbiome and innate immunity and interferons. We continue to gain insights from cancer therapy. Major initiatives are under way to identify a wide array of biomarkers in Sjögren's that will change the face of management and treatment. Regarding the treatment of dry mouth and dry eye, specific targets of new therapies and new systemic treatments are being identified. Finally, our experience with COVID-19 is raising new possibilities for the potential use of mRNA vaccinations in autoimmune diseases, and the long-term symptoms from COVID-19 that are shared with Sjögren's, such as fatigue, dysautonomia, and vasculitis, might shed new light on these difficult-to-treat symptoms in Sjögren's.

For Further Reading

Cankaya H, Alpöz E, Karabulut G, et al. Effects of hydroxychloroquine on salivary flow rates and oral complaints of Sjögren patients: A prospective sample study. *Oral Surg Oral Med Oral Pathol Oral Radiol Endod*. 2010;110(1):62–67. doi:10.1016/j.tripleo.2010.02.032

Choi SH, Oh JW Ryu JS, et al. IRT5 probiotics change immune modulatory protein expression in the extraorbital lacrimal glands of an autoimmune dry eye mouse model. *Invest Ophthalmol Vis Sci*. 2020;61(3):42.

Craig JP, Nelson JD, Azar DT, et al. TFOS DEWS II report: Executive summary. *Ocul Surf*. 2017;15(4):802–812. doi:10.1016/j.jtos.2017.08.003

D'Agostino C, Elkashty OA, Chivasso C, et al. Insight into salivary gland aquaporins. *Cells*. 202025;9(6):1547.

Fasano S, Isenberg DA. Present and novel biologic drugs in primary Sjögren's syndrome. *Clin Exp Rheumatol*. 2019;37 Suppl 118(3):167–174.

Garlapati K, Kammari A, Badam RK, et al. Meta-analysis on pharmacological therapies in the management of xerostomia in patients with Sjögren's syndrome. *Immunopharmacol Immunotoxicol.* 2019;41(2):312–318.

James JA, Guthridge JM, Chen H, et al. Unique Sjögren's syndrome patient subsets defined by molecular features. *Rheumatology.* 2020;59(4):860–868. doi:10.1093/rheumatology/kez335

Jeong SY, Choi WH, Jeon SG, et al. Establishment of functional epithelial organoids from human lacrimal glands. *Stem Cell Res Ther.* 2021;12:247.

Katsiougiannis S, Wong DT. The proteomics of saliva in Sjögren's syndrome. *Rheum Dis Clin North Am.* 2016;42(3):449–456.

McNamara NA, Ge S, Lee SM, et al. Reduced levels of tear lacritin are associated with corneal neuropathy in patients with the ocular component of Sjögren's syndrome. *Invest Ophthalmol Vis Sci.* 2016;57(13):5237–5243. doi:10.1167/iovs.16-19309

Odani T, Chiorini JA. Targeting primary Sjögren's syndrome. *Mod Rheumatol.* 2019;29(1):70–86.

Ramos-Casals M, Brito-Zerón P, Bombardieri S, et al. EULAR-Sjögren Syndrome Task Force Group. EULAR recommendations for the management of Sjögren's syndrome with topical and systemic therapies. *Ann Rheum Dis.* 2020;79(1):3–18. doi:10.1136/annrheumdis-2019-216114

Ramos-Casals M, Maria A, Suárez-Almazor ME, et al. Sicca/Sjögren's syndrome triggered by PD-1/PD-L1 checkpoint inhibitors. Data from the International ImmunoCancer Registry (ICIR). *Clin Exp Rheumatol.* 2019;37 Suppl 118(3):114–122.

Sène D, Ismael S, Forien M, et al. Ectopic germinal center-like structures in minor salivary gland biopsy tissue predict lymphoma occurrence in patients with primary Sjögren's syndrome. *Arthritis Rheumatol.* 2018;70(9):1481–1488. doi:10.1002/art.40528

Tsigalou C, Stavropoulou E, Bezirtzoglou E. Current insights in microbiome shifts in Sjogren's syndrome and possible therapeutic interventions. *Front Immunol.* 2018;9:1106. doi:10.3389/fimmu.2018.01106

Verstappen GM, Pringle S, Bootsma H, Kroese FGM. Epithelial-immune cell interplay in primary Sjögren syndrome salivary gland pathogenesis. *Nat Rev Rheumatol.* 2021;17(6):333–348.

49

Sjögren's Foundation Clinical Trials Consortium

Theresa Lawrence Ford

During its relatively short time in existence, the Sjögren's Foundation Clinical Trials Consortium (CTC) has already made a meaningful difference on clinical trials in Sjögren's. Since its inception by Drs. Elaine Alexander, the first Sjögren's Foundation CTC Chair, and Frederick Vivino, the Foundation's Medical and Scientific Advisory Board Chair at the time, the group has gone from no clinical trials for systemic therapies in Sjögren's to more than two dozen trials at the time of this book's publication, with many more in the planning stages. The CTC's vision, ultimately, is to improve the quality of life for Sjögren's patients by increasing the availability and accessibility of therapies to treat Sjögren's. To accomplish this, the CTC:

1. Supports and promotes objectives that facilitate the design of clinical trials through the development of biomarkers, novel diagnostics, internationally accepted classification criteria, and internationally accepted outcome measures
2. Increases partnerships between industry and the Sjögren's Foundation
3. Engages with government agencies, including the U.S. Food and Drug Administration (FDA), that oversee the approval of therapies

Initiatives

The CTC has developed and worked on a variety of initiatives to support its vision, which focus on education, communication, and building relationships.

Sjögren's Training & Education Platform

The Sjögren's Training & Education Platform (STEP) was created out of the need for better and more consistent training. STEP is the first ever online

Theresa Lawrence Ford, *Sjögren's Foundation Clinical Trials Consortium* In: *The Sjögren's Book*. Edited by: Daniel J. Wallace, Oxford University Press. © Sjögren's Foundation 2022. DOI: 10.1093/oso/9780197502112.003.0049 platform designed to train clinical trial investigators and educate clinicians from multiple specialties who treat Sjögren's. Our belief is that this program will encourage a greater interest in developing new therapies for Sjögren's and ensure higher-quality trials.

Currently, pharmaceutical companies must develop their own training programs for investigators leading their clinical trials, which can be very time-consuming and costly. Notably, this approach often falls short in terms of consistent training. By ensuring that clinical trial investigators receive consistent, easily accessible training, STEP helps train investigators more rapidly and ensures that data is being collected by all investigators in a consistent manner. This consistency is critical in allowing data to be compared between centers and trials to determine if a therapy is truly safe and effective.

This innovative platform helps to accomplish the following:

1. *Develop an online training program for current Sjögren's-specific outcome measures.* STEP participants are trained to use the European Alliance of Associations for Rheumatology (EULAR) Sjögren's Syndrome Disease Activity Index (ESSDAI) and the EULAR Sjögren's Syndrome Patient Reported Index (ESSPRI) for objective and patient-reported measurements, respectively. After the basic platform launched, the Foundation has worked to partner with individual pharmaceutical companies to develop personalized platforms for their clinical trials. Investigators take an online qualifying test to ensure that they meet the requirements for rating disease activity in Sjögren's according to standard testing developed by Foundation key opinion leaders and company-specific trials.

2. *Develop online training programs for additional outcome measures that can be used in Sjögren's trials.* In the future, offerings through STEP can be expanded to include training on multiple outcome measures that could potentially be used in a Sjögren's clinical trial. For example, fatigue and cognitive function are existing symptoms with outcome measures, and our hope is to add these, and others, to the online training, either as they are or slightly modified to better fit Sjögren's. These additional outcome measures will greatly expand the educational offerings and will help to ensure successful clinical trial design.

3. *Offer educational videos demonstrating how to perform Sjögren's-specific tests that can be used for clinical assessment of patients in a clinician's office and/or for use in clinical trials.* Healthcare professionals need to have the appropriate knowledge for consistently conducting Sjögren's-specific

tests. Properly and consistently performing these tests will help medical providers in their diagnosis and treatment of Sjögren's. Tests that will be covered in the STEP program include salivary gland ultrasound, small fiber biopsy for peripheral neuropathy, and ocular and oral testing.

Building Relationships with the FDA

The CTC recognizes the importance of having a productive and collaborative relationship with the FDA and has taken great strides to establish these relationships in recent years.

In 2016, the Sjögren's Foundation held an in-person meeting with FDA representatives from the Center for Drug Evaluation and Research, the Office of Professional Affairs and Stakeholder Engagement, and the Office of the Center Director to ensure that Sjögren's was on the FDA's radar and that they were aware of the current landscape in Sjögren's clinical trials and outcomes. In 2019, Foundation leadership and representatives from the medical and scientific community again met with FDA leadership to discuss key issues, such as patient-reported outcomes, broadening the patient base for trials, targeting patient subsets for clinical trials, and much more. These meetings were critical to establishing meaningful relationships within the FDA that the Foundation has and will continue to foster.

Additional efforts currently under way to help continue and grow these relationships include the Foundation being represented in various FDA-led groups, considerations for organizing a patient-focused drug-development meeting specifically for Sjögren's, and participating in a patient-focused drug-development meeting on xerostomia with partner organizations, and more. FDA members are invited to participate in the Foundation's CTC meetings and have presented on drug development at these meetings.

Classification Criteria

With the publication of the American College of Rheumatology (ACR)'s Sjögren's Syndrome Classification Criteria in 2012, the Sjögren's community was faced with the potential barrier of having multiple sets of published classification criteria, which were not in complete agreement. In this case, the other set of criteria was the American European Consensus Group criteria, published in 2002. This proved to be an impediment to a consistent definition of how a Sjögren's patient was defined, thus resulting in a barrier to forming clinical trials.

As one of the first major initiatives of the CTC, the Foundation worked to unite the international Sjögren's community to determine one set of criteria that would be used for clinical trials. To do this, the best aspects were taken from both the 2002 and 2012 criteria, which culminated in the publication of the 2016 ACR-EULAR classification criteria. This is now the most frequently used set of criteria in clinical trials for Sjögren's and is described throughout this book, including Chapter 17.

Global Reach

The Foundation and CTC's work is not exclusively for U.S. patients. As part of the International Sjögren's Network, the Foundation, along with numerous international representatives, works to ensure the involvement of Sjögren's patients throughout the world in clinical trials and the approval of new therapies. By broadening the patient base beyond the United States, pharmaceutical companies have greater access to Sjögren's patients at clinical sites around the world as well as partners to advocate for the approval of therapies from medical agencies beyond the FDA.

The Future

The CTC will continue to work for and support the development of new therapies for Sjögren's. As it was when the group first formed, its goal of identifying barriers to successful clinical trials and finding ways to bring the international community together to address these barriers will always be the top priority for the Sjögren's Foundation. Moving forward, the CTC will continue to work closely with all stakeholders—patients, industry, healthcare professionals, and government agencies—to accomplish its mission of (1) ensuring that clinical trials are patient-friendly; (2) ensuring that healthcare professionals are properly and consistently trained to carry out clinical trials; (3) identifying clinical trial sites that have both adequate Sjögren's populations and specialists with the appropriate knowledge on Sjögren's; (4) ensuring that government agencies are familiar with Sjögren's, the challenges for clinical trials, and best practices for conducting these trials; and (5) encouraging industry to engage in trials and partner with the Foundation to improve the opportunities for success.

For Further Reading

Lawrence Ford T. SSF advancing forward: Promoting clinical trial development. *Sjögren's Quarterly.* 2017;12(3):1–4.

Lawrence Ford T. Treating Sjögren's—the future! *Sjögren's Quarterly.* 2015;10(1):1–12.

Shiboski CH, Shiboski SC, Seror R, et al. 2016 American College of Rheumatology/European League Against Rheumatism classification criteria for primary Sjögren's syndrome: A consensus and data-driven methodology involving three international patient cohorts. *Ann Rheum Dis.* 2017;76(1):9–16. doi:10.1136/annrheumdis-2016-210571

50

Clinical Trials

What They Are, How to Get Involved, and the
Current State in Sjögren's

Matthew Makara and Daniel J. Wallace

Clinical trials are an important step in advancing medical treatment options for patients and are designed to determine if an intervention is safe and effective. A successful trial requires both the appropriate patient population and trained professionals to ensure the study is carried out and findings are interpreted correctly.

Although there are several agents approved for "dry eye," only two are approved by the U.S. Food and Drug Administration (FDA) for dry mouth related to Sjögren's. Pilocarpine (Salagen) and cevimeline (Evoxac) were approved 20 years ago. Since then no agent has been given an indication for Sjögren's, and no agent has been approved to date to treat the systemic manifestations of the disease.

This chapter will discuss some of the pros and cons of participating in a clinical trial for both patients and providers as well as the FDA approval process and where things stand regarding trials in Sjögren's.

Bringing a Drug to Market

Shepherding a new drug through the regulatory process requires a huge effort and substantial funding. In the United States, the average time for a drug to come to market is between 10 and 15 years, with average costs in the billions of dollars. For every 100 promising compounds that are studied in the test tube and in animal models, only a handful make it to the clinical trial stage. In the United States, the FDA oversees the process, while European efforts are coordinated through the European Medicines Agency (EMA). In other parts of the world, regional or national groups supervise drug development and discovery. When developing a potential drug for study, researchers will devise specific questions to which they plan to seek answers. Different trial phases are designed to answer such questions (Box 50.1).

Matthew Makara and Daniel J. Wallace, *Clinical Trials* In: *The Sjögren's Book*. Edited by: Daniel J. Wallace, Oxford University Press. © Sjögren's Foundation 2022. DOI: 10.1093/oso/9780197502112.003.0050

Box 50.1 Phases of a Clinical Trial

Phase 1: size: <100; duration: months; purpose: assess safety and dosage

Phase 2: size: 100–300; duration: months to a few years; purpose: assess safety and efficacy

Phase 3: size: hundreds to thousands; duration, 1–4 years; purpose: assess efficacy and adverse reactions

Phase 4: size: thousands; duration: years; purpose: assess long-term safety and efficacy, additional indications

---

Phase 1

Phase 1 trials always have safety as the primary endpoint. A candidate drug is usually tested in healthy subjects followed by a dose-escalation cohort where patients are given increasing, usually single, doses of the drug. The drug's pharmacokinetics, distribution, absorption, and excretion are carefully measured. Phase 1 usually involves fewer than 100 participants, though the number can be much less. Once the dose appears to be potentially efficacious and is believed to be safe, a phase 2 trial is initiated.

Phase 2

Phase 2 studies usually include 100 to 400 patients at 10 to 20 centers receiving two to four different doses, or placebo, over a period of 1 year. Post hoc (post-study) analyses are encouraged to ascertain which group of patients responded best to the options. Sometimes studies are halted if adverse effects or safety concerns arise. Approximately 25% of the drugs for rheumatic diseases studied over the last 10 years have gone onto a phase 3 trial.

Phase 3

Phase 3 trials usually enroll more than 1,000 patients from scores of centers and study the drug for at least 1 year. Often, patients are offered the opportunity for an open-label (no placebo) follow-up. If the primary endpoint is met, the sponsor may submit the drug to the FDA, EMA, or other regulatory agency depending on the country where approval is being sought. Once a drug is approved, there may be additional indications, or uses, that might help patients.

Phase 4

A phase 4 trial, sometimes referred to as a post-marketing surveillance trial, will assess the long-term safety and efficacy of a drug once it has become approved for use and is available on the market. Other factors, such as cost-effectiveness, may also be evaluated.

Getting Involved: Considerations for Patients

The prospect of participating in a clinical trial may be daunting for some and exciting for others; still others may not realize this option exists. Not everyone will be qualified to enroll in every trial, but in order for the medical and scientific fields to move forward, patients are needed for these studies. A 2017 report on public and patient perceptions of clinical research conducted by the Center for Information and Study on Clinical Research Participation noted the top two reasons for study participation were to help advance the science and treatment of the disease and condition (49%) and to obtain better treatment (44%). This same report noted that more than 90% of respondents said that they would participate in another clinical trial and that they would make a recommendation for others to participate, if relevant. Patients must know their rights and what to expect during the trial and must be comfortable with participating.

Classification and Inclusion/Exclusion Criteria

To be eligible for a Sjögren's study, patients must fulfill accepted classifications or definitions for the disease or have a specific area of involvement (e.g., dry eye, dry mouth, interstitial lung disease, fatigue) and activity that the sponsor is interested in studying. These parameters are part of the inclusion/exclusion criteria of a study, which are set at the beginning of the trial, prior to participant recruitment. Other common variables that may be considered are age and the presence of comorbid conditions.

During a trial, composite clinical indices are used to measure changes is symptoms, signs, and laboratory findings (perhaps using the European Alliance of Associations for Rheumatology [EULAR] Sjögren's Syndrome

Disease Activity Index [ESSDAI]). Patient-reported outcomes are measured as well. Participants usually are seen monthly so they can fill out forms and give a sample for blood testing.

Informed Consent and Other Safety Considerations

To enroll in a trial, patients must give informed consent. During this process, investigators will discuss the details of the trial, such as the potential benefits and risks, the study duration, the expected number of visits, and other information patients need to make an informed decision on whether they want to participate. This process also allows patients to ask any questions they may have to ensure they understand fully what their involvement entails. As part of the informed consent process, patients will learn that they have the right to withdraw from a study at any time and for any reason.

The FDA is the regulatory agency that oversees clinical trials taking place in the United States. As part of that oversight, investigators are required, in human trials, to receive approval from an institutional review board (IRB) before the trial can begin. This review helps ensure that the appropriate steps are being taken to protect the rights of study participants. For new medications being studied at multiple sites, or if the study involves certain risks, a data safety monitoring board will also be involved.

Potential Benefits and Risks of Participating in a Clinical Trial

Just as there are many potential benefits to participating in a clinical trial, so too can there be risks. However, these may be no greater than those related to normal medical care or the natural progression of disease. Box 50.2 outlines

---

Box 50.2 Benefits of Clinical Trial Participation

- Access to novel treatments at no cost
- Medical care, check-ups, and lab studies at no cost
- Financial reimbursement for participation (in some trials)
- Satisfaction that you are helping to advance the broader scientific and medical knowledge base and helping future patients

---

Box 50.3 Potential Risks of Clinical Trial Participation

- Treatment side effects are possible and might be serious.
- The treatment may not be effective.
- You could receive a placebo, depending on the study.
- Participation logistics may be inconvenient, time-consuming, and/or costly.

---

some of the benefits for patients to consider when deciding whether to participate in a clinical trial, while Box 50.3 outlines some of the potential risks or drawbacks.

Getting Involved: Considerations for Providers

When considering whether to participate in a trial, clinicians, similar to patients, must consider what their involvement entails and the subsequent benefits and potential risks.

As we stated previously, clinical trials are an important step in advancing science and medicine. Participating in a clinical trial offers clinicians a range of opportunities to acquire first-hand knowledge of novel treatments as well as contribute to the greater medical and scientific communities (Box 50.4).

On a professional level, participating clinicians can greatly expand their networks within their discipline, with other specialists, and with other sectors (e.g., researchers, industry, academia, etc.). These collaborations and relationships can help to expand a provider's knowledge base and allow them

---

Box 50.4 Potential Benefits of Clinical Trial Participation for Clinicians

---

- Expanding knowledge base and intellectual stimulation
- Expanding professional networks
- Gaining access to novel medications for patients and contributing to their development
- Contributing to the greater scientific and medical communities

---

to obtain perspectives from within and outside their field on important topics related to treatment and care, helping them to grow professionally and satisfy their intellectual curiosity.

Importantly, participating in a trial gives first-hand experience on the development of important treatments. This access, at times, may provide patients with effective therapies when no others exist. In addition to this improvement in care, experience working with a treatment under study can help provide clinicians with confidence in prescribing practices, as they have first-hand experience with a treatment prior to its approval.

Of course, there are logistical considerations for clinicians to take into account before becoming involved in a trial. Their site must meet certain standards, and there will be an increased administrative burden on staff. There are numerous resources that go into more depth on what is required and expected of a clinical trial site and its staff that can help those who want to make an informed decision.

Where Do Things Stand in Sjögren's?

As of this writing, only a handful of candidate drugs are being studied in phase 2 and 3 trials. Sjögren's experts are going through a learning process and still testing various methods of determining the best measure for disease improvement. Measures to determine how well a therapy is working (called "outcome measures") were only developed specifically for Sjögren's starting in 2007. Two indices were published to measure disease damage and activity, and since the ESSDAI was published in 2009 it has become the predominant disease activity measure for Sjögren's. However, it has been difficult to find a sufficient number of patients who meet the higher level of disease activity that is measured by ESSDAI and that is often required by companies, and some of the domains or areas rated by ESSDAI cannot improve with use of a therapy. This factor has hindered drug development. New measures for Sjögren's are currently in development and should increase the success of clinical trials in this disease. In addition, it can be very difficult to objectively measure fatigue, malaise, and aching. The Sjögren's Foundation is working with the National Institutes of Health and our international colleagues to streamline and stimulate the discovery process.

Agents for Sjögren's that have been evaluated in phase 3 or 4 trials are listed in Box 50.5.

Box 50.5 Drugs for Sjögren's and Related Dry Eye That Have Been Completed or Are Entering Phase 3 or 4 Studies

---

- VAY736 (ianalumab): an antibody targeting BAFF-R; successful completion of phase 2 and entering phase 3 as of this writing
- RSLV-132: an RNase Fc fusion protein aimed at reducing fatigue in Sjögren's; successful completion of phase 2 and entering phase 3 as of this writing
- Hydroxychloroquine: safe and appears to have modest benefits at 1 year
- Rituximab: safe, definite efficacy signals but did not meet primary endpoints
- Belimumab: safe, promising efficacy but needs further study
- Epratuzumab: in a lupus trial, subset with anti-SSA met endpoint in post hoc analysis
- Cyclosporine ophthalmic topical solution: approved for dry eye but not specifically Sjögren's
- Lifitegrast ophthalmic topical solution: approved for dry eye but not specifically Sjögren's

Clinical trials are rapidly evolving, so check https://www.sjogrens.org/living-with-sjogrens/clinical-trials/clinical-trial-locations for up-to-date information.

Summing Up

Clinical trials are used to evaluate new and existing treatments to determine proper usage and to ensure safety and effectiveness. They are divided into different phases. Before participating in a clinical trial, patients should understand their rights and the benefits and potential risks of participating. Safety is of the highest priority, and many safeguards are in place to monitor these studies. Participants often have access to extra care, novel medications, and testing at no cost and at times are reimbursed for their participation. However, with treatments that are under study, there are always risks of side effects, and the drug may not work. Logistical issues for participation can also be a burden to patients. For clinicians, getting involved in clinical trials can increase their knowledge, help them build networks and relationships, gain access to new treatments for their patients, and allow them to contribute to the scientific and medical communities. As of this writing, few treatments for Sjögren's and related symptoms have been studied, but continuing efforts are being made to stimulate and streamline this process.

For Further Reading

Baraf H. Clinical trials and this practicing rheumatologist. *Sjögren's Quarterly*. 2017;12(3):1–8.

Baraf H. Patient Education Sheet: Clinical trials—getting involved. https://www.sjogrens.org/files/brochures/ClinicalTrials2.pdf

Baraf H. Starting a clinical trials program. *Sjögren's Quarterly*. 2018;13(4):1–4.

Center for Information & Study on Clinical Research Participation. 2017 Perceptions & Insights Study: Report on the Participation Experience. https://www.ciscrp.org/wp-content/uploads/2019/06/2017-CISCRP-Perceptions-and-Insights-Study-Participation-Experience.pdf

ClinicalTrials.gov. Learn about clinical studies. https://clinicaltrials.gov/ct2/about-studies/learn#ClinicalTrials

DiMasi JA, Grabowski HG, Hansen RW. Innovation in the pharmaceutical industry: New estimates of R&D costs. *J Health Econ*. 2016 May;47:20–33. doi: 10.1016/j.jhealeco.2016.01.012. Epub 2016 Feb 12.

National Institutes of Health. NIH Clinical Research Trials and You: The Basics. https://www.nih.gov/health-information/nih-clinical-research-trials-you/basics

U.S. Food and Drug Administration. What are the different types of clinical research? https://www.fda.gov/patients/clinical-trials-what-patients-need-know/what-are-different-types-clinical-research

Wallace DJ. Epratuzumab: Reveille or requiem? Teachable moments for lupus and Sjögren's clinical trials. *Arthritis Rheumatol*. 2018;70(5):633–636. doi:10.1002/art.40427

51

International Collaboration and the Information Technology That Fuels It

Keys to a Brighter Future

Katherine M. Hammitt

Dramatic changes in the speed and ease of communication are leading to a more open international forum and collaborative approach in science and medicine. This movement will have a significant impact on Sjögren's. Collaboration, coupled with technological advances that offer vastly increased storage and speedier and more complex processing, is accelerating the pace of medical and scientific research that will expand our knowledge of Sjögren's far beyond anything we could have imagined only a few years ago.

Unlike the similarly transformative but slower-moving Industrial Revolution, the current Information Technology Revolution is moving so swiftly that it is hard to keep on top of changes. "Moore's law," a term originally used to describe the doubling of computer processing speed every 1.5 to 2 years, is now used to describe a similarly fast-paced transformation throughout the IT industry.

The recent rise of social media has made interaction with others easier and more immediate—for example, the opening of Facebook and the purchase of YouTube by Google in 2006 and a year later the first iPhone, Google's Android, Twitter, and Amazon's Kindle. In addition to new ways of receiving and sharing information, new platforms became available, enabling and encouraging collaboration via the internet. In 2007, GitHub launched the first such platform, inviting anyone and everyone to contribute to writing software. This collaborative, data-sharing effort allowed the international computing industry to come together and build on one another's ideas, ultimately revolutionizing computer software. The subsequent explosion in computer storage capacity and software development has led to the possibility of Big

Katherine M. Hammitt, *International Collaboration and the Information Technology That Fuels It* In: *The Sjögren's Book*. Edited by: Daniel J. Wallace, Oxford University Press. © Sjögren's Foundation 2022. DOI: 10.1093/oso/9780197502112.003.0051

Data, which is changing our ability to gather and analyze information and, most of all, truly understand massive amounts of data. These new possibilities are creating an exciting and dynamic world in science and medicine and have major repercussions for the future of Sjögren's.

The rapid speed of progress in Sjögren's that is projected to occur over the next several decades largely will come from international collaborative efforts in the Sjögren's community of medical and scientific researchers, healthcare professionals, patients, and the pharmaceutical and biotech industries. When we think about the possibilities that can come from initiatives such as the "Cancer Moonshot" and other major multi-institute and international efforts currently in progress, those of us with the Sjögren's Foundation asked, "Why not Sjögren's?"

Traditionally, medical and scientific researchers, and in parallel computer programmers, worked in silos, careful to protect proprietary information and eager to claim credit for their discoveries. As a result, progress was slow. Now, the collaborations that have led to the mind-boggling changes in the computer industry are spreading to medical research.

The Human Genome Project, which marked the world's largest biological collaboration when it was completed in 2003, is a prime example (https://www.genome.gov/11006944/whats-next-turning-genomics-vision-into-reality/). Funded in the beginning largely by the U.S. National Institutes of Health (NIH) and joined by numerous international groups and investigators, this project has allowed us to understand the full DNA sequencing in humans and has already led to discoveries in genes associated with Sjögren's and other diseases as well as the interactions of those genes with one another and our environment that lead to disease development. In late 2018, the NIH announced a new project, the Human BioMolecular Atlas Program (HuBMAP), which offers another open, global framework for mapping all human cells. Our cells can contribute to the emergence of disease and immune function, so providing a platform to understand all human cells and how they interact with one another and the immune system will lead to breakthroughs in our understanding of Sjögren's. These global collaborations will contribute to the development of "precision medicine," in which therapies will be targeted to individual patients based on their genetic and molecular makeup that will define risk factors and potential response to specific therapies.

Many efforts worldwide have recently been launched that will take advantage of new technology and our ability and willingness to collaborate on a global level. These efforts mark just the beginning of a new era and include the following.

Sjögren's Foundation Collaborative Initiatives

The Sjögren's Foundation has played a leadership role in bringing the international community and multiple specialists together to focus on initiatives to move the field of Sjögren's forward. Critical areas such as diagnosis, management, and treatment as well as criteria and outcome measures for clinical trials have been led by the Foundation to ensure progress in Sjögren's. Some examples:

- The Sjögren's Foundation Clinical Trials Consortium (see Chapter 49) is making a profound difference with the collaboration of Sjögren's experts as well as pharma and biotech companies to ensure successful clinical trial design.
- The Sjögren's Foundation Clinical Practice Guidelines have been taking specialists out of their too-often-siloed medical areas to work together in Sjögren's—something that is clearly needed in a disease that crosses almost every specialty area in medicine. This initiative is not only drawing different specialists together but is also bringing their professional organizations into Sjögren's to collaborate on diagnosis, management, and treatment. Specialists in fields such as rheumatology, ophthalmology, optometry, dentistry, and oral medicine as well as those in pulmonology, neurology, neuro-psychology, psychiatry, neuro-ophthalmology, oncology, and sleep medicine are interacting on these topics in Sjögren's. And organizations such as the American College of Rheumatology, the American Society of Clinical Oncology, and the American Association of Neurology are providing their support.
- Similarly, a Foundation-led team of multiple specialists and stakeholders was instrumental in securing change in the international diagnostic coding system for Sjögren's. This proposed U.S. coding change went into effect in October 2021 and is anticipated to increase accuracy in diagnosis, data-gathering, and patient identification for clinical trials.

Foundation for the NIH Biomarkers Consortium in Sjögren's and the NIH Accelerating Medicines Partnership®—Autoimmune and Immune-Mediated Disease (AMP®-AIM) Program

Discussed in Chapter 48, these major initiatives coordinated by the Foundation for the NIH (FNIH) will identify new biomarkers and potential therapeutic pathways and vastly increase our understanding of Sjögren's.

Sjögren's International Collaborative Clinical Alliance (SICCA)

Funded by the NIH and led by the University of California San Francisco, this major initiative comprises nine international sites and more than 3,500 Sjögren's patients. The alliance has established a data and biospecimen repository, has developed new classification criteria, and is working to better characterize phenotypes (physical and biochemical traits) and genetics in Sjögren's.

Sjögren's Genetics Network and Oklahoma Medical Research Foundation Laboratory

A current international collaboration in Sjögren's that is building on the Human Genome Project and the ability to collaborate internationally and share and process genetic samples is the Oklahoma Medical Research Foundation's Sjögren's Genetics Network (SGENE; omrf.org). This network has grown to a collaboration of 34 medical research centers worldwide that are working together to identify and isolate genes responsible for Sjögren's and understand how these genetic and environmental factors contribute to Sjögren's.

European League Against Rheumatism (EULAR) Big Data International Sjögren's Cohort

The ability to handle massive amounts of data, analyze this information, and visualize patterns led to the establishment of the Big Data initiative in 2014. Launched on behalf of EULAR, this project has established an international, multicenter registry to take a "high-definition" picture of the main features of Sjögren's at diagnosis, including epidemiology and clinical and immunologic characteristics of Sjögren's patients. By 2018, data-sharing had increased to 22 countries on five continents and more than 10,500 Sjögren's patients.

EULAR Sjögren's Syndrome Experimental and Translational Investigative Alliance (eSSential)

This initiative is aimed at creating a network of basic researchers and clinicians interested in Sjögren's and promoting research initiatives and facilitating international collaboration and interaction. Sub-groups have been formed to address translational and clinical research and the use of salivary ultrasound using cohorts across Europe.

Horizon 2020 and the Innovative Medicines Initiative

Horizon 2020 is the largest European Union research and innovation program to date, with €80 billion in funding, and is designed to encourage medical breakthroughs. The program started in 2014 and ended in 2020. The Innovative Medicines Initiative (IMI) grew out of Horizon 2020 as a public–private partnership between the European Union and the European Federation of Pharmaceutical Industries and Associations and is geared toward speeding the development of new therapies by supporting investigation into biomarkers, early-stage drugs, and the success of clinical trials. Several collaborative projects are in progress under the auspices of these initiatives:

- IMI PRECISESADS—molecular classification: This European initiative of the IMI involves 12 countries and aims to reclassify systemic autoimmune diseases, including Sjögren's, on a molecular level (https://www.imi.europa.eu/projects-results/project-factsheets/precisesads). A new classification system for autoimmune diseases will ultimately allow physicians to offer patients more personalized treatments and interventions at an earlier stage of disease. Current funding is from 2014 to 2019.
- IMI NECESSITY—outcome measures for clinical trials: Announced in 2017, funding for this IMI endeavor was generated to develop sensitive and validated endpoints for measuring the success of a therapy in clinical trials for Sjögren's. The NECESSITY project involves 12 countries in Europe as well as a partnership with the Sjögren's Foundation and aims to develop more meaningful objective measures that can improve with therapy and better measures for patient-reported symptoms (https://www.imi.europa.eu/projects-results/project-factsheets/necessity).
- Horizon 2020 HarmonicSS—Big Data analysis for improved stratification and treatment: This massive project, launched in 2017, involves 35 partners, including the Sjögren's Foundation and 13 countries (https://harmonicss.eu/). The goal is to harmonize and share data from international cohorts in Sjögren's and promote sustained and continued analysis of the data for improved stratification, treatment, and health policy. Core

information technology infrastructure has been devised to handle the massive amounts of data that will be integrated from the major international clinical and research centers in Sjögren's. Ultimately, this platform will allow Big Data mining via a cloud infrastructure and will be used to generate information on all areas of Sjögren's for many years to come.

Summing Up

The technology revolution might still be in its infancy, but the international collaborative initiatives already are taking off, and the future will see a sea change in Sjögren's. An important aspect of these initiatives is the cross-fertilization between and collaborations among projects. For example, eSSential plays into the translational work of HarmonicSS; progress in ultrasonography will inform the IMI NECESSITY; PRECISESADS, the FNIH Biomarkers Consortium in Sjögren's, and the NIH AMP-AIM* program will contribute to the development of new biomarkers and outcome measures in multiple endeavors. As the Foundation and others bring researchers, clinicians, patients, government, and industry together, advances in Sjögren's and the resulting benefits will occur at a pace never before seen in history.

For Further Reading

Forester T, ed. *The Information Technology Revolution*. MIT Press; 1985.

Friedman TL. *Thank You for Being Late: An Optimist's Guide to Thriving in the Age of Accelerations*. Farrar, Straus and Giroux; 2016.

Okin JR. *The Information Revolution: The Not-for-Dummies Guide to the History, Technology, and Use of the World Wide Web*. Ironbound Press; 2005.

Glossary

achlorhydria: Gastric acid deficiency.

acini: The small saclike dilations composing a compound gland.

ACR (American College of Rheumatology): A professional association of U.S. rheumatologists. Criteria (definitions) of many rheumatic diseases are called the *ACR Criteria.*

acupuncture: Procedure that involves inserting and manipulating needles into various points on the body to relieve pain or for therapeutic purposes.

adaptive immunity: Normally is functionally triggered after activation of the innate immunity system by foreign pathogens.

adenopathy: A swelling of the lymph nodes. In Sjögren's, this usually occurs in the neck and jaw region.

albumin: A protein that circulates in the blood and carries materials to cells. Levels are decreased in chronic disease.

allodynia: Pain due to a stimulus that does not normally produce pain.

alopecia: Hair loss.

alveoli: Small air sacs in the bronchi.

amylase: An enzyme present in saliva; another form of amylase is produced by the pancreas.

analgesic: A drug that alleviates pain.

androgen: A steroid hormone produced from cholesterol in the adrenal cortex, which is the primary precursor of natural estrogens.

anemia: Low numbers of red cells.

anhedonia: Loss of interest or pleasure in doing things.

anosmia: Loss of smell.

antibody: Substance in the blood that is normally made in response to infection. Also referred to as immunoglobulins such as IgG, IgM, etc.

anticardiolipin antibody: An antiphospholipid antibody.

anticentromere antibody: Antibodies to a cell nucleus associated with scleroderma.

anticholinergic: A class of medications that inhibit parasympathetic nerve impulses by selectively blocking the binding of the neurotransmitter acetylcholine to its receptor in nerve cells. A variety of these medications have side effects with resulting dry eyes and dry mouth.

anti-DNA (anti-double-stranded DNA): Antibodies to DNA; seen in half of patients with lupus.

anti-ENA (extractable nuclear antibodies): A group of antibodies that includes anti-Sm and anti-RNP.

antigen(s): A chemical substance that provokes the production of antibody. In tetanus vaccination, for example, tetanus is the antigen injected to produce antibodies and hence protective immunity to tetanus.

antimalarial drugs: Quinine-derived drugs, which were first developed to treat malaria and can manage Sjögren's, such as hydroxychloroquine (Plaquenil).

antimitochondrial antibodies (AMA): Antibodies (immunoglobulins) formed against mitochondria, primarily mitochondria in cells of the liver found in Sjögren's patients with biliary cirrhosis.

anti-muscarinic receptor antibody: This antibody is thought to block the action of the nerves that go to the salivary and lacrimal glands, thereby reducing the production of saliva and tears.

antinuclear antibodies (ANA): Autoantibodies directed against components in the nucleus of the cell. Screening test for lupus and other connective tissue diseases, including Sjögren's.

antiphospholipid antibody syndrome (APS): Thromboembolic events in a patient with antiphospholipid antibody.

antiphospholipid antibody: Antibodies to a constituent of cell membranes seen in a third of patients with lupus. In the presence of a cofactor, these antibodies can alter clotting and lead to strokes, blood clots, miscarriages, and low platelet counts. Also detected as the lupus anticoagulant.

anti-RNP: Antibody to ribonucleoprotein. Seen in lupus and mixed connective tissue disease.

anti-Sm: Anti-Smith antibody; found only in lupus.

antispasmodic drugs: Medications that quiet spasms. Usually used in reference to the gastrointestinal tract.

anti-SSA (Ro antibody): Associated with Sjögren's, sun sensitivity, neonatal lupus, and congenital heart block.

anti-SSB (La antibody): Almost always seen with anti-SSA.

apoptosis: Process by which a cell is programmed to self-destruct.

aqueous deficient dry eye: Disruption of the tear film because of inadequate tear production

arachidonic acid: An unsaturated fatty acid found in animal fats that is essential in human nutrition and is a precursor in the biosynthesis of some prostaglandins

arteriole: A very small artery.

arthralgia: Joint pain.

arthritis: Inflammation of a joint.

ascites: A collection of fluid in the abdomen due to certain liver and other disorders.

atelectasis: A collapse of lung tissue affecting part or all of one lung.

atrophic gastritis : Autoimmune destruction of acid-producing parietal cells of the stomach. May lead to vitamin B_{12} deficiency and pernicious anemia. Up to 20% of Sjögren's patients may have antibodies against parietal cells.

atrophic rhinitis: A nasal condition characterized by a foul smell, crusts, and even bleeding. As secretions become thick and occasionally foul-smelling, secondary infection may appear.

atrophic vaginitis : A condition characterized by dryness and inflammation of the vagina with thinning of the epithelial lining due to estrogen deficiency.

atrophy: A thinning of the surface; a form of wasting.

autoantibody: Antibody that attacks the body's own tissues and organs as if they were foreign.

autoimmune hepatitis: Inflammation of the liver that occurs when immune cells mistake the liver's normal cells for harmful invaders and attack them.

autoimmune pancreatitis: An increasingly recognized type of chronic pancreatitis that can be difficult to distinguish from pancreatic carcinoma but that responds to treatment with corticosteroids, particularly prednisone. Rare complication of Sjögren's.

autoimmune thyroiditis : Disease of the thyroid gland due to autoimmunity in which the patient's immune system attacks and damages the thyroid.

autoimmunity: A state in which the body inappropriately produces antibody against its own tissues. The antigens are components of the body.

autonomic neuropathy: Nerve dysfunction that affects the autonomic nervous system, which controls digestive, bladder, bowel, cardiac, and sexual function.

BAFF (B-cell activating factor of the TNF family), also called BLyS: A powerful driver of B-cell development.

basal (resting) rate: Unstimulated (used in reference to both tears and salivary flow).

B cell or B lymphocyte: A white blood cell that makes antibodies.

biologic therapies: Treatment to stimulate or restore the ability of the immune (defense) system to fight infection and disease.

biosimilar: A biologic medical product highly similar with no clinically meaningful differences to an already approved biologic product.

blepharitis: Common, persistent, and sometimes chronic inflammation of the eyelids, resulting from bacteria that reside on the skin.

bolus: A morsel of food, already chewed, ready to be swallowed.

brain fog: Impaired concentration and memory that can be due to various causes.

bronchi: Branches of the trachea.

buffer: A mixture of acid or base that, when added to a solution, enables the solution to resist changes in the pH that would otherwise occur when acid or alkali is added to it.

calcification: A process in which tissue or noncellular material in the body becomes hardened as the result of deposits of insoluble calcium salts.

Candida: A yeast-like fungal organism.

candidiasis : A condition affecting the skin or oral mucosa caused by overgrowth of the common yeast (fungus) *Candida*. Formerly called moniliasis.

cariostatic: Having the ability to help prevent dental caries.

cartilage: Tissue material covering bone. The nose, outer ears, and trachea consist primarily of cartilage.

celiac spruce: An inherited, autoimmune disease in which the lining of the small intestine is damaged from eating gluten and other proteins found in wheat, barley, rye, and possibly oats. Also known as gluten enteropathy. May be 10 times more prevalent in Sjögren's patients than in general population.

central nervous system: The brain and spinal cord.

cheilitis: Sores at the corners of the mouth (angles of the lips).

chemokines: One of a large group of proteins that act as lures and were first found attracting white blood cells.

chilblains: inflammation of small blood vessels usually brought on by cold temperatures

chronic active hepatitis: A disorder that occurs when viral hepatitis proceeds in an active state beyond its usual cause.

chronic fatigue syndrome : Best defined as a low-energy state characterized by physical or mental weariness.

collagen vascular disease: *See* connective tissue disease.

commensal bacteria: A part of the normal flora in the body.

complement: A protein consumed with inflammation; levels may be decreased in Sjögren's.

complementary medicine : Nonprescription use of products found in nature to treat medical conditions. Also includes noninvasive mind–body techniques such as biofeedback, acupuncture, yoga.

complete blood count (CBC): A blood test measuring the amount of red cells, white blood cells, and platelets in the body.

congenital heart block: A dysfunction of the rate/rhythm conduction system in the fetal or infant heart caused by antibodies to SSA or SSB.

conjunctiva: The mucous membrane covering the outside of the eyeball and the inner lining of the eyelids.

connective tissue disease: A disorder marked by inflammation of the connective tissue (joints, skin, muscles) in multiple areas. In most instances, connective tissue diseases are associated with autoimmunity.

constitutional symptoms: A symptom that affects the general well-being or general status of a patient. Examples include weight loss, shaking, chills, fever, and vomiting.

contrast sialography: A test that assesses the structure of the major salivary glands.

cornea: The central transparent part of the eyeball that helps focus the entering light rays. The clear "watch crystal" structure covering the pupil and iris (colored portion of the eye). It is composed of several vital layers, all of which are functionally important. The surface layer, or epithelium, is covered by the tears, which lubricate and protect the surface.

corticosteroid: A hormone produced by the adrenal cortex gland. Natural adrenal gland hormones have powerful anti-inflammatory activity and are often used in the treatment of severe inflammation affecting vital organs. The many side effects of corticosteroids should markedly curtail their use in mild disorders.

costochondritis: An irritation of a rib and adjoining cartilage that causes chest pain.

C-reactive protein (CRP): Protein produced by the liver. Levels rise when there is inflammation throughout the body.

CREST syndrome: A limited form of scleroderma characterized by C (calcium deposits under the skin), R (Raynaud's phenomenon), E (esophageal dysfunction), S (sclerodactyly or tight skin), and T (a rash called telangiectasia).

crossover syndrome: An autoimmune process that has features of more than one rheumatic disease.

cryoglobulinemia: Condition in which blood vessels become inflamed (vasculitis) and protein complexes circulating in the blood become deposited during cold weather.

cryptogenic cirrhosis: Liver disease of unknown etiology (origin) in patients with no history of alcoholism or previous acute hepatitis.

cystic lung disease: condition when multiple cysts in the lungs are identified; suggests presence of amyloid or MALT lymphoma in Sjögren's

cytokine: A group of chemicals that signal cells to perform certain actions.

demineralization: The process of removing hard minerals (calcium) from the tooth surface. Progressive removal of these minerals results in a progressive dental cavity. This is part of the dental caries process.

demyelination: Areas of damage to the coatings of the nerve fibers.

dendritic cells: Immune cells that form part of the mammalian immune system.

dental caries : A process in which the tooth is gradually dissolved (demineralized) by acids from bacteria attached to the surface, which leads to progressive cavitation. If the caries process is allowed to continue without treatment, it will progress through the tooth into its pulp (containing the nerve of the tooth). Also known as dental decay or cavity.

dermatomyositis: An autoimmune process directed against muscles that is associated with skin rashes.

diuretics: Medications that increase the body's ability to rid itself of fluids.

docosahexaenoic (DHA): An omega-3 fatty acid.

double-blind study: A study in which neither the physician nor the patients being treated know whether patients are receiving the active ingredient being tested or a placebo (an inactive substance).

dysautonomia: dysfunction of the autonomic nervous system

dysbiosis: A microbial imbalance or maladaptation on or inside the body, such as an impaired microbiota.

dysorexia: Impaired or deranged appetite.

dyspareunia: Painful sexual intercourse.

dyspepsia: Painful, difficult, or disturbed digestion; may be accompanied by symptoms such as nausea and vomiting, heartburn, bloating, and stomach discomfort.

dysphagia: Swallowing difficulty. In Sjögren's, this may be attributable to several causes, including a decrease in saliva, infiltration of the glands at the esophageal mucosa, or esophageal webbing.

dyspnea: Air hunger resulting in labored or difficult breathing, sometimes accompanied by pain.

dysuria: Pain on urination.

ecchymosis: A purplish patch caused by oozing of blood into the skin; ecchymoses differ from petechiae in size.

edema: Swelling caused by retained fluid.

eicosapentaenoic acid (EPA): An omega-3 fatty acid found in fish oils.

electromyography (EMG) : A technique for evaluating and recording the electrical activity produced by skeletal muscles.

ELISA (enzyme-linked immunosorbent assay): A sensitive blood test for detecting the presence of autoantibodies.

endoscopy: A procedure in which a small, flexible tube (an endoscope) is inserted to view the esophagus, stomach, and duodenum.

eosinophilic esophagitis: build-up of eosinophils, a type of white blood cell, in the lining of the esophagus

epigenetics: An emerging field that studies how heritable modifications that do not involve changes in the nucleotide sequence lead to altered gene expression.

epistaxis: Nosebleed; may be caused by dryness of the nasal mucous membrane in Sjögren's.

epithelial: The outside layer of cells that covers all the free, open surfaces of the body, including the skin, and mucous membranes that communicate with the outside of the body.

erythema: A red color, usually associated with increased blood flow to an inflamed area, often the skin.

erythrocyte sedimentation rate (ESR): A laboratory test that measures the degree to which a specimen of whole blood separates into plasma (the upper layer) and packed red cells (the lower layer) over the course of one hour. The blood is collected in tubes containing a chemical that prevents clotting (anticoagulant). ESR is elevated with inflammation.

erythrocyte: Red blood cell.

esophageal dysmotility: Muscular incoordination of the esophagus; may affect up to a third of Sjögren's patients with dysphagia.

esophagitis: Chronic irritation of the esophagus resulting from prolonged reflux of acid.

esophagus: A narrow tube with muscular walls allowing passage of food from the pharynx (the end of the mouth) to the stomach.

ESSDAI (EULAR Sjogren's Syndrome Disease Activity Index): Used in clinical studies to assess Sjogren's disease activity.

ESSPRI (EULAR Sjogren's Syndrome Patient Reported Inventory): Used in clinical studies to measure how a Sjögren's patient feels.

estrogens: Any of several steroid hormones produced chiefly by the ovaries and responsible for promoting estrus and the development and maintenance of female secondary sex characteristics.

etiology: The cause(s) of a disease.

eustachian tube: The tube running from the back of the nose to the middle ear.

exocrine glands: Glands that secrete outside the body (e.g., lacrimal, salivary, or sweat glands).

exocrinopathy: Disease related to the exocrine glands.

extraglandular: Outside of the glands.

fecal microbial transplant (FMT): A procedure in which fecal matter, or stool, is collected from a healthy donor and placed in the gastrointestinal tract of a patient.

fibromyalgia: A pain amplification syndrome seen in Sjögren's patients that reflects sensory afferent sensitization.

fibrosis: Abnormal formation of fibrous tissue.

filamentary keratopathy: Condition in which mucous strands stick to the cornea at sites of focal desiccation and surface cells extend onto the strand, making it adherent to the cornea and causing discomfort or even pain when blinking pulls on the strand.

fissure: A crack in the tissue surface (skin, tongue, etc.).

fluorescein stain: A dye that stains areas of the eye surface where cells have been lost.

focal lymphocytic sialoadenitis: A characteristic pattern of inflammation.

gastritis: Stomach inflammation.

gastroesophageal reflux (GERD): Condition in which muscle tone in the wall of the esophagus is reduced, allowing gastric juice to move up the esophagus, producing a burning sensation behind the breastbone (heartburn) and chest pain.

genes: Units of heredity that control the physical traits that are passed from parents to their offspring.

gene therapy: A method of treating disease by introducing normal DNA directly into cells to correct a genetic defect that is causing the disease.

genetic factors: Traits inherited from parents, grandparents, and so on.

genetics: The study of genes.

gene transfer: The insertion of unrelated genetic information in the form of DNA into cells.

genome: All of the genetic information possessed by an organism.

genome-wide association study (GWAS): Method by which the complete set of DNA, or genome, of many individual people can be rapidly scanned to find genetic variations associated with a complex disease, such as Sjögren's.

gingiva: The gums.

gingivitis: Inflammation of the gums.

globulin: A protein whose levels are increased in inflammation.

glomerulonephritis: Inflammation of the kidney; seen in 10% of Sjögren's patients.

goblet cell: Specialized epithelial cells found in the mucous membranes of the stomach, intestines, and respiratory passages.

granulocytes: A type of white blood cell.

granuloma: A nodular, inflammatory lesion.

Graves disease: An autoimmune thyroid disease.

halitosis: Bad breath.

Hashimoto's thyroiditis: The most common form of thyroiditis and the most frequent cause of hypothyroidism.

Helicobacter pylori: A common chronic bacterial infection of the stomach. Associated with an increased risk of gastrointestinal (MALT) lymphoma.

hematocrit: blood test measuring red blood cells and included in the complete blood count (CBC)

hepatitis: Inflammation of the liver; seen in Sjögren's patients who have biliary cirrhosis.

hepatitis C virus: Not associated with Sjögren's, but can present with sicca symptoms mimicking it.

homeopathy: A method of treating disease by administering tiny amounts of remedies that, in large amounts in healthy people, produce symptoms similar to those being treated.

hormone replacement therapy (HRT): Treatment in which estrogen and progesterone are administered to menopausal women to relieve severe hot flashes, disrupted sleep, and in some cases mild depressive symptoms.

hormones: Chemical messengers made by the body, including thyroid, insulin, steroids, estrogen, progesterone, and testosterone.

human leukocyte antigens (HLA): A group of genes that governs the ability of lymphocytes, such as T cells and B cells, to respond to foreign and self substances.

hydroxychloroquine: Anti-inflammatory drug (trade name Plaquenil) used to treat autoimmune conditions such as rheumatoid arthritis, Sjögren's, and systemic lupus erythematosus.

hyperalgesia: An extreme reaction to a stimulus that is not normally painful.

hypergammaglobulinemia: Condition in which levels of gamma globulin are elevated.

hypergammaglobulinemic purpura: A purple-brown skin rash.

hypokalemia: Low potassium levels.

hypothyroidism: A condition in which the thyroid gland does not make enough thyroid hormone.

idiopathic: Of unknown cause.

immunogenetics: The study of genetic factors that control the immune response.

immunoglobulin E (IgE): Antibody associated with allergies.

immunoglobulins (gamma globulins): The protein fraction of serum responsible for antibody activity. Measurement of serum immunoglobulin levels can serve as a guide to disease activity in some patients with Sjögren's.

immunomodulators: Medications that affect the body's immune system.

immunosuppressive agents: Drugs used to treat malignant disease and severe autoimmune disease and to prevent transplant rejection.

incisal: Cutting edge of a tooth.

indigestion (dyspepsia): A painful or burning feeling in the upper abdomen; usually accompanied by nausea, bloating or gas, a feeling of fullness, and, sometimes, vomiting.

innate immunity: Primitive responses to bacteria and viruses via a pattern recognition mechanism.

interferon: A protein made to protect the body from infection; it is overactive in Sjögren's.

interstitial: of the connective tissue supporting an organ or tissue.

interstitial cystitis: Condition in which the bladder becomes inflamed.

interstitial lung disease (ILD): Condition in which the lung becomes inflamed.

interstitial nephritis: Condition in which the connective tissue of the kidney becomes inflamed; may be associated with Sjögren's.

interstitial pneumonitis: Condition in which the supporting tissue around the alveoli (air sacs) of the lungs becomes inflamed due to an autoimmune process.

intraoral: Inside the mouth.

intrathoracic: Within the chest cavity.

irritable bowel syndrome: inflammation of the intestine causing diarrhea/constipation, pain, bloating, and cramping .

IV immunoglobulin (IVIg): A blood product made from the plasma component of blood pooled from thousands of donors. It contains immunoglobulins, which interact with the immune system in order to suppress it.

jaundice: Yellowing of the skin.

keratoconjunctivitis sicca: Dry eye; a condition that most frequently occurs in women in their forties and fifties.

lacrimal: Relating to the tears.

lacrimal glands: Glands that produce tears. Smaller accessory glands in the eyelid produce the tears needed from minute to minute. The main lacrimal glands, located just inside the bony tissue surrounding the eye, produce large amounts of tears.

laryngopharyngeal reflux (LPR): Reflux of gastric contents and acids to the level of the throat; can lead to hoarseness, chronic cough, throat clearing, mild pharyngeal dysphagia, or globus sensations (sensation of a lump or foreign body in the throat).

laryngotracheobronchitis: An acute respiratory infection involving the larynx, trachea, and bronchi. Also called *croup*.

larynx: Voice box.

latent: Not manifest but potentially discernible.

leukemia: a type of blood cancer most often affecting white blood cells and involving the bone marrow and lymphatic system

leukopenia: Low level of white blood cells.

leukorrhea: A whitish, viscid discharge from the vagina and uterine cavity.

lichen sclerosus: a condition of the skin and mucosa that appears in white patches; can affect mucosal lining of mouth and genitals

lip biopsy: Procedure in which an incision of approximately 1 cm is made on the inside surface of the lower lip and minor salivary glands are removed for microscopic examination and analysis.

lissamine green: A vital stain that is similar to rose bengal but causes less discomfort. It stains dead or degenerated epithelial cells green and facilitates the diagnosis of keratoconjunctivitis sicca, xerophthalmia, etc.

lymph: A fluid collected from the tissues throughout the body; it flows through the lymph nodes and is eventually added to the circulating blood.

lymphadenopathy: Abnormally enlarged lymph nodes; commonly called "swollen glands."

lymphocyte: A type of white blood cell responsible for antibody production and regulation. Collections of lymphocytes are seen in the salivary glands of Sjögren's patients.

lymphoma: A condition involving abnormal (malignant) lymphocytes. Two types develop in a small proportion of Sjögren's patients: mucosa-associated lymphoid tissue (MALT) lymphoma (also called extra-nodal marginal zone lymphoma), which is very slow-growing, may cause progressive salivary gland enlargement, and is rarely fatal; the other type, large B-cell lymphoma, occurs even less frequently but can be aggressive.

lymphoproliferation: Excessive production of lymphocytes.

macrophage: A cell that kills foreign material and presents information to lymphocytes.

MALT (mucosa-associated lymphoid tissue): Tissue that most often develops in the mucosa, the moist lining of some organs and body cavities.

manometry: Test in which the pressure inside the wall of the esophagus is measured during swallowing; used to diagnose dysmotility.

matrix: The section of the tooth enamel that holds calcium and phosphate minerals.

Meibomian glands: Fat-producing glands in the eyelids that produce an essential component of tears.

MHC: Major histocompatibility complex. In humans, it is the same as HLA.

microbiome: The genetic material of all microbes inside the human body.

mixed connective tissue disease: A connective tissue disease that manifests as an overlap of other connective tissue disorders.

monoclonal antibody: A single antibody designed to uniquely recognize a specific target, such as a lymphocyte or cytokine.

mononeuritis multiplex: Inflammation of multiple nerves.

mucin: Thinnest layer of the tear film; layer closest to the cornea.

mucolytic agents: Medications that dissolve mucus. Most patients with dry eye complain of excess mucous discharge. Some patients may benefit from these medications if other eye drops that enhance the tear film are ineffective.

multiple myeloma: a blood cancer that arises in plasma cells, a type of white blood cell

myalgia: Muscle pain.

necrosis: Tissue death.

neonatal lupus syndrome: A rare autoimmune disorder that is present at birth in patients with anti-SSA or SSAB; usually manifests with a rash or heart block.

nephritis: Kidney inflammation.

nerve conduction study: Test used to evaluate the function (especially electrical conduction) of the motor and sensory nerves.

neutrophil: A granulated white blood cell involved in bacterial killing and acute inflammation.

nonspecific: Caused by other diseases or multiple factors.

nonsteroidal anti-inflammatory drugs (NSAIDs): Medications that block the action of prostaglandins and are used to treat pain in patients with rheumatoid arthritis and other connective tissue disorders. Examples include ibuprofen (Motrin, Advil) and naproxen (Aleve).

norepinephrine: A hormone and neurotransmitter secreted by the adrenal medulla and the nerve endings of the sympathetic nervous system; causes vasoconstriction and increases in heart rate, blood pressure, and the sugar level of the blood.

olfactory: Relating to the sense of smell.

ophthalmologist: A physician who specializes in diseases and surgery of the eye.

optic neuritis: Inflammation of the optic nerve; may cause vision loss.

oral lichen planus: inflammation of the mucosa lining of the mouth; causes burning mouth

oral soft tissue: Tongue, mucous lining of the cheeks, and lips.

orthostasis: Maintenance of an upright standing posture.

otalgia: Ear pain.

otitis: Inflammation of the ear; may be marked by pain, fever, hearing abnormalities, deafness, tinnitus (a ringing sensation), and vertigo. In Sjögren's, eustachian tube blockage due to infection can lead to conduction deafness and chronic otitis.

otolaryngology: The medical specialty that deals with diseases of the ear, nose, and throat.

palpable purpura: Rashes, particularly small red raised eruptions on the extremities in Sjögren's patients.

pancreatitis: Acute inflammation of the pancreas.

parasympathetic nervous system: The part of the autonomic nervous system whose functions include constriction of the pupils of the eyes, slowing of the heartbeat, and stimulation of certain digestive glands. These nerves originate in the midbrain, the hindbrain, and the sacral region of the spinal cord; impulses are mediated by acetylcholine.

parasympathomimetic agents: Systemic agents that can stimulate salivary output.

paresthesias : Abnormal sensations such as tingling, constriction, and discomfort.

parotid gland flow: Measurement of the amount of saliva produced over a certain period of time. Normal parotid gland flow rate is 1.5 mL/min. In Sjögren's, the flow rate is approximately 0.5 mL/min, with the flow rate correlating inversely with the severity of disease.

parotid glands: The major salivary glands that are along the jaw line.

parotid scintigraphy: A nuclear medicine test that evaluates the function of the parotid and submandibular glands.

pathogenesis: The development of a disease.

peptides: Various natural or synthetic compounds containing two or more amino acids linked by the carboxyl group of one amino acid to the amino group of another.

perforation: A hole.

pericarditis: Inflammation of the lining around the heart (the pericardium).

perimenopause: The time period that starts a few years before menopause during which menses are irregular.

periodontitis: Inflammation of the gums and soft tissue and bone surrounding and supporting the teeth.

peripheral nerves: Nerves outside the central nervous system.

peripheral neuropathy: Condition involving pain, loss of sensation, and inability to control muscles that is due to a problem with the nerves that carry information to and from the brain and spinal cord.

pernicious anemia: A blood disorder caused by inadequate vitamin B_{12} in the blood.

petechiae: A small, pinpoint, non-raised, perfectly round, purplish-red spot caused by intradermal or submucosal hemorrhaging.

phagocytic cells: Cells such as white blood cells that engulf and absorb waste material, harmful microorganisms, or other foreign bodies in the bloodstream and tissues.

pharmacodynamics: The way in which a drug works.

pharmacokinetics: The movement of a drug within the body.

pharynx: Throat.

photosensitivity: Sensitivity to ultraviolet light; present in most patients with antibodies to SSA (Ro).

placebo: An inactive substance used as a "dummy" medication in clinical trials.

plaque: A thin, sticky film that builds up on the teeth, trapping harmful bacteria.

plasma: The fluid portion of the circulating blood.

plasmapheresis: Procedure in which blood plasma is filtered through a machine to remove proteins that may aggravate Sjögren's.

platelet: a blood component involved in clotting

pleura: A sac lining the lung.

pleurisy: Inflammation of the lining around the lung.

polychondritis: Inflammation and destruction of the cartilage of various tissues of the body.

polyclonal: Derived from different cells.

polymyositis: A connective tissue disorder characterized by muscle pain and severe weakness secondary to inflammation in the major voluntary muscles.

polysomnography: A sleep study.

Postural Tachycardia Syudrome (POTs): A potential manifestation of autonomic nervous system dysfunction leading to dizziness upon standing, orthostatic hypotension, and/or heart arrhythmias

primary biliary cirrhosis (PBC): Impairment of bile excretion secondary to liver inflammation and scarring.

probiotics: The administration of "good" bacteria that kill harmful gut bacteria.

progestins: Steroid hormones that have the effect of progesterone.

prostaglandins: Substances produced by the body that are responsible for the features of inflammation, such as swelling, pain, stiffness, redness, and warmth.

protein: A collection of amino acids. Antibodies are proteins.

proteinuria: Excess protein levels in the urine (also called albuminuria).

proteomics: The study of proteins.

pruritus : Itching.

psoralen: A drug administered orally or topically to treat vitiligo (white patches caused by loss of pigment).

pulse steroids: High doses of corticosteroids given intravenously over several days to critically ill patients.

puncta: Small holes in the eyelids that normally drain tears. Patients with severe dry eye benefit from punctal closure, which allows maximal tear preservation.

punctal plugs: Plugs inserted into the tear ducts to increase the volume of tears retained on the surface of the eye

purpura: A condition characterized by hemorrhage into the skin, appearing as crops of petechiae (very small red spots).

radioactive isotope: Material used in diagnostic tests.

radionuclide studies: Tests in which radioactive isotopes, such as radiolabeled human serum albumin, are injected into an organ. A gamma scintillation camera, coupled with a digital computer system and a cathode ray display, detects the radioactive emissions. Areas of perfusion will show marked radiographic emissions; areas of obstruction will show no activity.

Raynaud's phenomenon: Painful blanching of the fingertips on exposure to cold; may be seen alone or in association with a connective tissue disease.

reflux: Regurgitation of gas, fluid, or a small amount of food from the stomach.

regulatory immunity: Needed to evolve to facilitate termination of a no-longer-needed adaptive response and, as well, to limit responses to 'self' (auto) antigen.

remineralization: The process of restoring minerals (calcium and phosphate) to the tooth surface.

renal: Related to the kidneys.

renal tubular acidosis: Damage to the kidney tubules involving a decreased pH level.

restless legs syndrome: Condition characterized by unpleasant sensations in the limbs, usually the legs, that occur at rest or before sleep and are relieved by activity such as walking.

rheumatoid arthritis (RA): An autoimmune disease characterized by inflammation of the joints, stiffness, swelling, synovial hypertrophy, and pain. Sjögren's frequently occurs in conjunction with RA.

rheumatoid factor: An autoantibody whose presence in the blood usually indicates autoimmune activity.

rheumatologist: A physician skilled in the diagnosis and treatment of rheumatic conditions.

Ro antibody: *See* anti-SSA.

rosacea: A chronic dermatitis of the face, especially of the nose and cheeks, characterized by a red or rosy coloration with deep-seated papules and pustules. It is caused by dilation of capillaries. Can be mistaken for lupus or anti-SSA-associated rashes.

rose bengal : A dye that stains abnormal cells on the surface of the eye. When used for diagnosis in patients with significant dry eyes (keratoconjunctivitis sicca), it is very irritating and has been generally replaced by lissamine green, an equivalent dye that is not irritating.

salicylates: Aspirin-like drugs.

salivary flow rate: The amount of saliva naturally produced by the salivary glands.

salivary glands: Exocrine glands (parotid, submandibular, and sublingual) that produce saliva.

salivary scintigraphy: Test used to measure salivary gland function that involves intravenous injection of a radioactive material.

sarcoidosis: A systemic disease with granulomatous (nodular, inflammatory) lesions involving the lungs and sometimes the salivary glands, with resulting fibrosis.

Schirmer test: The standard objective test to diagnose dry eye. Small pieces of filter paper are placed between the lower eyelid and eyeball and soak up the tears for five minutes. The value obtained is a rough estimate of tear production in relative terms. Lower values are consistent with dry eye.

scleroderma: A connective tissue and autoimmune disease characterized by thickening and hardening of the skin. Sometimes internal organs (intestines, kidneys) are affected, causing bowel irregularity and high blood pressure. Sjögren's is not uncommon in patients with scleroderma.

sclerosing cholangitis: A chronic disorder of the liver in which the ducts carrying bile from the liver to the intestine, and often the ducts carrying bile within the liver, become inflamed, thickened, scarred (sclerotic), and obstructed.

sclerosing sialadenitis: Swelling and inflammation of the salivary glands with scarring.

secretogogue: A medication that can stimulate salivary flow.

serotonin: A chemical produced by the brain that functions as a neurotransmitter. It plays a part in the regulation of mood, sleep, learning, and constriction of blood vessels (vasoconstriction).

serum: The fluid portion of the blood (obtained after removal of the fibrin clot and blood cells), distinguished from the plasma in the blood.

serum protein electrophoresis: A laboratory test that examines specific proteins in the blood called globulins.

serum sickness: a delayed allergic reaction to the injection of an antiserum; caused by an antibody reaction to an antigen in the donor serum.

sialochemistry: Measurement of the constituents in saliva.

sialography: X-ray examination of the salivary duct system by use of liquid contrast medium. Radiologically sensitive dye placed into the duct system outlines the system clearly.

sicca: An autoimmune disease, also known as Sjögren's, that classically combines dry eyes, dry mouth, and another disease of the connective tissue such as rheumatoid arthritis (most common), lupus, scleroderma, or polymyositis.

signs: Changes that can be seen or measured.

sinusitis: Sinus inflammation.

Sjögren's : A systemic multi-organ autoimmune disease that generally has a chronic or progressive course and is characterized by secretory dysfunction. It may occur alone or precede or follow other autoimmune diseases in the same patient.

Sjögren's antibodies: Abnormal antibodies found in the sera of Sjögren's patients. These antibodies react with the extracts of certain cells, and a test based on this principle can be helpful in the diagnosis of Sjögren's. *See also* SSA and SSB.

Sjögren's Foundation: The principal U.S. organization for Sjögren's patients and professionals; supports research, education, and advocacy.

SSA: Sjögren's syndrome-associated antigen A (anti-Ro).

SSB: Sjögren's syndrome-associated antigen B (anti-La).

steatorrhea: Presence of large amounts of fat in the feces; occurs in pancreatic disease and malabsorption syndrome.

steroids: Cortisone-derived medications.

subacute cutaneous lupus (SCLE): Set of photosensitive rashes originally described in patients with lupus. The rashes may occur in Sjögren's patients and are common in patients with anti-SSA (Ro) and anti-SSB (La) antibodies.

sublingual glands: Major salivary glands located in the floor of the mouth under the tongue.

symptoms: Changes that patients feel.

synovitis: Inflammation of the tissues lining a joint.

synovium: Tissue that lines a joint.

systemic: Involving multiple organ systems throughout the body.

systemic lupus erythematosus (SLE): An autoimmune disease that is closely related to Sjögren's syndrome. It occurs frequently in conjunction with Sjögren's and can damage any body organ or system.

T cell: A lymphocyte (white blood cell) responsible for immunologic memory.

tear breakup test: A standard part of the evaluation of dry eye.

tear osmolarity test: Test that measures the concentration of the tear film, which can be elevated in either aqueous deficient or evaporative dry eye.

thrombocytopenia: Low platelet count.

thrombosis: recurrent arterial and venous thromboses (blood clots) and/or recurrent spontaneous abortions (miscarriages) associated with the presence of antibodies to phospholipids.

thrush: Infection of the oral tissues with *Candida albicans.*

thymus: A gland in the neck responsible for immunologic memory.

thyroiditis: A disease in which autoantibodies cause immune system cells (lymphocytes) to destroy the thyroid gland.

tinnitus: Ringing in the ears.

titer: The strength or concentration of a particular substance; usually refers to amount of antibody present.

TMJ (temporomandibular joint): The joint of the lower jaw where a ball-and-socket arrangement is formed by the condyle of the lower jaw (the ball) and the fossa of the temporal bone (the socket). The joint space is filled with synovial or lubricating fluid. This joint and the surrounding synovial tissues may become inflamed if rheumatoid arthritis accompanies Sjögren's and involves the joint.

tolerance: The failure to make antibodies to an antigen.

Toll receptor: A pattern recognition feature of the innate immune system.

trachea: Windpipe.

tracheobronchial tree: The windpipe and the bronchi into which it subdivides.

trigeminal nerve: The chief nerve of sensation for the face and the motor nerve controlling the muscles of mastication (chewing).

tumor necrosis factor (TNF): A cytokine produced primarily by monocytes and macrophages that promotes inflammation.

UCTD (undifferentiated connective tissue disease): Conditions with features of autoimmunity such as inflammatory arthritis or Raynaud's in a patient who does not meet the ACR criteria for lupus, rheumatoid arthritis, or other disorders.

ultraviolet light (UV light): A spectrum of light including UVA (320–400 nanometers), UVB (290–320 nanometers), and UVC (200–290 nanometers).

urinalysis: Examination of urine under a microscope.

urticaria: Hives.

uveitis: inflammation inside the eye, causing pain, redness and blurred vision

vasculitis: Inflammation of a blood vessel.

venous thromboses: Clots in veins of the lower extremities and less frequently the lungs.

venule: A very small vein.

viscera: The organs of the digestive, respiratory, urogenital, and endocrine systems, as well as the spleen, heart, and great vessels (blood and lymph ducts).

vitamin B$_{12}$ deficiency: A reduction in vitamin B$_{12}$ due to inadequate dietary intake or impaired absorption.

vitamin D: A fat-soluble vitamin that enhances the absorption of calcium and phosphorus from the intestine and promotes their deposition onto the bone.

vitiligo: White patches on the skin due to loss of pigment.

WBC: White blood cell.

xerophthalmia: Dry eyes.

xerosis: Abnormal dryness of the skin (xeroderma), the conjunctiva of the eye (xerophthalmia), or the mucous membranes such as dry mouth (xerostomia).

xerostomia: Dryness of the mouth. It is usually associated with decreased salivary secretion but may occur in some individuals with normal secretion. It can be caused by many different prescription drugs, Sjögren's, radiation therapy, uncontrolled diabetes, and other diseases.

xylitol: An acceptable sweetener that has been shown to reduce dental caries.

Index

For the benefit of digital users, indexed terms that span two pages (e.g., 52–53) may, on occasion, appear on only one of those pages.

Tables, figures, and boxes are indicated by *t*, *f*, and *b* following the page number.